AEU 9953
B-00
29.95

LEVI BRANCH LIBRARY
3676 S. THIRD ST.
MEMPHIS, TN. 38109
789-3140

W9-AOV-582

DISCARDED BY
MEMPHIS PUBLIC LIBRARY

The A-to-Z of
Pregnancy and Childbirth

Here is the latest information on childbirth and pregnancy, in an easy-to-use A-to-Z format. Throughout are expert, concise definitions of terms from "AFP screening" to "zygote intrafallopian transfer" and everything in between. Find out:

* the best time to conceive

* questions to ask about assisted reproductive technology

* how sexually transmitted diseases and alcohol can affect pregnancy and unborn babies

* the pros and cons of both standard and alternative delivery procedures

* the likelihood of having a cesarean section—and how to avoid one

* important ways to care for yourself after the baby's birth

Enlightened and authoritative, *The A-to-Z of Pregnancy and Childbirth* provides instant answers to questions and concerns that all expectant parents may have during one of the most profound experiences of their lives.

Other books in this series from Hunter House

The New *A-to-Z of Women's Health*
by Christine Ammer

The A-to-Z of Women's Sexuality
by Ada P. Kahn and Linda Hughey Holt, M.D.

Ordering information

Orders by individuals or organizations
Hunter House books are available through most bookstores or can be ordered directly from the publisher by calling 510-865-5282

Quantity sales
Hunter House books are available at special quantity discounts when purchased in bulk by corporations, associations, and others. For details, call the number above or write to Special Sales, Hunter House Inc., P.O. Box 2914, Alameda CA 94501

Orders for college textbooks/course adoptions
Please contact Hunter House at the address and phone number above

Orders by U.S. trade bookstores and wholesalers
Please contact Publishers Group West, Box 8843, Emeryville CA 94608 telephone 800-788-3123; fax 510-658-1834

The
A-to-Z
of
Pregnancy
and Childbirth

A Concise Encyclopedia

by

NANCY EVANS

Foreword by Celeste Phillips, R.N., Ed.D.
President, Phillips+Fenwick

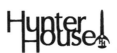

Copyright © 1994 by Nancy Evans

All rights reserved. No part of this publication may be reproduced or transmitted in any form or by any means, electronic or mechanical, including photocopying or recording, or introduced into any information storage and retrieval system without the written permission of the copyright owner and the publisher of this book. Brief quotations may be used in reviews prepared for inclusion in a magazine, newspaper, or broadcast.
For further information contact:
Hunter House Inc., Publishers
P.O. Box 2914
Alameda CA 94501-0914

The author is grateful for permission received to reprint or adapt from those works listed below or acknowledged elsewhere in the text: foldout chart from *Maternal Newborn Nursing,* Fourth Edition, by Olds, et al. © 1992 by Addison-Wesley Nursing, used by permission of the publisher; illustrations on pages 55–56 by Ken Miller from *The Informed Women's Guide to Breast Health,* by Kerry A. McGinn, Palo Alto CA: Bull Publishing, © 1992, used by permission.

Library of Congress Cataloging-in-Publication Data
Evans, Nancy (Nancy Jane)
The A-to-Z of pregnancy and childbirth : a concise encyclopedia / Nancy Evans.
p. cm.
Includes bibliography and index.
ISBN 0-89793-136-X (hard cover) : $29.95
ISBN 0-89793-129-7 (soft cover) : $16.95
1. Pregnancy—Dictionaries. I. Title.
RG525.E824   1993
618.2'003 — dc20   93-2247

Cover design by Tamra Goris Design   Book design by *Qalagraphia*
Copyeditors: Mary Lou Sumberg, Bobbie Sumberg   Proofreader: Susan Burckhard
Project editor: Lisa E. Lee   Production Manager: Paul J. Frindt
Marketing: Corrine M. Sahli   Promotion: Robin Donovan
Customer Service: Laura O'Brien   Fulfillment: Sergio Gaspari
Publisher: Kiran S. Rana
Set in Times Roman and Falstaff by 847 Communications, Alameda CA
Printed by Publishers Press, Salt Lake City UT
Manufactured in the United States of America

9   8   7   6   5   4   3   2   First edition

Contents

Acknowledgments vi

Foreword by Celeste Phillips, R.N. Ed.D. vii

Important Note to the Reader viii

How to Use This Book xi

Alphabetical Entries 1

Bibliography 313

Resources 315

Subject Index 320

Month-by-Month Chart of Maternal and
    Fetal Development .... inside back cover

Acknowledgments

Though writing is a solitary activity, publishing a book is seldom a solo performance. Thus I would like to acknowledge my gratitude to the following friends and associates who have helped make this book possible:

The maternity nurse authors whose books and whose friendship have enriched my life and work immeasurably: Margaret Jensen, Irene Bobak, Sally Olds, Marcia London, Patricia Ladewig, Persis Hamilton, Joy Ingalls, and Connie Salerno;

Celeste Phillips and Loel Fenwick, courageous agents of change, whose understanding and advocacy of true family-centered maternity care continue to transform clinical practice;

Jack Tandy, longtime colleague and artist, whose excellent illustrations on the foldout chart depict month-by-month changes in mother and baby throughout pregnancy;

Catherine Way, whose helpful review of the manuscript late in her second pregnancy offered the double benefit of professional and personal expertise;

Marilyn McGregor and Linda Reyes, who offered valuable comments and suggestions on the material on breast health and breast cancer, based on research and real-life experience;

Leslie Cleveland and Marie Dolcini, whose editorial assistance made an overwhelming task possible;

Kerry McGinn, nurse author, who referred me to Hunter House;

Betty-Lou Harmon, best friend and housemate, who continues to support my efforts and endure the agony and unpredictability of my writing life with grace and patience and understanding;

Lisa Lee, editor, and Kiran Rana, publisher, and all the other Hunter House publishing professionals, who have helped make this book a reality.

My deepest thanks and appreciation to all.

Nancy Evans
San Francisco CA

Foreword

Women having babies today have many choices. As our knowledge has grown, the technology and procedures surrounding infertility, pregnancy, and birth have proliferated.

At the same time, hospitals, in their competition for patients, are increasing their offerings of consumer-friendly alternatives to the traditional hospital birth environment. Some advertise homelike rooms for labor and birth and numerous amenities, including private jacuzzi tubs. Continuous epidurals for pain relief during labor are standard in some facilities. In some hospitals, infant and mother stay together from delivery, while in other hospitals this practice is discouraged.

What is a woman to do? What are the benefits and potential risks of today's reproductive technology and obstetric procedures? What is placenta abruptio, previa, etc.?

Is there one source that can provide the answers to these questions? Yes, there is. You are reading it now.

Nancy Evans has diligently conducted the library research and has compiled this encyclopedia on the "a" to "z" of pregnancy and birth for you.

Of all the books written about pregnancy and birth, this one is different; it explains the language of childbirth that is often reserved for obstetrical professionals.

This is not a book that begins with preconception and leads you step by step through pregnancy and postpartum. Nor is it a primer on how to breathe through contractions or how to provide infant care.

It is first and foremost a resource that can help you interpret what you read and what you are told about pregnancy and birth. If you are concerned about particular obstetrical procedures, you will find their explanations in this book.

Instead of being confused or intimidated by obstetrical jargon, you will find that you understand the physical and psychological aspects of birth and the procedures and techniques used by your care providers.

Here is your resource. . . your own personal encyclopedia of pregnancy and birth. Keep it handy. Refer to it often. Knowledge is power. When you can speak the language of childbirth, you can decide what kind of maternity care is right for you.

Celeste Phillips, R.N., Ed.D.
President, Phillips+Fenwick

Important Note to the Reader

The material in this book is intended to provide an overview of the issues and terminology surrounding pregnancy and childbirth. Every effort has been made to provide accurate and dependable information and the contents of this book have been compiled in consultation with medical professionals. The reader should be aware that professionals in the field may have differing opinions and change is always taking place. Therefore the author, publisher, and editors cannot be held responsible for any error, omission, or outdated material.

The author and the publisher have made every effort to ensure that all drug dosages and schedules of treatment are correct and in keeping with current recommendations and practice at the time of publication. However, because of new research, changes in government regulation, and the continuing flow of information related to drug therapy, the reader is advised to consult the package insert for each drug for the latest information. The author and publisher disclaim any liability, loss, injury, or damage incurred as a consequence, directly or indirectly, of the use and application of any of the contents of this volume.

If you have any questions or concerns about the information in this book or the care and treatment of yourself or your pregnancy, please consult a licensed health practitioner.

The author welcomes comments and suggestions from readers for ways that the book might be improved in succeeding editions. If you do not find terms in here that are needed, or if anything is unclear, please write to me at the address below.

Nancy Evans
c/o Hunter House, Inc.
P.O. Box 2914
Alameda CA 94501-0914

The A-to-Z of
Pregnancy and Childbirth

Dedicated to
Eric, Joyce, Dylan, and Nicole,
my joy today,
my hope for tomorrow.

How to Use This Book

Pregnancy and birth are at once unique and universal life experiences. Each woman and each couple bring unique needs, desires, and meaning to the process, from pre-conception through the postpartum period. Choosing a caregiver and a facility that acknowledge the uniquely personal aspects of pregnancy and birth can provide both immediate and long-term benefits.

Fortunately, today's health care system offers many choices and options concerning when, how, where, and with whom our children are born. Choosing wisely from those options depends on understanding: what are the physiologic, psychosocial, and political dimensions involved in pregnancy and birth? The better we understand human growth and development, nutrition, exercise, and the kinds of support and care available, the more likely we are to choose caregivers and institutions that will meet our own individual needs.

The A-to-Z of Pregnancy and Childbirth: A Concise Encyclopedia can help you gain new understanding of pregnancy and birth because it explains the medical language used by caregivers. Organized alphabetically for convenience and accessibility, this book helps you interpret the information you get from your caregiver and from your own research. Some definitions are brief; others are lengthy. All are written in a clear, concise style, reflecting current research findings.

Identical or related terms with different meanings are defined under a single heading. For example, *anesthesia* includes definitions of both general and regional anesthesia, as well as four types of regional anesthesia: *epidural, pudendal, spinal,* and *caudal.* Definitions of terms that have several common names as well as scientific names include all the important variations of the term, even slang usage.

Terms that are mentioned in one definition but explained in more detail in another location are printed in small capital letters, for example, LABOR, CESAREAN DELIVERY, or PLACENTA.

A subject index is provided at the back of the book, and lists all relevant terms by major category, such as birth control and sterilization, breastfeeding, drugs, and medications. For readers who want more detailed information, the Bibliography lists current references on various topics. The Resources section provides the names of organizations that offer information and referral, categorized by topic area such as childbirth education, infertility, grief and loss.

Few life experiences hold greater excitement, anxiety, and potential than pregnancy and birth; this process lets us participate in a miracle. Understanding the process enables us to enjoy the fullest possible participation, and to realize our full potential in preparing for parenthood. This book can help build that understanding.

abdomen The lower part of the trunk of the body, extending from the lower chest to the MONS PUBIS (pubic mound), containing the stomach, the large and small intestines, the liver, spleen, kidneys, appendix, pancreas, and other organs. During pregnancy the expanding uterus pushes up into the abdomen, crowding all other organs.

abdominal effleurage Light stroking of the abdomen, used during LABOR to help relax abdominal muscles and relieve mild to moderate pain.

abnormal presentation Any position of the FETUS in which the top of the head (the crown) will not be the first body part to emerge from the BIRTH CANAL. Principal types of abnormal presentation are BREECH, BROW, FACE, POSTERIOR, and SHOULDER; each is defined in a separate entry.

abortion The loss or interruption of a PREGNANCY before the FETUS attains a weight of 500 grams (1 pound 1½ ounce), the minimum weight considered viable (capable of living outside the UTERUS).

spontaneous abortion Unintentional loss of pregnancy, commonly called MISCARRIAGE. Expulsion of the entire PLACENTA, membranes (AMNIOTIC SAC), and contents of the uterus is termed *complete* abortion; partial expulsion of these tissues is called *incomplete* abortion, a problem that can lead to serious infection. For this reason, incomplete abortion should be followed by DILATATION AND CURETTAGE (D&C), a surgical scraping of the uterine lining to remove all extraneous tissue. Unexplained and persistent BLEEDING, CRAMPING, and backache during pregnancy signal *threatened* abortion. Death of the fetus in utero (within the uterus or womb), without expulsion, is called *missed* abortion and requires prompt medical intervention. Spontaneous abortion occurring in three or more consecutive pregnancies is called *habitual* abortion.

induced abortion   The *elective* or intentional termination of pregnancy. If performed legally, it is called a *therapeutic* abortion; if performed illegally, it is termed a *criminal* abortion. Procedures for elective abortion vary according to the length of pregnancy. In most pregnancies of 12 weeks or less, surgical D&C has been replaced by VACUUM ASPIRATION (removal of placental and fetal tissue from the uterus using suction). In pregnancies of 13 to 16 weeks, DILATATION AND EVACUATION is used, and in pregnancies of 16 to 24 weeks, AMNIOINFUSION or HYSTEROTOMY is used.

    Even although elective abortion is legal in the United States and Canada, it remains highly controversial with deeply held beliefs on either side of the issue.

abruptio placentae   Also *placental abruption, premature separation.* The detachment of all or part of the PLACENTA from the uterine wall after the 20th week of PREGNANCY but before birth. When such detachment occurs prior to the 20th week, it often causes MISCARRIAGE. Later detachment is a medical emergency requiring immediate treatment to avoid life-threatening HEMORRHAGE, shock, infection, or other complications for both mother and INFANT.

    Abruptio placentae and PLACENTA PREVIA are the two most common causes of hemorrhage in late pregnancy, although both are relatively rare. Abruptio placentae occurs primarily in women who have borne six or more children, women who smoke, use cocaine, or have high blood pressure (hypertension). The symptoms vary according to the degree of separation. About one-third of separations are small, producing few or no symptoms, and are noticed only when the placenta is inspected after birth. Larger separations, however, cause abdominal or back pain; uterine irritation and tenderness; FETAL DISTRESS, including absence of a fetal heartbeat; and hemorrhage, either visible or concealed. Bleeding generally begins just under the placenta, which is normally attached to the FUNDUS (the topmost portion of the UTERUS) at either the front or rear uterine wall. As blood accumulates, the placenta starts to separate from its fragile connection. Depending on the position of the placenta and the FETUS, the blood may exit through the CERVIX and VAGINA (visible hemorrhage) or be retained inside the uterus (concealed hemorrhage). While profuse vaginal BLEEDING clearly signals the need for treatment, concealed hemorrhage is more dangerous because it masks the severity of the problem.

Emergency treatment for abruptio placentae includes transfusions to replace lost blood and to fight shock, and antibiotics to prevent or control infection. The fetus must be delivered promptly (within six hours of diagnosis, according to most authorities). Delivery may be either vaginal, inducing labor by RUPTURING THE MEMBRANES and/or administering OXYTOCIN; or surgical, by CESAREAN section. Prompt treatment will almost always save the mother's life; the fetus, however, dependent on the placenta for OXYGEN, has a much slimmer chance for survival—from 20% in the most severe cases to 50% in more moderate cases. Many clinicians believe that immediate cesarean delivery offers the best outcome for both mother and baby.

abscess   A localized collection of pus, caused by bacterial infection. Abscesses can occur in many external and internal parts of the body.

breast abscess   Also *submammary abscess.* An abscess that develops most frequently when BREASTFEEDING leads to dry, cracked NIPPLES, which admit bacteria present on the skin or in the baby's mouth. Initial symptoms include swelling, inflammation, and tenderness, followed by fever, chills, and formation of a large, hard lump. Oral antibiotics are the usual treatment, possibly followed by surgical drainage. If antibiotics are given at the first signs of inflammation and swelling, the formation of such abscesses can often be prevented. See MASTITIS.

pelvic abscess   An abscess found most often in the genital tract, usually following childbirth, ABORTION, or gynecologic surgery, or less frequently, in the OVARIES or FALLOPIAN TUBES; related to PELVIC INFLAMMATORY DISEASE. These abscesses are generally caused by bacterial infection, either from vaginal bacteria or from contaminated external sources such as nonsterile instruments. Initial symptoms are fever and pelvic pain. Severe infection may produce any or all of the following: high fever, chills, vomiting, abnormally rapid heartbeat. Intravenous antibiotics are the treatment of choice, followed by surgical drainage of the abscess and irrigation with sterile saline solution. See PUERPERAL FEVER.

abstinence, periodic
     See under NATURAL FAMILY PLANNING.

acceleration   Periodic increases in the baseline FETAL HEART RATE, caused by CONTRACTIONS and/or fetal movement.

acme   The period of highest intensity of a uterine CONTRACTION.

acrocyanosis   A description of newborn skin coloration in which the extremities are bluish (cyanotic) and the rest of the body is pink, at one minute after birth. This condition is typical in 85% of normal newborns.

acrosin test   A test that evaluates the ability of SPERM to penetrate the egg (oocyte) and thereby achieve FERTILIZATION.

active acquired immunity   Formation of maternal ANTIBODIES or IMMUNOGLOBULINS (Ig) during PREGNANCY in response to disease or immunization. These include IgG, IgA, and IgM. Only one of these immunoglobulins—IgG—crosses the PLACENTA to the FETUS. This transfer occurs primarily in the third TRIMESTER; thus premature infants are more susceptible to infections than full-term newborns.
   See also PASSIVE ACQUIRED IMMUNITY.

adnexa   Adjoining parts of a larger structure. For example, the uterine adnexa are the OVARIES and FALLOPIAN TUBES.

adolescence
   See PUBERTY.

adolescent pregnancy   PREGNANCY before the age of 19, a phenomenon repeated more than one million times each year in the United States. The rate of adolescent pregnancy in the United States is more than double that in Canada, England, or France, and seven times higher than in the Netherlands, even though the numbers of sexually active teenagers are comparable. The rate of ABORTION for U.S. adolescents exceeds that in all Western countries for which data are available. Many factors are believed to contribute to these figures: inadequate emphasis on sex education, cost and confidentiality issues surrounding contraceptives, sexual innuendo throughout the popular media without emphasizing sexual responsibility issues, and the declining influence of the family. As teenage sexual activity becomes more commonplace, the teen pregnancy rate continues to soar, despite

the additional danger of AIDS and other SEXUALLY TRANSMITTED DIS-
EASES that can result from unprotected sex.

Adolescent pregnancy puts both mother and baby (and the father,
if he chooses to assume responsibility in the pregnancy and childbearing) at risk for many reasons, both physical and psychosocial. The
risks of PREMATURE births, low-BIRTH-WEIGHT babies, PREGNANCY-IN-
DUCED HYPERTENSION (PIH), and iron-deficiency ANEMIA are much
greater for pregnant adolescents than for women 20 years old or older.
As children having children, they face a possible lifetime of social,
emotional, educational, and economic vulnerability.

adolescent mother   Adolescence means change—physical, psychological, and social. Hormonal changes trigger a growth spurt, weight
change, the development of BREASTS and pubic hair, the beginning of
menstruation. Hormonal changes also put adolescents on an emotional
roller coaster at a time when they are struggling with issues of depend-
ence versus independence, same and opposite sex relationships, economic and social stability, peer group pressures, body image, and
personal versus family values. Adolescence proves doubly difficult
when compounded by the physical and psychological impact of pregnancy.

PRENATAL CARE, important for every expectant mother, is critical
to the well-being of the adolescent mother and her baby. Many pregnant adolescents, however, do not seek early prenatal care, and those
who do may not follow the recommendations concerning DIET, SMOK-
ING, use of ALCOHOL and other DRUGS, or SEXUALLY TRANSMITTED DIS-
EASES. Because many pregnant teenagers come from disadvantaged
backgrounds, their general health may be poor and their level of understanding inadequate to promote healthful behaviors during pregnancy. Concern about body image may take precedence over proper
nutrition, leading to inadequate WEIGHT GAIN (less than 20 pounds) and
increased probability of a low-birth-weight infant.

Many adolescents face pregnancy without the support of a partner or a parent, thus increasing the all-too-common feelings of loneli-
ness and isolation. Often, pregnant teenagers drop out of school, thus
limiting their own development and earning power. Studies show that
the younger an adolescent is at the time of her first pregnancy, the
more likely she is to become pregnant again during adolescence.
Many of these young women establish single-parent, matriarchal family units with little stability. Those who choose to marry the baby's

father, usually also an adolescent, frequently divorce. Becoming parents too soon means interrupted personal and educational development, inability to become self-supporting, and emotional immaturity in intimate relationships—all ingredients for failed marriage.

adolescent father   Although the adolescent father is spared the physical changes and discomforts of pregnancy, if he elects to participate in the childbearing process he is just as unprepared socially and emotionally as his partner. He is often the target of anger and disappointment from his partner, their families, and their peer group. His minimal job skills, limited education, and emotional immaturity are generally no match for the overwhelming moral and economic responsibility of supporting a family. Thus, he faces risks similar to that of the adolescent mother: less formal education, decreased economic success and job satisfaction, and higher probability for divorce. The conscientious adolescent father can benefit from prenatal counseling and education about pregnancy, birth, childrearing, and parenting, and thereby better support his partner through this difficult time. Educational and vocational counseling are equally important if the new family is to survive and thrive.

adrenal glands   Also *suprarenal glands*. Two small ENDOCRINE GLANDS located at the top of each kidney (*ad* means "on," *renal* means "related to the kidney"). The right adrenal is triangular, the left more rounded and crescent-like, and covered on its lower surface by the pancreas. Each gland is made up of a cortex, a firm outer part that constitutes most of the gland, plus a medulla, a soft inner part. The medulla secretes adrenalin (epinephrine) and other substances; the cortex secretes many different steroid HORMONES, including the sex hormones (ANDROGEN, ESTROGEN, and PROGESTERONE). These hormones act in various ways to maintain physiologic equilibrium or balance (homeostasis), and to aid survival during fight-or-flight situations, fasting, injuries, shock, and other stressors.

The adrenal glands can be affected by a number of diseases, including ADRENOGENITAL SYNDROME, which causes genital abnormalities and menstrual irregularities.

adrenogenital syndrome   Also *adrenal virilism, adrenal hyperplasia*. A disorder, usually congenital (present from birth), in which the ADRENAL GLANDS produce excess ANDROGENS (male sex hormones).

This condition can also be caused in an adult by an ovarian or adrenal tumor, or by administration of synthetic PROGESTINS during PREGNANCY to prevent miscarriage. This syndrome causes females to develop male SECONDARY SEX CHARACTERISTICS and males to evidence precocious sexual development (abnormally early development of secondary sex characteristics). The effects are more pronounced in females; even mild cases are characterized by HIRSUTISM (excess body hair). Even though the sex CHROMOSOMES and internal organs are female, the genitalia are masculinized to some degree, particularly the CLITORIS. Other symptoms include baldness, acne, deepening of the voice, cessation of menstruation, uterine atrophy, decreased BREAST size, and increased muscularity. Surgical treatment is necessary to correct sexually ambiguous genitalia, whereas treatment with cortisone generally eliminates the other symptoms. If the disorder is congenital, however, cortisone treatment must be continued for life.

afterbirth
See PLACENTA.

afterpains   Cramping pains caused by uterine CONTRACTIONS after the birth of a baby, most acute during BREASTFEEDING, lasting several days.
See under CONTRACTION, UTERINE.

agalactia   A rare disorder in which the mother is unable to secrete breast milk after childbirth. Generally, the secretion of breast milk can be increased by more frequent nursing.
See also BREASTFEEDING; LACTATION.

age, childbearing   Technically, the years between the first ovulation after MENARCHE (average age, 12.6) and MENOPAUSE (average age, between 45 to 53), when menstruation ceases. The physiologically ideal time for childbearing is from the late teens up to age 30. Females under age 16 or over 34 are at high risk for complications.
See also ADOLESCENT PREGNANCY; BIRTH DEFECTS; HIGH-RISK PREGNANCY.

AIDS   Acquired Immune Deficiency Syndrome, a fatal viral infection first diagnosed in 1981, believed to be caused by the Human Immunodeficiency Virus (HIV), identified in 1983. By attacking the immune system, HIV decreases the body's ability to resist opportunistic infections (OIs) and cancers that, while ordinarily not life-threatening, prove fatal to the HIV-infected person.

HIV enters the body through blood (including menstrual blood), blood products, and other body secretions such as SEMEN, vaginal fluid, urine, feces, and breast milk. Tears and saliva also contain very weak concentrations of the virus, but the concentration is so low that exposure is not considered to be a risk.

HIV can live in the body for as long as nine years or more before causing any symptoms. Thus, the infected person can unknowingly infect others through unprotected sexual intercourse or sharing needles during intravenous DRUG USE, and the symptoms of those thus infected may appear earlier in others than in the carrier of the infection.

Early symptoms include swollen glands, aches, pains, and fever, mimicking mononucleosis, but in some cases no symptoms appear until the intermediate stage, known as AIDS-related complex (ARC). The most common symptom of ARC is lymphadenopathy, or swollen lymph nodes in the neck, armpits, and/or groin; these nodes may be either painless or tender. Other symptoms of ARC include anorexia (loss of appetite) and weight loss of more than 10 pounds in two months; unexplained fever; night sweats; weakness, particularly in the legs when climbing stairs; persistent unexplained diarrhea; persistent dry cough; oral or vaginal THRUSH (candidiasis), a yeast infection characterized by white spots and blemishes in the mouth and throat or in the vagina; herpes zoster (shingles); hairy leukoplakia, a precancerous condition causing white sores and a thickened MUCOUS MEMBRANE in the mouth and vagina; and lymphoma, a cancer of the lymphatic system.

The diagnosis of full-blown AIDS is based on the patient's having one or more life-threatening OIs, such as pneumocystis pneumonia; cytomegalovirus (CMV) infection, a HERPES VIRUS that can cause blindness, pneumonia, colitis, and esophagitis; candidiasis; cryptosporidiosis; cryptococcosis; toxoplasmosis; Kaposi's sarcoma, a skin cancer; tuberculosis; infection of the brain or lungs caused by *Mycobacterium avium intracellulare;* herpes simplex infections of various organs; cervical carcinoma; and dementia.

Once considered a disease of homosexual and bisexual men, HIV-AIDS is now among the 10 leading causes of death in American women of childbearing age. In New York City, it is the leading cause of death in women of childbearing age. More than 25,000 women have been diagnosed with AIDS, contracted primarily through sharing needles with an infected intravenous drug user (51%), or through unprotected HETEROSEXUAL intercourse (32%). The highest numbers of women with AIDS are concentrated in New York, New Jersey, Florida, and California (ranked from highest to lowest numbers of cases). Women of color are disproportionately affected: 53% of U.S. women with AIDS are African-American; 21% are Latina.

HIV-infected women can infect their babies during PREGNANCY or through BREASTFEEDING; thus they are advised to avoid pregnancy. HIV, however, limits a woman's choice of contraceptive methods: ORAL CONTRACEPTIVES may speed the progression of the disease and INTRAUTERINE DEVICES may increase the transmission of the virus to a woman's sexual partners. Therefore, the CONDOM remains the most effective method of reducing the risk of both pregnancy and the transmission of the virus.

Women who suspect they are pregnant often seek confirmation from a healthcare provider. The U.S. Centers for Disease Control (CDC) recommend HIV-testing for any woman at risk of HIV infection through either intravenous drug use or unprotected sex with an HIV-positive partner. Since both pregnancy and HIV are characterized by such nonspecific symptoms as fatigue, anorexia, and weight loss, women who were unaware that their sexual partners put them at risk may not know they are infected until they seek PRENATAL CARE.

Between 30% and 50% of infants born to HIV-infected mothers are also infected, and thereby doomed to early death from AIDS. The rate of HIV infection is the same whether babies are delivered vaginally or by CESAREAN section. Women with HIV are advised not to breastfeed unless there is no other food source available. A woman who is HIV-positive may want to terminate her pregnancy, if diagnosed early. Many women with HIV, however, are poor, uninsured, and forced to rely on Medicaid funds for abortions, thus limiting this option.

Prenatal care of the HIV-positive woman who chooses to carry her pregnancy to term depends on her stage of infection. If she experiences few or mild symptoms, her care is no different from that of a healthy woman. Unfortunately, however, other infectious and blood-borne diseases often accompany an HIV-positive diagnosis: GONORRHEA, SYPHILIS, HEPATITIS B, CHLAMYDIA, herpes simplex virus (HSV), papilloma virus (genital WARTS), and mycobacterium tuberculosis. Because pregnancy can depress immune function, such latent infections as HSV, CMV, and toxoplasmosis can become much more serious and even life-threatening for mother and fetus.

Treatment of these secondary diseases is limited by the potential toxic effects on the developing FETUS. Acyclovir, one of the antiviral drugs approved for use in HIV patients, is not considered safe. Zidovudine (Retrovir), the other major antiviral drug, crosses the PLA-CENTA and may have toxic effects on the fetus similar to those in young infants; its effects, however, are not completely understood. Treatment to prevent pneumocystis pneumonia may decrease the risk of hypoxic damage to the fetus, but drugs such as trimethoprim and most antiviral agents should be avoided unless the mother has a life-threatening illness. Pentamidine isethionate (NebuPent), a drug used to treat pneumocystis carini pneumonia, should not be given to a pregnant woman unless the potential benefits outweigh the known risk.

Authorities believe that pregnancy may be complicated in the woman with advanced HIV disease. Women with T4 (T-cells, which are white blood cells formed in lymphatic tissue that help fight infection) lymphocyte counts of fewer than 300 have a much greater risk of infection during pregnancy. In addition, HIV impairs the function of lungs, heart, kidneys, and liver, limiting the use of medication during LABOR and DELIVERY and the woman's ability to tolerate the physical effort of labor. If she has HIV-associated dementia, her thinking process will be impaired. ANEMIA, common in HIV-infected persons, could increase the impact of blood loss during delivery.

Research indicates that the more advanced the mother's HIV illness and the more premature the birth, the more likely is the transmission of infection to the baby. Many questions about HIV in pregnant women remain unanswered, however, such as: Does HIV infection have an impact on the overall health of the mother? Does pregnancy influence disease progression? Do HIV-infected women, whose offspring develop AIDS and die, experience a faster disease progression than HIV-positive women with healthy offspring?

Scientists caution that both a preventive vaccine and a cure for HIV infection remain only a distant hope. Until either or both are available, prevention through education and safer sex habits is the only effective measure. Guidelines for safer sex are summarized in Table A-1.

Women with AIDS need information about living with their disease. The following may be helpful: *The Guide to Resources on Women*

Table A-1   Sexual Practices That Reduce the Risk of HIV Transmission

Completely safe	Abstinence
	Monogamous sexual activities with monogamous, non-infected partner
Probably safe	Non-insertive sexual practices
	Insertive sexual practices with condoms and spermicides
Risky	All other sexual behaviors, particularly with intravenous drug users

with AIDS provides a state-by-state listing of many available services and can be obtained from the Center for Women's Policy Studies (202-872-1770). Other sources include the hotline for AIDS Clinical Trials Information (800-874-2572); the National AIDS Hotline (800-342-2437); and Project Inform (800-822-7422), which provides information about the latest treatment recommendations.

albumin, urinary   Also *albuminuria*. A protein found in the urine, indicating any of a variety of kidney diseases. Normal urine contains no albumin. During PREGNANCY, albumin in the urine signals developing preeclampsia; thus each prenatal visit includes testing the urine for albumin.

See also ECLAMPSIA; HYPERTENSION.

alcohol use   Drinking of alcoholic beverages. Moderate use of alcohol—three to five drinks per week—is not considered harmful for most women who are *not* pregnant. However, **the safest course for pregnant women is to abstain from all alcohol**. Research has shown that women are affected more quickly by alcohol than men because their stomachs are less able to digest or neutralize alcohol. In alcoholic women, it appears that the stomach stops digesting any alcohol. This means that a much greater portion of the alcohol women drink enters their bloodstream as pure ethanol; if a woman is pregnant, the alcohol crosses the PLACENTA to the FETUS. Even moderate alcohol use can harm the developing fetus, particularly early in pregnancy before a woman knows she is pregnant. Women who are trying to conceive should abstain from all alcohol consumption. Heavy drinking (six or more drinks daily) can produce a baby with *fetal alcohol syndrome* (FAS), a cluster of severe BIRTH DEFECTS including mental retardation, growth retardation, heart defects, malformed facial features, a small head, and problems with fine motor coordination. Even having two drinks daily has been associated with low-birth-weight babies and may contribute to other long-range problems, such as learning disabilities.

The number of babies born with birth defects because their mothers used alcohol and/or other drugs is rising dramatically, perhaps by as much as 3,000% over the past 10 years. According to one study, more than 11% of all INFANTS born in the United States in 1988 tested positive for alcohol or cocaine the first time a blood sample was obtained. Such damaged children represent a national tragedy—a tragedy that every woman who is pregnant or planning to become pregnant can help prevent.

alpha-fetoprotein test   A BLOOD TEST used to evaluate fetal development and the possibility of BIRTH DEFECTS. Alpha-fetoprotein (AFP) is found in the fetal circulation, AMNIOTIC FLUID, and maternal blood. Abnormally high levels of AFP can indicate NEURAL TUBE DEFECTS, such as spina bifida and anencephaly; multiple gestation (twins, triplets, and so on); incorrect gestational age; a dead FETUS; FETAL DISTRESS; abdominal wall defects; or Rh-sensitization. Low levels of AFP suggest a high risk of DOWN SYNDROME. The test is performed at 15 to 18 weeks' gestation; if AFP levels are abnormal, a second test is done one week later. If the second test shows high AFP levels, further evaluation using ULTRASOUND or AMNIOCENTESIS is necessary to determine whether birth defects are present.

amenorrhea   Absence of menstrual periods at an age when regular menstruation is to be expected and when a female is neither pregnant nor lactating. It may be either *primary* or *secondary amenorrhea,* and is not a disease but a symptom of a disruption in normal function of the female body.

primary amenorrhea   Failure to begin menstruating by age 16. In the United States, more than 97% of females begin normal MENSTRUAL CYCLES by age 16. However, the age at which menstruation begins varies from 10 to 18 years, depending on nutrition, lifestyle, and family history. Failure to begin menstruating by age 16 may not be cause for concern unless no other signs of puberty are present (such as a growth spurt, development of BREASTS, and/or growth of underarm or pubic hair). It is important to rule out *cryptomenorrhea,* a condition in which menstrual bleeding is retained inside the vagina by an anatomical obstruction such as imperforate hymen (a condition in which the hymen, the membrane that normally covers part of the vaginal opening, completely covers the opening to the vagina).

Primary amenorrhea most often results from dysfunction of the PITUITARY GLAND and/or the OVARIES, rather than an anatomic abnormality (such as lack of a VAGINA or UTERUS). Diagnosis begins with a detailed medical and family history, the possibility of unsuspected PREGNANCY, recent fluctuations in body weight, and symptoms of other metabolic disorders such as DIABETES or thyroid deficiency. History-taking is followed by physical examination, including a pelvic examination. If no abnormalities are detected in the uterus or ovaries, the next step is an X-ray of the skull to rule out tumors of the pituitary gland, and cytologic tests of vaginal and buccal (oral) smears and of the urine to detect HORMONES and any abnormalities of the CHROMOSOMES.

If thorough testing and examination do not indicate disease or abnormality, the diagnosis is likely delayed puberty or slow maturation. Some adolescent girls, particularly those who are very athletic, diet-conscious, or anorexic, may not have reached critical weight: the proportion of body fat tissue required to initiate and maintain normal menstrual cycles. Many physicians prefer not to treat primary amenorrhea until age 18, recommending only careful follow-up once or twice each year to assess the situation.

If menstruation has not begun by age 18, one of several endocrine disorders may be the cause. These include diabetes mellitus; acromegaly (a disorder caused by excess secretion of pituitary growth hormone, sometimes related to a pituitary tumor) or other pituitary problems; STEIN-LEVENTHAL SYNDROME, or other ovarian disorders; or dysfunction of the THYROID or ADRENAL GLANDS. Except for DIABETES, these are relatively rare and usually can be corrected by medication and/or surgery. Chromosomal disorders such as TURNER'S SYNDROME, HERMAPHRODITISM, and ANDROGEN INSENSITIVITY SYNDROME can also cause primary amenorrhea. Eating disorders, increasingly common in adolescent girls, such as anorexia nervosa (a type of self-starvation practiced largely by teenage girls) and OBESITY, can also delay menstruation, as can heart disease, tuberculosis, use of tranquilizers and/or barbiturates, and emotional stress.

primary amenorrhea and pregnancy   Women with primary amenorrhea who wish to become pregnant have various treatment options, depending on the cause of the amenorrhea. Hormonal imbalance can be corrected with medication; imperforate hymen or closed CERVIX can be surgically repaired. A woman with a normal uterus but dysfunctional ovaries may have a donor embryo, fertilized by her partner's SPERM, implanted in her uterus (see EMBRYO TRANSFER). A woman without a uterus but with normal ovarian function may choose to engage the services of a SURROGATE MOTHER to nurture the fertilized egg and carry the pregnancy to term. This is a highly controversial practice with emotional and ethical implications; in some states it is illegal to pay a surrogate mother for her services.

secondary amenorrhea   The absence of menstrual periods for six months in a woman who has established a normal menstrual cycle, or for three cycles in a woman with *oligomenorrhea,* menstrual periods occurring more than 35 days apart. Menstrual cycles vary widely among healthy women and within the life experience of the same woman, so unless symptoms suggest underlying disease or INFERTILITY, it is not an urgent problem. Pregnancy is a major cause of secondary amenorrhea; therefore it should be ruled out, as should early MENOPAUSE, before further testing.

The diagnostic process is similar to that in primary amenorrhea, but may also include an endometrial biopsy if hormonal tests indicate a high probability of endometrial cancer. If tests rule out serious disease, no treatment is necessary unless the woman wants to become pregnant. Then, hormone therapy may be effective in inducing menstruation and ovulation. Such therapy might include PROGESTERONE, perhaps combined with ESTROGEN to stimulate the pituitary and initiate bleeding, followed by the FERTILITY PILL, to stimulate OVULATION.

Other causes of secondary amenorrhea include, in addition to those listed for primary amenorrhea (see above), damage to the pituitary caused by POSTPARTUM HEMORRHAGE and/or shock (SHEEHAN'S SYNDROME); damage to the ENDOMETRIUM by excessive CURETTAGE (ASHERMAN'S SYNDROME); radiation therapy; ovarian cysts and/or tumors; and drugs, including ORAL CONTRACEPTIVES. Excessive weight loss and/or vigorous physical exercise, such as that of professional dancers or athletes, can also be responsible for amenorrhea.

Amenorrhea following childbirth is termed *postpartum* amenorrhea if it lasts for more than three months after delivery in a woman who does not breastfeed. *Lactation amenorrhea* (AMENORRHEA-GALACTORRHEA SYNDROME) is the absence of menstrual periods more than six weeks after breastfeeding is discontinued. These conditions may disappear spontaneously. Many women rely on herbal remedies to induce delayed menstruation. See EMMENAGOGUE.

amenorrhea-galactorrhea syndrome   Also *inappropriate lactation syndrome, lactation amenorrhea.* A disorder involving failure to menstruate and inappropriate secretion of breast milk. Two types of this syndrome occur, one after a pregnancy (Chiari-Frommel syndrome) and the other unrelated to pregnancy (Ahumada del Castillo syndrome). Both types result from absence of the PROLACTIN-INHIBITING FACTOR (PIF), a substance normally produced by the HYPOTHALAMUS. Because this disorder can be triggered by a pituitary tumor, such a lesion must be ruled out before proceeding with hormonal treatment. It can also be caused by hypothyroidism (decreased secretion of THYROID hormones), or use of ORAL CONTRACEPTIVES, phenothiazines (a class of tranquilizers), tricyclic antidepressants, narcotics, or antihypertensive drugs (to correct high blood pressure). Treatment may be surgical (removal of a pituitary tumor), or medical (discontinuing the causative drug) or administering bromocryptine, a drug that suppresses prolactin production. Chiari-Frommel syndrome often resolves without treatment, although it frequently recurs after subsequent pregnancies.

amniocentesis   A procedure involving removal and analysis of fluid from the AMNIOTIC SAC that surrounds the FETUS to evaluate fetal maturity and detect genetic abnormalities and BIRTH DEFECTS, including DOWN SYNDROME, TAY-SACHS DISEASE, NEURAL TUBE DEFECTS, Rh incompatibility, and SICKLE CELL ANEMIA. Developed in the mid-1960s, this test cannot be performed before 16 weeks' GESTATION. Thus, it has been replaced in many medical centers by CHORIONIC VILLUS SAMPLING (CVS), a newer and equally reliable procedure that can be performed during the first TRIMESTER. If a serious problem is detected during the first trimester, termination of the PREGNANCY at that time carries less risk than during the second trimester.

Amniocentesis is usually recommended to pregnant women over age 35 since the risk of birth defects increases with age. Down syn-

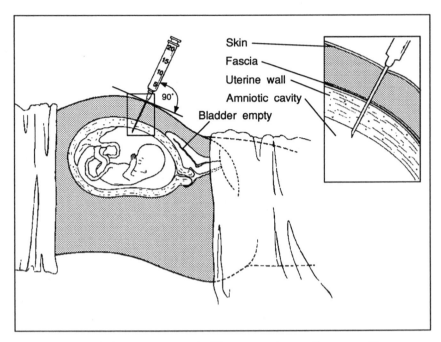

Figure A-1   Amniocentesis. The woman is usually scanned by ultrasound to determine the placental site and to locate a pocket of amniotic fluid. As the needle is inserted, three levels of resistance are felt when the needle penetrates skin, fascia, and uterine wall. When the needle is within the uterine cavity, amniotic fluid is withdrawn.

(From Maternal Newborn Nursing, *Fourth Edition, by S. Olds, M. London, and P. Ladewig. ©1992 by Addison-Wesley Nursing. Reprinted by permission.)*

drome, also called trisomy 21, is the most common birth defect, occurring in one of every 400 births to women age 35 and in one of every 100 births to women age 40. Amniocentesis is also recommended to women who have had a previous child with a birth defect or three or more spontaneous ABORTIONS, and for those whose previous experience or family history suggest the risk of CHROMOSOME abnormalities, metabolic disease, or neural tube defects.

The procedure is performed on an outpatient basis, either in a hospital or physician's office. It consists of ULTRASOUND examination to determine the position of PLACENTA and fetus, followed by insertion of a needle through the abdomen and uterine wall into the amniotic sac, and withdrawal of 15 to 20 milliliters (1 to 1.5 ounces) of amniotic fluid (Figure A-1). The fetal cells from the fluid are cultured in a special medium, after which the chromosomes are analyzed and metabolic studies done, a process that takes two to four weeks. In about 10% of cases, cells fail to grow and the procedure must be repeated.

Amniocentesis carries little risk to the mother but greater risk to the fetus because the test can bring on premature labor (in less than 1% of cases). Therefore, it is important to select a facility and personnel who are experienced in amniocentesis. It is also important for the woman and her partner to consider before the test whether she would choose to have an abortion if the test indicates the presence of serious birth defects. Even if her personal or religious beliefs prevent having an abortion, knowing that her baby will be born with a defect may allow her to better prepare for the changes this will make in her life.

amniography   A special X-ray procedure used to detect structural abnormalities in the FETUS. This procedure is usually delayed until late in PREGNANCY to avoid radiation damage to the baby. It involves injecting radiopaque dye into the AMNIOTIC SAC and taking an X-ray. The dye shows the shape of the fetus more clearly than an ordinary X-ray. The technique has limited use, however, because it must be done late in the pregnancy, making ABORTION of a severely malformed fetus much more difficult.

See also FETOSCOPY.

amnioinfusion   Also *amniocentesis abortion, intra-amniotic infusion, late abortion, midtrimester abortion, premature induction of labor.* Terminating a PREGNANCY of 13 to 24 weeks by injection (infusion) of a foreign substance into the amniotic fluid to induce CONTRACTIONS. Within a few hours after injection, contractions begin and eventually the FETUS and PLACENTA are expelled. Prior to 1975, amnioinfusion was performed using a concentrated saline (salt) solution (saline abortion); now, however, many clinicians prefer to inject either UREA (a nitrogen compound found in urine; urea abortion), or one of the PROSTAGLANDINS (hormones; prostaglandin abortion).

Several hours before beginning amnioinfusion, many clinicians use LAMINARIA to "soften" and help dilate the CERVIX. Then a local anesthetic is injected into the lower abdomen, followed by a thin hollow needle into the AMNIOTIC SAC for withdrawal of amniotic fluid and infusion of the solution (saline, urea, or prostaglandin). The solution is infused slowly over a period of 10 to 15 or more minutes.

During this time, the woman remains awake so she can report any pain, dizziness, or other sensation that could indicate an adverse reaction to the drug being used. After the needle is withdrawn, the woman waits for uterine contractions to start, usually within 12 hours. At some point, the woman may be given an injection of OXYTOCIN to speed up the process or to increase the strength of contractions. Saline solution takes from 8 to 12 hours to initiate contractions and may make the woman very thirsty. Prostaglandins cause contractions to start more quickly but can result in NAUSEA, vomiting, and/or diarrhea.

Once contractions begin, they increase in intensity and frequency, and the fetus and placenta are expelled. During the final hours of this process, the woman may need drugs for relief of pain or anxiety; however, general ANESTHESIA is not used. Some physicians administer SCOPOLAMINE to the woman just before expulsion of the fetus, in order to induce amnesia. Saline solution usually causes FETAL DEATH immediately upon injection. In rare cases of prostaglandin abortion, a fetus may emerge alive; in this instance, the law requires that it be treated as a PREMATURE INFANT, even though it has only a slight chance of survival. Within an hour after the fetus emerges, the placenta usually will be expelled. With prostaglandin abortion, however, the placenta may need to be extracted, increasing the risk of HEMORRHAGE and retained fragments of placenta that will need to be surgically removed (CURETTAGE).

Amnioinfusion carries greater physical and emotional risk for the woman than either first trimester abortion using suction or surgical curettage or second trimester DILATATION AND EVACUATION (D&E) abortion. Because of the potential for complications, the procedure requires hospitalization from 24 to 48 hours. Some hospitals may ask that patients return home after the injection and return only after contractions are well established, a practice that increases patient risk.

The woman who chooses amnioinfusion faces a risk equal to that of full-term birth. Saline solution accidentally injected into a blood vessel can cause shock or even death. Prostaglandin abortion involves sharper, more painful contractions and greater risk of cervical tearing and hemorrhage, in addition to nausea, vomiting, and/or diarrhea. It also increases the likelihood of a fetus that shows signs of life, making the experience extremely painful emotionally for the woman and for the hospital staff.

Amnioinfusion is absolutely contraindicated for some patients. Any woman with heart, liver, or kidney disease, HYPERTENSION (high blood pressure), or SICKLE CELL ANEMIA should *not* have a saline abortion. Any woman with heart or lung disease, asthma, hypertension, epilepsy, a history of convulsions, glaucoma, or a known allergy to prostaglandins, should *not* have a prostaglandin abortion. When amnioinfusion is contraindicated, surgery remains the only option. See HYSTEROTOMY.

Amnioinfusion is sometimes performed during labor to relieve cord compression in women with ruptured membranes or decreased amniotic fluid.

amnion   The inner layer of membranes forming the sac or bag of waters containing the amniotic fluid and the FETUS. The outer layer is the CHORION.

amnionitis   Also *chorioamnionitis*. Infection within the AMNIOTIC SAC caused by bacterial invasion and inflammation of the membranes before birth. When the bag of waters breaks prior to the onset of labor, it is termed *premature rupture of membranes (PROM)*. Amnionitis is only one cause of PROM; others include INCOMPETENT CERVIX, urinary tract infection, HYDRAMNIOS, trauma, and MULTIPLE PREGNANCY. Symptoms of amnionitis include fever, uterine tenderness, and rapid maternal and/or FETAL HEART RATE. The first priority is to deliver the FETUS within 24 hours, either through INDUCTION OF LABOR or CESAREAN SECTION.

See also RUPTURE OF MEMBRANES.

amniotic fluid embolism   A life-threatening emergency occurring during LABOR or DELIVERY in which amniotic fluid is released into the mother's circulatory system and enters her lungs. It can be caused by a tear in the amniotic membrane high in the UTERUS, tears in the CERVIX, or separation of the PLACENTA from the uterine wall. Pressure from the contracting uterus forces the fluid into the maternal system. Only 20% of women with this complication survive; fetal mortality and morbidity are also high.

amniotic sac   Also *bag of waters, membranes*. A sac that surrounds a fertilized egg within one week after FERTILIZATION, gradually expanding to enclose the entire EMBRYO (called the FETUS after 12 weeks GESTATION). It is made up of two membrane layers: the CHORION (a thick outer layer with many fingerlike projections, called *chorionic* *villi,* on the surface) and the AMNION (inner layer). As the fetus develops, the amniotic sac expands and fills with a clear liquid called *amniotic fluid.*

The *amniotic fluid* cushions the embryo/fetus as it grows and develops; helps regulate body temperature; permits freedom of movement, aiding musculoskeletal development; and, prevents the amnion from adhering to the fetus. It also inhibits the growth of bacteria, helping to protect the fetus from infection.

At 10 weeks' gestation, the amniotic sac contains about 30 milliliters of fluid, increasing rapidly to 350 milliliters at 20 weeks. After 20 weeks, the volume of fluid ranges from 500 milliliters up to 1 liter (slightly more than 1 quart) at 36 to 38 weeks. As the 40th week approaches, the volume decreases, averaging 800 milliliters at birth. If pregnancy is prolonged beyond 40 weeks, the amount of fluid may become quite scanty. The volume of fluid changes continually as it · moves back and forth across the placental membrane. Every 24 hours the fetus swallows up to 400 milliliters of the fluid and excretes about the same volume of urine. Abnormally high volume of amniotic fluid is called HYDRAMNIOS (also *polyhydramnios)* and may indicate MULTIPLE PREGNANCY (especially identical twins), fetal abnormalities, or maternal disease such as DIABETES. Abnormally low volume of fluid is termed *oligohydramnios* and nearly always indicates the presence of abnormalities such as a fetus SMALL FOR GESTATIONAL AGE (SGA), or with kidney or urinary tract abnormalities.

During pregnancy, the fetus sheds cells from the skin, amnion, and gastrointestinal and urinary tracts into the amniotic fluid. Analysis of these cells can detect more than 100 different BIRTH DEFECTS. See AMNIOCENTESIS.

Normally, the amniotic sac ruptures spontaneously during early LABOR, releasing a gush of clear, amber-colored amniotic fluid through the mother's VAGINA. When the sac ruptures before labor begins, it is termed *premature rupture of membranes (PROM),* indicating the need for treatment to prevent infection. Rarely, the membranes remain intact throughout delivery and the infant is born within the sac. In this case, the infant's head is covered with a portion of the membranes termed the caul, believed by some to endow the child with psychic ability or "second sight." Labor is sometimes induced by artificial rupture of membranes (AROM), either surgically or manually. See AMNIOTOMY; RUPTURE OF MEMBRANES.

amniotomy   Also *artificial rupture of membranes (AROM), break-ing the bag of waters.* Intentional rupture of the membranes, or AM-NIOTIC SAC, to induce LABOR. Wearing a sterile glove, the clinician inserts an index finger or two fingers into the dilated CERVIX until the baby's head can be felt. Then, with an amnihook or other surgical instrument, the membranes are penetrated or torn near the cervix. The clinician then elevates the baby's head slightly to allow the amniotic fluid to escape. Labor generally begins within an hour or two of this procedure, although it may take as long as six to eight hours. If labor has not begun within 24 hours of amniotomy, the clinician may admin-ister OXYTOCIN to start the contractions. Amniotomy does not require ANESTHESIA, but it does increase the risk of maternal infection.

See also INDUCTION OF LABOR.

analgesic   Any drug or other remedy that relieves pain. Analgesic drugs are classified as either narcotic or nonnarcotic. The principal narcotic analgesics are opium and its alkaloids (such as morphine and codeine) and synthetic narcotics, such as meperidine (DEMEROL), methadone, and propoxyphene (Darvon). All narcotics are potentially habit-forming; they can create both physical and psychological de-pendence in the user, which results in withdrawal symptoms when the drugs are discontinued.

The principal nonnarcotic analgesics are the salicylates, such as aspirin; ibuprofen (Advil, Medipren, Nuprin); the pyrazolone deriva-tives, such as phenylbutazone (Azolid, Butazolidin) and indomethacin (Indocin); and the aniline derivatives, such as acetaminophen (Ty-lenol, Datril, Panadol, Liquiprin, Anacin-3). In addition to relieving pain, most of these drugs (except for the aniline derivatives) also decrease fever and inflammation.

Use of any drug, either over-the-counter (OTC) or prescription, carries the risk of harming the FETUS, particularly in the first TRIMES-TER. Even aspirin, usually considered harmless for most people, is not recommended for women who are pregnant or BREASTFEEDING because it can cause ulcers, ANEMIA, or impaired blood clotting, increasing the risk of HEMORRHAGE. Ibuprofen has similar effects. See DRUG USE AND PREGNANCY.

Both analgesics and anesthetics may be given to relieve discom-fort and pain during childbirth. However, all must be carefully evalu-ated based on their effects on the mother, the fetus, and uterine CONTRACTIONS. All systemic drugs given during LABOR cross the placental barrier, some more easily than others, and may depress fetal respiration. Normally, these drugs are given by intravenous or intramuscular injection to increase their effectiveness. Timing is critical: given too early, analgesics can prolong labor and depress the fetus; given too late, analgesics fail to relieve the mother's pain but still depress the fetus.

See also ANESTHESIA.

androgen   Any HORMONE that produces masculine characteristics in either sex. The major androgen is TESTOSTERONE, produced by the male TESTES and, in small quantities, by the female OVARIES and ADRENAL GLANDS.

androgen insensitivity syndrome   Also *testicular feminization.* A CONGENITAL ABNORMALITY in which females appear to have normal female genitals, except for a lump or swelling in each groin, sparse pubic and underarm hair, and a VAGINA too short for sexual intercourse. Their UTERUS and FALLOPIAN TUBES are not fully developed; thus they do not menstruate and cannot become pregnant. The disorder is caused by insufficient androgen-binding protein in the cells of the FETUS, resulting in partially developed masculine organs that then prevent normal development of female organs. Genetic testing will show that the sex chromosomes are all XY, as in normal men, rather than XX, as in normal women. When the individual reaches puberty, BREAST development and overall body contours appear female, resulting from ESTROGEN produced in the rudimentary TESTES. Although no treatment exists to make PREGNANCY possible for women with this condition, surgery can lengthen the vagina sufficiently to permit vaginal intercourse.

anemia   A scarcity of red blood cells, diagnosed through a blood count (see under BLOOD TEST). If red blood cells constitute less than 37% of total blood volume, or if the blood's hemoglobin value is below 12 grams per 100 milliliters of blood, a woman is termed anemic. Symptoms of anemia include fatigue, dizziness, heart palpitations or rapid heartbeat, seeing spots, HEADACHES, difficult breathing, and pale skin. Iron deficiency is the most common cause of anemia; other causes include HEMORRHAGE, vitamin B_{12} or FOLIC ACID deficiency, bone marrow disease, and blood disorders such as SICKLE CELL ANEMIA. *Pernicious anemia* due to vitamin B_{12} deficiency rarely occurs during PREGNANCY. However, *folic acid deficiency anemia* (also *megaloblastic anemia*) is common in women with poor diets and carries serious consequences for the developing FETUS, particularly NEURAL TUBE DEFECTS such as spina bifida and anencephaly. Recent studies recommend that all pregnant women receive daily supplements of 0.4 milligram of folate. Women with folic acid deficiency nearly always are iron deficient as well.

During pregnancy, blood volume increases progressively, beginning in the first TRIMESTER and peaking in the third trimester at about 45% above normal levels. This increased blood flow primarily benefits the additional workload of the UTERUS and the kidneys. Although the red blood cell volume also increases 18 to 30%, the proportion of whole blood composed of red cells decreases by an average of about 7%. This decrease is referred to as the physiologic anemia of pregnancy (pseudoanemia).

Since iron is essential to the production of red blood cells, the pregnant woman's need for iron increases from 15 to 18 milligrams per day (the maximum that can be absorbed from the DIET) to 30 milligrams. Although gastrointestinal absorption of iron increases somewhat during pregnancy, it is usually necessary to supplement dietary iron with an additional 30 to 60 milligrams daily, particularly during the second half of pregnancy when the fetus is growing rapidly. Iron supplements are usually not given during the first trimester since they may increase NAUSEA.

It is important for the pregnant woman to have an iron-rich diet; the best sources of dietary iron are lean meats; dark green, leafy vegetables (spinach, broccoli, watercress, parsley, escarole—also good sources of folic acid); whole-grain cereals and breads; eggs; dried fruits; legumes (also contain folic acid); shellfish; and molasses. Cooking in large volumes of water or in the microwave can destroy much of the folic acid content of foods.

Since many women begin pregnancy with slight anemia, it is important to ensure that the problem is corrected. The normal blood loss during childbirth can increase risk for the anemic woman.

anesthesia   Loss of touch and pain perception caused by drugs called anesthetics. Anesthesia may be *topical* (affecting a small surface area), *regional* or *local* (affecting segments of the nervous system in a particular section of the body), or *general* (affecting the entire body and causing unconsciousness). Anesthesia is used to eliminate pain during surgery, dentistry, other traumatic medical procedures, and childbirth.

topical anesthesia   Many topical anesthetics are available without prescription; they include sunburn creams and lotions, throat spray or lozenges, and creams or lotions to relieve the pain and itching of insect bites or poison ivy.

general anesthesia   General anesthesia must be administered by a physician, certified nurse, anesthetist, or dentist. In procedures performed in hospitals or clinics, anesthesia should be administered by an anesthesiologist, a physician with advanced education in use of anesthesia; a nurse anesthetist; or a specially-prepared technician working under the supervision of an anesthesiologist.

General anesthesia rarely is given during childbirth because it crosses the PLACENTA and anesthetizes the baby as well, increasing the risk of serious respiratory problems in the infant. It also slows uterine CONTRACTIONS and increases the risk of vomiting, which can lead to respiratory arrest if vomited material is aspirated (breathed into the lungs). If used at all during birth, it is administered at the end of LABOR, just before DELIVERY of the baby. Nitrous oxide (laughing gas) offers pain relief but not true anesthesia, and it can seriously delay development of the baby's motor skills (sitting, standing, walking).

The use of anesthesia in childbirth gained popularity after Queen Victoria inhaled chloroform during delivery of one of her children. Later *inhalation anesthetics* included ether, cyclopropane, and halothane, all of which were used effectively in surgery. The intravenous anesthetic, thiopental sodium (Pentothal) was also effective. The use of these anesthetics in childbirth, however, resulted in sleepy babies with slowed reflexes, impaired sucking response, and sometimes serious respiratory problems.

regional anesthesia   Regional anesthesia, also called *conduction anesthesia,* has proved much more satisfactory in childbirth than general anesthesia. Given by injection, regional anesthetics do not cause unconsciousness but only eliminate the pain in a specific region of the body by blocking conduction of pain impulses to the brain. These agents have minimal effect on the baby since they are only slightly absorbed into the mother's bloodstream. However, they can lower the mother's blood pressure, slow or weaken contractions, and cause postpartum HEADACHES. The anesthetic agents most commonly used in childbirth are lidocaine (Xylocaine), chloroprocaine (Nesacaine) and bupivacaine (Marcaine).

All anesthesia has risks as well as benefits, which women need to understand. Many women now realize that with psychological preparation and coaching by a supportive birth partner, anesthesia may be unnecessary during birth (see PREPARED CHILDBIRTH). However, since every birth is unique for both mother and baby, women should not feel that they have "failed" if they need or want regional anesthesia during labor and delivery.

The four most widely used forms of regional anesthesia (regional nerve blocks) are *caudal, epidural, pudendal,* and *spinal* anesthesia, usually injected in small amounts as needed.

caudal anesthesia Also *caudal block.* Numbing of the area from belly to knees by means of injection in the sacral canal at the base of the back, providing pain relief to the CERVIX, VAGINA, and PERINEUM. Caudal anesthesia is usually administered on a continuing basis through an in-dwelling catheter rather than a single injection, beginning about halfway through the first stage of labor and continuing until just before delivery. The term caudal is derived from a Latin word meaning "tail." This procedure requires a larger dose of anesthetic than either a spinal or an epidural, thus posing greater risk for mother and baby. For that reason, it is used less often today. Advantages include a conscious mother able to witness the entire birth, minimal blood loss, and a relaxed perineum less likely to tear when the baby emerges. Disadvantages include less effective contractions, thus prolonging labor, dropping maternal blood pressure, postpartum backache, and increased need for FORCEPS delivery since the mother cannot feel the urge to push. Because of the risk of shock, caudal anesthesia cannot be used if the woman is hemorrhaging or subject to a condition such as preeclampsia.

epidural anesthesia Also *lumbar epidural.* Numbing of the area from belly to knees by continuous infusion through a small catheter in the epidural space between the bony vertebrae and the base of the spinal cord. Epidurals are generally started when the cervix has dilated to 4 centimeters and no more than 9 centimeters. The most popular regional block for both vaginal and CESAREAN births, the epidural requires a smaller dose of anesthetic than the caudal and is easier to administer and monitor. However, it carries risks similar to the caudal: maternal hypotension (sudden drop in blood pressure), reducing the baby's oxygen supply, and sometimes slowing the FETAL HEART RATE.

Epidural anesthesia can also impede the progress of labor, slowing the strength and effectiveness of contractions. Because of these risks, choosing an epidural means choosing an array of devices and procedures that may further complicate the birth process, including: external or internal FETAL MONITORING, an intravenous solution for hydration and possible addition of PITOCIN to speed up contractions, a blood pressure cuff, artificial rupture of membranes (AROM), a urinary CATHETER. An epidural blocks the mother's urge to push, thus increasing the likelihood that a VACUUM EXTRACTOR or forceps will be needed to help the baby be born. Recent studies suggest that epidurals also increase the need for cesarean delivery.

Epidural anesthesia is contraindicated when there is danger of hemorrhage, such as PLACENTA PREVIA, preeclampsia, or ECLAMPSIA, or during fetal distress. In some areas of the country, choosing to give birth in a hospital may almost automatically mean choosing epidural anesthesia. However, this need not be the case; each woman has the right to make an informed choice of whether to have any anesthesia, and if so, what kind.

pudendal anesthesia   Numbing of the vulva by means of injection in the perineal or vaginal area. Pudendal anesthesia is used primarily just before or immediately following delivery, in order to perform or repair an EPISIOTOMY or use forceps. This procedure carries the lowest risk of complications but has been reported to cause decreased oxygen saturation in the newborn.

spinal anesthesia   Also *saddle block, subarachnoid block.* Numbing of the entire body below the rib cage by means of a single injection into the spinal fluid in the spinal canal just before delivery. High spinal anesthesia is usually used for cesarean section, while low spinal or saddle block is used for forceps-assisted vaginal delivery. Spinal anesthesia totally arrests the labor process, eliminating all sensation, including the need to push. It can cause nausea and vomiting, with the additional risk of aspiration (sucking the vomitus fluid into the lungs by gasping, thereby impeding breathing), and requires that the mother lie flat on her back for at least eight hours after delivery. Spinal anesthesia also causes post-anesthesia headaches in many women, and holds the greatest risk of serious and even fatal complications. Thus it is used much less frequently than in the past.

antepartum

See PRENATAL CARE.

antibody   A protein in the blood that identifies a substance foreign to the body, called an ANTIGEN, reacts to and neutralizes it. Antibodies are one of the immune system's two major defenses against invading substances (such as viruses and bacteria). The second defense comes from body cells, such as T cells, that surround and attack foreign substances.

See also RH FACTOR.

antigen   A substance that elicits ANTIBODY production and reacts specifically with antibodies.

See also ANTIBODY; RH FACTOR.

Apgar score   A scoring system to evaluate a newborn's physical condition and need for possible resuscitation, based on five measurements: heart rate, respiratory effort, muscle tone, reflexes, and skin color. The newborn is rated at one minute after birth and again at five minutes after birth, with a possible total score ranging from 0 to 10 each time. An Apgar score of 8 to 10 indicates a newborn in good condition. A score below 8 may indicate the need for resuscitation. A score of 3 or less means the infant's survival is in jeopardy. The test is named for Virginia Apgar, an American anesthesiologist who developed the test in 1952.

Table A-2   Apgar Scoring

	Points scored		
Signs	0	1	2
Heartbeats per minute	Absent	Slow (<100)	Over 100
Respiratory effort	Absent	Slow, irregular	Good, crying
Muscle tone	Limp	Some flexion of extremities	Active motion
Reflex irritability	No response	Grimace	Cry or cough
Color	Blue or pale	Body pink, extremities blue	Completely pink

apnea   An interruption of breathing for more than 20 seconds; or for less than 20 seconds when accompanied by cyanosis (bluish discoloration of the skin caused by insufficient oxygen in the blood), irregular heartbeat, and limpness. Apnea is a common problem in PREMATURE INFANTS (less than 36 weeks' gestation) and thought to result from immaturity of the nervous system.

apocrine glands   One of two types of sweat glands, located under the arms and in the pubic area. The other type is the *eccrine glands,* located in the palms of the hands and soles of the feet. They are important in regulating body temperature. Apocrine glands begin to function at PUBERTY, influenced by ANDROGENS, producing an odorless secretion that takes on a musky, unpleasant scent when decomposed by bacteria on the skin. Women have more than twice as many apocrine glands as men.

areola   The dark pigmented area around the NIPPLE of the BREAST. Highly sensitive nerve endings in the areola and the nipple make this part of the breast an area of sexual arousal. Small, rudimentary sebaceous glands on the nipple and areola are called *Montgomery's tubercles* or *Montgomery's follicles;* during PREGNANCY, these glands become more pronounced. During BREASTFEEDING, these glands secrete a fatty substance that helps lubricate and protect the breast. During pregnancy, some women may develop a *secondary areola,* a ring of faint color just outside the true areola, which becomes fainter or disappears after birth.

artificial insemination   Depositing of SEMEN at the cervical os or in the UTERUS of a woman by mechanical means in order for her to become pregnant. A couple chooses this procedure only after tests have shown that the woman is fertile but the man is producing problem SPERM (too few or not enough MOTILITY to achieve FERTILIZATION). It also is sometimes used when factors such as infection, inadequate ESTROGEN secretion, or antisperm ANTIBODY production make the woman's CERVIX inhospitable to sperm. In these cases, the sperm are deposited directly into the uterus *(intrauterine* insemination); however, this treatment remains controversial for women with antibodies. Artificial insemination is also used by women who are part of a LESBIAN couple and by single women who want to bear a child without HETEROSEXUAL intercourse.

Two types of artificial insemination are available: artificial insemination with the husband's or regular partner's sperm (AIH), also called *homologous* insemination; and artificial insemination by donor (AID), also called *heterologous* insemination. AIH can be an effective treatment for INFERTILITY when the man produces healthy sperm but in insufficient quantity (see OLIGOSPERMIA), or in the case of cervical disorders. It proves successful in about 15% of cases.

The conception rate for AID is twice that of AIH; estimates are that more than 30,000 babies are conceived each year by means of AID. Although the actual procedure is simple, the ethical, religious, legal, economic, and emotional implications can be difficult and complex. For example, the Roman Catholic and Orthodox Jewish faiths consider AID a form of adultery. Men may experience grief, guilt, and even shame, equating infertility with failed masculinity. They may have concern about being able to accept the child. Both partners need to consider what they will tell their friends and family, and most important, what they will tell the child. Many clinicians recommend that women and couples considering AID talk with others who have chosen this procedure and perhaps also with counseling or educational groups such as Resolve, Inc. before making a decision (see Resources). It is important that the man truly want the procedure and not just allow the woman her desire because she wants to bear a child.

Many couples prefer that AID be a completely anonymous process, arranged through a physician; this helps avoid legal and psychological difficulties over custody, visitation rights, and financial responsibility. Others, especially lesbian couples, may want the donor to be a friend who could be involved in the child's life. Anonymity can create problems later on for the child conceived by AID who needs or wants to locate his biological father. It is also important to protect the legal rights of children conceived by AID because not all states in the United States recognize them as "legitimate" offspring. Working with an attorney, these issues can and should be resolved before the procedure.

In choosing a donor, fertility and general good health are most important. The donor should be free of any hereditary or transmittable illness, (particularly in the age of AIDS), emotionally stable, and similar in intelligence to the couple. Ideally, his physical characteristics should be similar to those of the male partner, and his blood group and type compatible with the female partner. If AID is arranged without physician involvement, it is possible to have the donor screened by an independent clinician.

The American Fertility Society recommends the use of frozen rather than fresh SEMEN. However, freezing makes the sperm less motile and can increase the number of inseminations necessary to achieve conception, while fresh sperm must be used within an hour of ejaculation. Costs range from $750 to $1,000 per insemination, so this decision has economic consequences as well.

The procedure for AID is relatively simple. After determining the time of OVULATION, a SPECULUM is used to dilate the VAGINA and expose the CERVIX. The semen is then inserted into the vagina while the woman is lying on her back, using a syringe without a needle. She remains in this position for at least 30 minutes, and may use a CERVICAL CAP or tampon to help hold the semen close to the cervical os. Clinicians usually repeat this process two days later with another semen sample. If CONCEPTION does not occur, the process is repeated at the next ovulation, and so on, for a period of six months. More than half of women using AID become pregnant within six months. However, women over age 30 or those with ENDOMETRIOSIS, pelvic disorders, or ovulatory problems are not as successful in conceiving.

See also SPERM BANK; TEST-TUBE BABY.

artificial rupture of membranes (AROM)
See AMNIOTOMY.

Ascheim-Zondeck test
See under PREGNANCY TEST.

Asherman's syndrome Also *uterine synechiae*. Extensive scar tissue (adhesion) in the uterine wall that can prevent regular menstruation and cause INFERTILITY. The usual cause is a complicated DILATATION AND CURETTAGE (D&C) following a pelvic infection, but it can also result from surgical removal of uterine tumors (myomectomy), CESAREAN DELIVERY, and tuberculous ENDOMETRITIS.

aspartame An artificial sweetener (brand names: Equal®, NutraSweet®) that is nearly 200 times as sweet as sugar, and is used in many so-called "diet" drinks and foods (often with many other additives and empty calories). Aspartame is made up of two amino acids: aspartic acid and phenylalanine. Although some clinicians may suggest that moderate amounts of aspartame can be included in a prenatal DIET, caution is advisable. Because phenylalanine can cross the PLA-

CENTA to the FETUS and cause brain damage, aspartame is CONTRAINDICATED for women with PHENYLKETONURIA (PKU). It has been suggested that some women may be unable to metabolize phenylalanine even though they show no symptoms of PKU; these women may risk damaging their babies by consuming large amounts of aspartame.

aspermatogenesis   Failure to produce SPERM, resulting in STERILITY.

aspiration
    See VACUUM ASPIRATION.

asymptomatic   Showing no symptoms, that is, no apparent evidence of a particular disease. For example, an HIV-positive man may be asymptomatic and thus may unknowingly infect his partner.

atony   Lack of muscle tone. Uterine atony can be life-threatening in the POSTPARTUM period because it results in HEMORRHAGE, either slow and steady or sudden and massive. This condition generally can be anticipated and either prevented or managed successfully, beginning with adequate nutrition, good PRENATAL CARE, and early diagnosis and management of any complications. Factors contributing to uterine atony include over-distention of the UTERUS (by twins, for example), dysfunctional LABOR signaling abnormal patterns of CONTRACTION, OXYTOCIN use during labor, and the use of ANESTHESIA that produces uterine relaxation. Treatment ranges from uterine massage to injection of oxytocin or PROSTAGLANDINS, blood transfusion, or possible HYSTERECTOMY.

attachment   A kind of bonding or close intimate relationship between people, usually parent and child, and particularly parent and newborn.

attitude, fetal   The position of the fetal body parts in relation to each other. The normal fetal position is with the neck flexed slightly forward, the arms flexed onto the chest, and the legs flexed onto the abdomen. When fetal attitude changes, particularly the position of the head, it can contribute to difficult LABOR.

autosome   Any CHROMOSOME that is not a sex chromosome.

azoospermia The absence of SPERM in SEMEN, causing male STERIL-ITY. Depending on the cause of azoospermia, the condition may be treatable. Men with azoospermia related to hypothalamic or pituitary insufficiency may be given hormone replacement therapy. If the condition is related to vasectomy, microsurgery may be successful in reversing the earlier operation.

B

back labor   Labor pain in the lower back, usually intensified during uterine CONTRACTIONS, caused by POSTERIOR PRESENTATION of the FETUS, in which the head exerts pressure against the mother's back. This pain can sometimes be relieved by changing positions: either walking, squatting, or getting down on all fours; and/or by having the birth attendant apply heat, cold, or counterpressure on the lower back, whatever offers greatest relief. An acupressure technique of pressing firmly with a finger just below the center of the ball of the foot may also relieve back labor.

back pain   Also *backache*. Pain or discomfort in the lower back that, during PREGNANCY, results from the enlarged abdomen and the changes in posture caused by the additional weight and by relaxation of the pelvic joints. Maintaining good posture, keeping weight gain within recommended guidelines, wearing properly fitted shoes with wide heels, minimizing standing for long periods of time, and sitting with feet elevated sometimes helps relieve pain. Sleeping on a firm, comfortable bed and using a heating pad are also helpful. When sitting, it helps to elevate the feet.

bag of waters
   See AMNIOTIC SAC.

ballottement
   See QUICKENING.

barrier methods   Contraceptive devices or substances that prevent contact between SPERM and OVUM. These include the CONDOM, DIAPHRAGM, CERVICAL CAP, CONTRACEPTIVE SPONGE, and various SPERMICIDES (in jelly, foam, or suppository form).

basal body temperature (BBT) method   One of several FERTILITY awareness methods used to predict the time of OVULATION to either avoid or encourage conception. This method involves measuring the woman's basal body temperature (the initial body temperature before any activity, such as smoking, drinking, or urinating) every day for three or four months, and recording it on a graph to determine her normal cycle. It requires an especially sensitive thermometer, called a basal body thermometer, and is based on the fact that a woman's temperature often drops just before ovulation and usually rises just after, remaining elevated for several days. To avoid PREGNANCY, intercourse must be avoided on the day her temperature rises and for at least three days thereafter. The BBT method is a more effective contraceptive than the calendar method but it is still highly unreliable, even for women with very regular MENSTRUAL CYCLES. Many factors can invalidate the results, including fatigue, stress, fever, a cold, or other infection.

See also NATURAL FAMILY PLANNING.

baseline rate   The average FETAL HEART RATE measured over a period of ten minutes between CONTRACTIONS.

baseline variability   The irregularity of the FETAL HEART RATE as recorded by electronic monitor. The heart rate of a healthy FETUS includes some irregularity of the BASELINE RATE. Sustained variability can indicate fetal distress. Variability can be either short-term or long-term; both types are important in evaluating fetal status.

battering   Also *spouse abuse, woman abuse, domestic violence.* Physical abuse of a woman by her husband or lover. According to U.S. Federal Bureau of Investigation (FBI) statistics, every 15 seconds a woman is beaten by her husband or lover. Nearly one-third of all female homicide victims are killed by their husbands or boyfriends. Wife battering is the most frequently committed but least reported violent crime in the United States. Studies estimate that battering occurs in one out of three marriages, and is more common among lower socioeconomic groups, urban families, minority racial groups, families where the husband is unemployed, or families with more than three children. Some authorities suggest, however, that the problem cuts across all of society and is simply better concealed among more affluent women who have access to private physicians, therapists, and attorneys.

Battering often begins or increases during PREGNANCY, particularly if the man is unemployed or perceives the child as an extra financial burden or as a competitor for the woman's time and attention. Unless the woman leaves an abusive relationship, battering may not only injure her but result in MISCARRIAGE, PRETERM LABOR, a low-BIRTH-WEIGHT baby, or injury or death of the FETUS. Women often remain in abusive relationships because they feel economically vulnerable, and this feeling can intensify during pregnancy. However, it is important to realize that help is available. Almost every community now has emergency shelters for battered women, as well as police, legal, social, and counseling services. Many communities offer job training and placement programs that can help women become economically independent.

Women in abusive relationships need to recognize that the battering is not their fault, but the fault of the batterer. Each person is responsible for his or her own behavior and no one else's. No one deserves to be beaten and no one has the right to beat someone else. Leaving an abusive relationship is not easy but it is possible and it is essential for any woman who values her own life and the life of her unborn child.

bimanual examination
See GYNECOLOGIC EXAMINATION.

biophysical profile An ultrasound test performed at 18 and 28 weeks to evaluate fetal well-being, based on five factors: breathing movement, body movement, tone, amniotic fluid volume, and FETAL HEART RATE reactivity. This test may also be performed when pregnancy continues more than 42 weeks after the LAST MENSTRUAL PERIOD (LMP).

birth attendant Someone who assists a woman during LABOR and DELIVERY, usually a health professional such as a physician, nurse-MIDWIFE, nurse practitioner, or other obstetrical nurse, but sometimes a nonprofessional "labor coach." Some couples who choose to give birth at home may choose a birth attendant who does not have professional training, such as a lay midwife, a husband or other relative, or a friend.
See also MIDWIFE; PREPARED CHILDBIRTH.

birth canal   The passage through which a baby normally emerges from its mother. This includes the UTERUS and bony PELVIS, the CERVIX, and the VAGINA.

birth center   A facility for LABOR and DELIVERY that emphasizes birth as a normal, healthy, family-centered event, rather than an illness requiring obstetric technology and treatment. Birth centers can be found within hospitals or as separate, freestanding facilities.

birth control
    See CONTRACEPTION.

birth defects   Also *congenital abnormalities (anomalies, defects)*. Abnormalities in INFANTS that are present at birth, but may or may not be inherited. Some birth defects, such as PHENYLKETONURIA (PKU), maple syrup urine disease, and homocystinuria, can be diagnosed immediately after birth and treated successfully with dietary management. Other defects, such as TAY-SACHS DISEASE and SICKLE CELL ANEMIA, may go undetected for months or years and prove untreatable and even fatal. Chromosomal abnormalities such as DOWN SYNDROME can vary in their effects from slight to severe.
    Birth defects are caused either by external causes, such as the mother's use of ALCOHOL or other DRUGS, or by internal causes, such as abnormalities in the infant's genes or CHROMOSOMES (genetic disorders). Some genetic disorders may be inherited, such as Marfan's syndrome; others, such as Down syndrome, are not.
    External causes of birth defects include: maternal exposure to alcohol, nicotine, and other drugs, as well as chemicals, radiation, and viruses; malnutrition; traumatic injury to the mother, either accidental or deliberately inflicted (see BATTERING); and injuries during the birth process. External causes that interfere with fetal development are called TERATOGENS. Table B-1 lists a number of substances to avoid during PREGNANCY. As a general rule, pregnant women should avoid all medications, unless prescribed by a physician aware of the pregnancy. This includes over-the-counter medications such as aspirin, laxatives, and megavitamins. All alcoholic drinks should be avoided since the effects of alcohol on the FETUS are incompletely understood. See *fetal alcohol syndrome* under ALCOHOL USE.

***Table B-1   Precautions During Pregnancy
to Help Avoid Birth Defects***

Avoid consuming	Alcoholic beverages
	Tobacco in any form
	Illegal drugs (marijuana, cocaine, crack, and others)
	Caffeine (coffee, tea, cola drinks, chocolate)
	All vitamins *except* those recommended by physician
	Medications prescribed before pregnancy
	Over-the-counter medications
	Vaccines
Avoid handling	Paint, especially oil-based paints and/or turpentine
	Pesticides and herbicides (weed killers)
	Cat litter
	Raw meat
Avoid	X-rays
	General anesthesia
	Infection, particularly rubella, measles, mumps, HIV or other sexually transmitted diseases
	Solvents, such as those used in arts and crafts

Women who smoke should stop when they become pregnant; otherwise, they risk MISCARRIAGE, bleeding problems such as PLACENTA PREVIA or ABRUPTIO PLACENTAE, and birth of PREMATURE, low-BIRTH-WEIGHT babies. Second-hand smoke (from cigarettes, pipes, or cigars) can also cause problems for the mother and fetus; thus the pregnant woman should encourage her partner and others close to her to refrain from smoking.

Although caffeine has not been shown to cause birth defects, its effect on the pregnant woman is increased threefold during the last TRIMESTER of pregnancy. The same level of caffeine intake (from coffee, tea, cola drinks, and chocolate) triples the amount of caffeine in the blood, making it advisable to restrict consumption of caffeine or eliminate it entirely.

RUBELLA and other viral infections may have only mild effects on the mother but cause severe birth defects in the baby. It is important for pregnant women to avoid persons with these diseases, as well as to avoid immunization with any live virus vaccine, even flu vaccines. Unless X-RAYS are essential, they should be avoided also. If they cannot be avoided, the abdominal area should be shielded with a lead apron during exposure.

There are three types of genetic disorders that cause birth defects: *chromosome defects, single-gene disorders,* and *multifactorial (polygenic) disorders. Chromosome defects* involve either an abnormality of number (too many or too few) or of structure. Down syndrome is the most common chromosome defect (1 in 700 live births), and usually results from an extra chromosome. The risk of this condition increases with the age of the mother, as is typical with most chromosome defects. Occasionally Down syndrome is caused by an abnormal rearrangement of chromosomes. Some chromosomal defects affect only the sex chromosomes, resulting in ambiguous genitalia (the sex organs do not clearly indicate gender), such as TURNER'S SYNDROME and KLINEFELTER'S SYNDROME. Prospective parents can learn whether they have chromosomal defects by consulting a geneticist for chromosomal analysis. This test is based on a buccal smear, an examination of cells scraped from the membrane that lines the mouth.

Single-gene disorders may be caused by one or a pair of mutant genes. A mother or father with a dominant mutant gene has a 50% chance of passing the mutant gene to each child. Researchers have identified more than 1,200 dominant gene disorders, among which are Huntington chorea (a progressive, ultimately fatal neurologic condition) and achondroplastic dwarfism (short-limb dwarfism). When both parents have a mutant gene that is recessive, their children have a 25% chance of inheriting it. Nearly 1,000 such disorders have been identified, including Tay-Sachs disease, sickle cell anemia and phenylketonuria. A mutant recessive gene present only on the X-chromosome in the mother has a 50% chance of being passed from mother to son. The clotting disorder HEMOPHILIA A is one of the more than 150 such genetic disorders. Duchenne MUSCULAR DYSTROPHY, a progressive wasting of the muscle fibers, and color blindness are also X-linked chromosome defects. A recently identified chromosome defect is the fragile-X syndrome, a central nervous system disorder characterized by mental retardation, large protuberant ears, and abnormally large TESTES following PUBERTY. It is caused by a "fragile site" on the X chromosome.

Multifactorial or *polygenic disorders* stem from the combination of genes interacting with each other and being acted upon by environmental factors. Most birth defects fall into this category, including such conditions as cleft palate, spina bifida, congenital heart defects, and clubfoot. Other diseases that are believed to be multifactorial in origin include DIABETES, some types of heart disease, HYPERTENSION, and mental illness.

Many birth defects can be detected by tests in the first TRIMESTER of pregnancy, offering the woman the choice of terminating the pregnancy. AMNIOCENTESIS was the first such test, developed in the late 1960s; more recent tests include CHORIONIC VILLUS SAMPLING and the ALPHA-FETOPROTEIN TEST. Parents concerned about the possibility of inherited disorders or other birth defects can seek GENETIC COUNSELING for recommendations on tests to determine their risks. Recently developed technology also makes it possible to treat the fetus in utero (within the uterus) for certain life-threatening diseases. One such method involves assessing the fetus by analyzing blood withdrawn through the UMBILICAL CORD and administering a transfusion through the same route.

birth rate   The number of live births per 1,000 population. The birth rate has been increasing in the United States since 1986, from 15.6 in 1986 to 16.7 in 1990.

See also FERTILITY RATE.

birth weight   The weight of a newborn INFANT at birth. This weight reflects the infant's maturity and, in many cases, chances for survival. The average birth weight is 3,420 grams (7 pounds, 9 ounces) for white babies and 3,180 grams (7 pounds) for Black babies. Newborns weighing less than 2,500 grams (5½ pounds) usually are considered high-risk. Often these low-birth-weight babies are PREMATURE (born before 37 weeks' gestation) and will not survive without intensive care (some will not survive even with intensive care). Because some low-birth-weight babies are full-term or even POSTMATURE, however, GESTATIONAL AGE is also used in evaluating each infant and the need for care, as are the APGAR SCORE and other factors.

Low-birth-weight can be caused by genetic factors (parents of small stature or transmission of a genetic disorder causing small stature), or, more commonly, by malnutrition. The baby's malnutrition can result from maternal disease, such as severe DIABETES, kidney disease, or HYPERTENSION, which inhibits the passage of nutrients across the PLACENTA, or from inadequate maternal DIET. Inadequate diet can be related to poverty or to an effort not to gain too much weight. Proper nutrition can become a low priority in the presence of ALCOHOL or other drug abuse.

See also GESTATION.

birthing bed   A special multi-position bed that allows the woman to LABOR and DELIVER in the same bed, rather than transferring from a labor bed to a conventional inflexible delivery table. The laboring woman controls the bed, changing positions (of her body and the bed) during labor for maximum comfort. Thus she is able to choose from a variety of positions in which to give birth, including squatting and other upright positions. When the baby's head becomes visible (CROWNING), the bottom portion of the bed can be detached to give the BIRTH ATTENDANT easier access to "catch" the baby. Many of these beds include bars that support the woman's upper body when she is in a squatting position, the most physiologically and psychologically beneficial position for birth. Modern research has confirmed the wisdom of many ancient birthing practices, such as walking about during early labor, changing positions frequently during labor, and giving birth in an upright position. This allows the emerging FETUS to work with the forces of gravity, making uterine CONTRACTIONS more efficient and shortening the period of labor. Until these research results were available, however, most U.S. women delivered in the DORSAL LITHOTOMY position (lying on their backs with their feet in stirrups). For more than half-a-century, physicians treated PREGNANCY and childbirth as an illness requiring medical and sometimes surgical intervention. During the women's movement of the 1960s and 1970s, consumers began to demand a more natural, less technological approach to pregnancy and birth, ultimately changing birth environments, equipment, and practices.

birthing chair   A low chair with a portion of the seat cut away to give the BIRTH ATTENDANT access to the pelvic area. Birthing chairs were used in ancient Egyptian, Greek, Roman, and Incan civilizations

but fell into disfavor during the 1800s due to the high rate of PUER-
PERAL FEVER ("childbed fever"). Modern methods of infection control
have made it possible to use birthing chairs again and women are
finding that these chairs can help reduce or eliminate back pain. In this
sitting position the woman can see the baby being born, and can help
lift the baby out and up to her face. Short women, however, may find
that sitting with their legs spread increases pressure on the PERINEUM,
which could lead to tearing. In addition, the chair does not afford the
variety of positions available with the BIRTHING BED.

birthing room   A hospital room designed to provide a natural,
homelike setting for family-centered maternity care. Also called "single purpose" rooms, these rooms are equipped to meet the needs of the
woman and her family throughout LABOR, DELIVERY, recovery, and in
some cases, the POSTPARTUM PERIOD. Designed with room enough for
the father or other birth partner and close friends, these rooms include
easy chairs as well as a bed, and often a television set. They eliminate
the need for multiple transfers of mother from labor to delivery to
recovery to postpartum room, reducing the risk of infection and offering a more relaxed, private birthing environment. In response to consumer demand for a more human approach to the birth process,
hospitals began to use birthing rooms in the 1970s as a safer alternative to HOME BIRTH or to the conventional maternity unit designed like
a surgical suite. Initially, only low-risk couples could choose birthing
rooms; those at higher risk were confined to the conventional unit.
Recently, however, some hospitals have adopted SINGLE ROOM MATER-
NITY CARE (SRMC) as standard practice, so that all women, except
those whose conditions demand CESAREAN DELIVERY, can enjoy the
benefits of this homelike birthing environment.
   See also LDRP.

birthing stool   A low, backless stool designed much like the birthing
chair, with similar advantages and disadvantages.
   See also BIRTHING CHAIR.

birthmarks   Congenital discolorations of the newborn's skin,
caused by an overgrowth of one or more of the normal components of
the skin: pigment cells, blood vessels, lymphatic cells, and so forth.
Most birthmarks fade by the age of two years. *Telangiectatic nevi* or
"stork bites" are flat, pale pink or red patches, frequently found on the

eyelids, nose, and nape of the neck. Although they usually fade by age two, they sometimes reappear when the child cries. *Cafe au lait* spots are flat, light brown patches that can appear anywhere on the body. They occur in 10% of white children and 22% of Black children, and remain throughout life. The presence of six or more cafe au lait spots larger than 1.5 centimeters in their longest diameter can indicate *neurofibromatosis,* a genetic disorder involving tumors along the nerves, the spinal column, or in the eye.

See also NEVUS FLAMMEUS; NEVUS VASCULOSUS.

bladder   Also *urinary bladder.* Muscular sac located in the lower abdomen that holds urine. The bladder receives urine from the kidneys through the ureters, and releases it through the URETHRA. Made up of layers of involuntary muscle fibers, the bladder is highly expandable, changing from a triangular shape when empty to an oval form when full. A full bladder creates a feeling of pressure, signaling the need to urinate. During PREGNANCY, the expanding UTERUS enhances this pressure, creating a frequent need for urination.

Women are subject to frequent infections of the bladder or urinary tract because the urethra can easily become contaminated with bacteria from the nearby VAGINA or rectum (see CYSTITIS). It is important to always wipe from front to back after urination or bowel movements, and to urinate immediately after sexual intercourse. Urinary tract infection (UTI) can have serious consequences for the pregnant woman; amniotic fluid infection can develop and retard growth of the PLACENTA. Untreated UTI can also be life-threatening if it ascends to the kidneys.

Pregnancy and birth sometimes cause sufficient relaxation of the muscles supporting the bladder that it projects all the way into the vagina.

See also CYSTOCELE; FREQUENCY, URINARY; STRESS INCONTINENCE.

bleeding, vaginal   Between MENARCHE and MENOPAUSE, bleeding that originates in the UTERUS and emerges by way of the VAGINA, constituting either normal menstruation or a disturbance of the menstrual cycle, called *breakthrough bleeding* (also *spotting, staining, metrorrhagia).* Any vaginal bleeding before menarche (a woman's first menstrual period) or after menopause (one year after her final period) is abnormal and should be investigated at once. Vaginal bleeding during PREGNANCY also signals potential problems and should be diagnosed promptly. Bloody discharge can also be a symptom of vaginal infection.

See also HEMORRHAGE, VAGINAL; POSTPARTAL HEMORRHAGE; VAGINITIS.

blended family   A family created by remarriage; it may include children from previous marriages of one or both partners, plus children of the current marriage.

bloating
> See EDEMA.

blood clot
> See THROMBUS.

blood count
> See under BLOOD TEST.

blood pressure
> See HYPERTENSION.

blood sugar
> See DIABETES MELLITUS.

blood test   A laboratory analysis of a blood sample to help diagnose a disease or disorder, such as AIDS, SYPHILIS, RUBELLA, THYROID dysfunction, liver dysfunction, mononucleosis, prostate cancer, and many other conditions. Most states in the United States require that couples pass a blood test for syphilis before they are granted a marriage license.

The most common blood test is a *blood count* to detect ANEMIA, using a small amount of blood taken from the finger or earlobe. Most other blood tests require a larger specimen drawn from a vein in the arm or elsewhere. The blood count can be determined by either the *hemoglobin method* or the *hematocrit method*. The *hemoglobin method* measures the concentration of hemoglobin (oxygen-carrying red pigment) in the blood; any concentration less than 12 grams per 100 milliliters of blood signals anemia. The *hematocrit method* measures the concentration of red blood cells in the blood; an elevated hematocrit indicates dehydration.

Patients admitted to hospitals are routinely screened using a *complete blood count (CBC)* which measures the number, size, and oxygen-carrying capacity of the components that make up the blood. In adults, the number of mature red and white cells remains fairly constant; as old cells die, they are replaced by new cells produced in the bone marrow. The CBC monitors this function, as well as the oxygen-carrying function of hemoglobin. A rise in the number of white blood cells indicates infection. The CBC also counts the blood platelets, which help clotting, and describes the structure of all blood cells in the sample.

Patients' blood is also analyzed to determine to which *blood group* or *blood type* it belongs. This is important in the event a transfusion becomes necessary. The system in widest use is the ABO system, in which blood cells are classified as A, B, AB, and O, according to their ability to produce specific antibodies. This system has been used in paternity disputes, but is now being replaced by more reliable genetic testing. Pregnant women are also screened for the RH FACTOR. An Rh-negative woman carrying an Rh-positive FETUS is subject to Rh sensitization, in which the mother's blood produces antibodies that attack the red blood cells of the fetus. This can be life-threatening for the fetus.

bloody show
    See MUCUS PLUG.

bonding
    See ATTACHMENT.

bottle feeding   Also *formula feeding*. Using commercially prepared formula rather than breast milk to nourish a baby. Many different kinds of infant formula are available that adequately meet the nutritional needs of the healthy infant; however, none of these provides the natural immunity against infection that breast milk offers. Commercial formula has a higher protein and saturated fat content than breast milk, causing bottle-fed babies to gain weight almost twice as fast as those who are breastfed. Some formulas also contain higher concentrations of calcium, sodium, and chloride than breast milk, possibly creating problems for the newborn's immature kidneys. Table B-2 compares the pros and cons of BREASTFEEDING versus bottle feeding.

(text continued on page 46)

Table B-2   Comparison of Breast and Bottle Feeding

Breast	Bottle
Newborn's health	
Colostrum is rich in antibodies until baby's own immune system is established.	Some babies are allergic to certain formulas. Trial and error necessary.
Mother's milk is almost always tolerated by baby. Breast milk proteins are easily digested and fats are well absorbed.	Formula is linked to an increased number of GI and respiratory infections.
Baby cannot overeat, limits self to natural weight. No need to empty bottle.	More air may be ingested into stomach.
Composition	
Breast milk contains higher levels of lactose, cystine, and cholesterol, which are necessary for brain and nerve growth.	Made to be as close to human milk as possible, but nutrients are not as biodegradable. Contains adequate vitamins and minerals.
Perfect balance of proteins, carbohydrates, fats, vitamins, and minerals.	
Purity	
Pure and as free from foreign materials as whatever the mother consumes.	Formula companies comply with federal guidelines for sterility and quality.
No storage, sanitation, or spoilage unless pumped milk is not refrigerated. Frozen milk can be safely kept for at least one month.	Ready-to-drink formula has an expiration date and shelf half-life even if unopened. Once mixed, powdered formula should be used within 24 hours.
Cost	
Costs are minimal, including the cost of two or three nursing bras, cloth or disposable nursing pads used for about first six weeks, breast	Expenses include cost of bottles or disposable nursers with plastic liners, nipples, nipple caps, and a heat-resistant mixing container.

Table B-2   Comparison of Breast and Bottle Feeding (continued)

Breast	Bottle
cream to prevent and/or treat sore and cracked nipples, manual or electric breast pump, and the cost of a well-balanced diet for the mother. No waste with breast milk.	Formula is a major expense, especially when baby takes 24 oz. or four bottles a day.

Convenience

Breast	Bottle
Mother can feed whenever baby needs; milk is at perfect temperature.	Mother has more freedom to come and go rather than timing her trips from home based on baby's feeding schedule.
If baby is only on breast milk, mother is tied down and cannot miss too many feedings. She risks decreasing her supply if she supplements.	Requires frequent trips to store or buying formula in large quantities.
Engorgement can cause discomfort. Certain clothes may make discreet nursing difficult.	Night feedings are more disruptive. Preparation time is about the same as for making iced tea.

Emotional aspects

Breast	Bottle
Pleasant way to nurture—skin-to-skin contact enhances closeness. Nursing has calming effect on baby, who hears familiar sound of mother's heartbeat and smells her scent.	Same degree of intimacy as with breast if mother or father holds baby close, smiles, and snuggles during feedings.
Mother may be embarrassed, nervous, or have aversion to breastfeeding, especially in public.	Mother may be more at ease with bottle than with offering breast.
Father is left out of nurturing experience if baby is breastfed exclusively.	Father equal partner in nurturing and feeding experience.

Source: Adapted from Lesko W., and Lesko M.: *The Maternity Source Book.* New York: Warner Books, 1984, pp 284–87.

Whether the mother chooses to breastfeed or bottle feed her infant, she should not feel guilty about her choice. Either method of feeding can help form positive parent-child relationships. The American Academy of Pediatrics recommends that infants be fed either breast milk or formula rather than cow's milk until one year of age. Neither unmodified cow's milk nor skim milk should be substituted for newborn feeding because the protein content in cow's milk is 50 to 75% higher than in human milk, making it hard to digest.

brachial palsy   A birth injury resulting in partial or complete paralysis of portions of the arm, causing it to hang limply at the side. Brachial palsy occurs most often when the BIRTH ATTENDANT exerts strong traction on the baby's head while its shoulder is lodged behind the mother's pubic bone, or during a BREECH birth when the arm becomes trapped over the infant's head and strong traction is applied.

Bradley method   Also *partner-coached birth*. One method of PREPARED CHILDBIRTH promoted in the 1940s by Robert A. Bradley, an American obstetrician, in which a trained husband coaches his wife in achieving a spontaneous DELIVERY without medication. Although Bradley later conceded that a mother, sister, or friend might prove just as effective a coach, he believed the husband was the ideal person. Like the method devised by Grantley DICK-READ, the Bradley method is based on use of relaxation and breathing techniques, changing positions during LABOR, and reassurance. Couples usually attend a series of eight classes, the first during the third or fourth month, and the remainder during the last TRIMESTER. Originally intended for hospital births, the method has been successfully used in alternative settings such as BIRTH CENTERS or homes.

Braxton Hicks contractions   Irregular, uterine CONTRACTIONS occurring throughout PREGNANCY but most noticeably during the final weeks. Although not painful, these contractions aid the EFFACEMENT and DILATATION OF THE CERVIX. Late in pregnancy, they can become uncomfortable and are mistaken for true labor.

See also FALSE LABOR.

Brazelton's neonatal behavioral assessment   An evaluation tool designed by Dr. T. Berry Brazelton, a pediatrician, to assess the newborn's behavioral responses to the environment as well as his neurologic adequacy and capabilities. Usually administered by a nurse or other trained professional, it takes about 30 minutes and involves about 30 tests, including response to auditory and visual stimuli, motor activity, self-quieting activity, and cuddliness or social behaviors.

breast Also *mammary gland*. One of two modified sebaceous glands located on either side of the chest in both men and women, above the pectoral muscle. While men's breasts have no function, women's breasts enable them to secrete milk for their INFANTS.

The breast is made up of about one-third fat and connective tissue, and two-thirds breast tissue. Breast tissue extends from the collarbone down to the fifth or sixth rib, and from the breastbone in the center of the chest to the back of the armpit. Most of the breast tissue is located near the armpit and in the upper breast, referred to as the upper outer quadrant. Sometimes a small section of breast tissue extends from this quadrant into the armpit; this is called the *axillary tail,* or *tail of Spence*. The fat is mainly in the middle and lower part of the breast. Two principal structures comprise breast tissue: *lobules,* where milk is produced, and *ducts,* the tubes that carry the milk to the NIPPLE. The breast also contains a network of blood vessels and lymphatic vessels that transport nutrients and remove waste.

HORMONES control the growth and development of the breast, principally ESTROGEN and PROGESTERONE secreted by the OVARIES, and PROLACTIN secreted by the PITUITARY. Estrogen and progesterone promote growth and maturation of the milk ducts and fibrous tissues, and intensify the pigmentation (coloring) of the AREOLA, the ring of darker skin around the nipple. Prolactin stimulates milk production. Two additional hormones, somatotropin and adrenocorticotropin, influence breast development, but their function is not completely understood.

By the end of the second month of PREGNANCY breast changes are obvious, particularly during the first pregnancy. The areola darkens, nipples are more erectile when touched, and superficial veins become more prominent. STRIAE (stretch marks) may develop as pregnancy progresses.

During the last TRIMESTER of pregnancy, the breasts may begin to leak *colostrum,* a yellowish secretion rich in antibodies, which changes to milk within the first few days after childbirth. Many women find it helpful to use absorbent breast pads inside their bra to prevent staining their clothing.

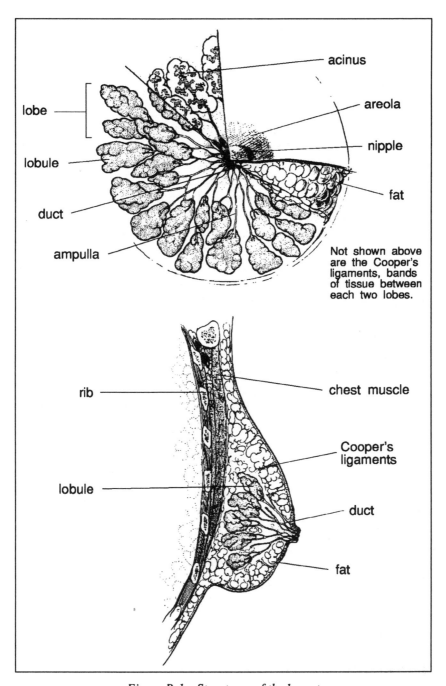

Figure B-1   Structures of the breast

(*courtesy of* Breast Cancer Digest, *National Cancer Institute*)

Breast size depends largely on heredity, which determines the proportion of fat to breast tissue. When women lose weight, their breast size decreases because the fat content changes. During pregnancy, weight gain and hormonal activity combine to increase breast size dramatically, even in women with small breasts.

There is no single normal size for breasts, and, in most women, one breast is usually larger than the other. Unfortunately for some women, American society places great importance on breast size and shape; thus many women resort to plastic surgery to either enlarge their breasts using implants filled with saline or silicone, or reduce them. In 1992, however, the number of complications related to breast implants resulted in restrictions by the Food and Drug Administration (FDA) on the use of these devices, except for women who had reconstructive surgery following BREAST CANCER. The issue remains controversial and will not be resolved until extensive long-term studies are conducted. Prior to the FDA restriction, the use of breast implants had not been adequately researched; it had, however, developed into a $400 million-a-year industry.

Wearing a bra is optional; some women are uncomfortable wearing one, others uncomfortable without. Women with large, heavy breasts may want the extra support provided by a bra; the same holds true during pregnancy and BREASTFEEDING. The only medical reason to wear a bra, however, is to provide support following breast surgery. Unsupported breasts are more painful, heal more slowly, and heal with larger scars.

Breasts are subject to several problems, ranging in severity from minor pain or infection to cancer. These include: tenderness, swelling, and lumpiness related to menstrual periods; MASTALGIA (severe breast pain), infections and inflammations; discharge and other nipple problems; lumpiness or nodularity; and dominant lumps, such as CYSTS and fibroadenomas. The term "fibrocystic disease" is a catch-all term that doctors have used to describe any breast problem that is not cancerous; however, it is becoming outmoded, replaced by more specific descriptions of the various problems.

See also BREAST CANCER; BREASTFEEDING; BREAST SELF-EXAMINATION; LACTATION; MASTALGIA; MASTITIS; PAGET'S DISEASE.

breast cancer   The most common kind of cancer in women and of epidemic proportions in the United States. Thirty years ago, one woman in twenty could expect to develop breast cancer some time during her life; in 1993, the odds have narrowed to one in eight. Breast cancer competes with lung cancer as the leading killer of women. More than 180,000 new cases were diagnosed in 1992 and 46,000 women died from breast cancer—one every 12 minutes. Breast cancer is the leading cause of cancer death in African-American women.

Risk factors for breast cancer include: age (over age 50); family history of premenopausal breast cancer; PREGNANCY after age 35 or no pregnancy; early MENARCHE (first menstrual period before age 11); late MENOPAUSE (after age 55); and OBESITY. Although these are proven risk factors, 70% of women diagnosed with breast cancer have none of these risk factors, so many unanswered questions remain. Some authorities discuss the "estrogen window" as a major factor in breast cancer; that is, the longer the woman's exposure to high estrogen levels—the interval between menarche and menopause when she is not pregnant—the greater her risk of breast cancer. Some research suggests that a high fat diet increases the risk of breast cancer; however, some authorities state that the fat itself is not the source but is a carrier of HORMONES injected into animals, and the pesticides from plants and grains consumed by animals. These pesticides are stored in the animals' fat that is then consumed by humans. Still other studies suggest a connection between breast cancer and ORAL CONTRACEPTIVES and/or hormone replacement therapy in postmenopausal women.

Breast cancer is a complex, systemic disease with many variations. There are more than a dozen different kinds of breast cancer; each has a unique rate of growth and tendency to spread (metastasize) to other areas of the body. Because most cancers grow slowly, authorities estimate that most breast cancers have been in the body for nine years before they can be seen on a mammogram, and ten years before they can be felt as a lump. Thus breast cancer can spread beyond the breast, by way of the lymphatic network, before it can be detected. That is why surgery for breast cancer usually includes removal of axillary (underarm) lymph nodes on the affected side. If no cancer cells are evident, the patient is said to be node negative; if cancer cells are present in the nodes (node positive), it indicates metastasis, which necessitates some form of systemic therapy (chemotherapy or hormones) to treat the disease throughout the body. Most often, breast cancer spreads to the lungs, liver, and bones.

Because the multiple and interacting causes of breast cancer are incompletely understood, there is no sure way to prevent the disease. This means that early detection holds the best hope for successful treatment and long-term survival. The simplest, most convenient, least expensive detection method is BREAST SELF-EXAMINATION (BSE), performed at the same time each month, preferably a few days after menstruation ceases. More than 90% of breast cancers are found by women themselves either in the course of showering, applying deodorant, or performing regular self-examination. This is the only effective method for young women (under age 40) to use since their breast tissue normally is too dense for mammography to penetrate; in fact, since mammography is radiation, a known carcinogen (cancer-causing agent), it may be harmful for women under age 40 to have MAMMO-GRAMS; however, this remains controversial.

Breast self-examination is important during PREGNANCY as well, since, in rare instances, breast cancer is detected during pregnancy or LACTATION. Because of the breast changes that occur during pregnancy, including more than normal "lumpiness," breast cancers are sometimes overlooked by women and misdiagnosed by their doctors. However, it is reassuring to know that most breast lumps (80%) are benign (noncancerous) CYSTS or fibroadenomas.

In addition to breast lumps, other symptoms of breast cancer are irregular shape of the breast, retraction of the NIPPLE, discharge from the nipple, puckering, enlarged pores, inflammation, flaking, or other skin changes. Breast cancer is ordinarily not painful unless it is very advanced. Cysts are often painful, particularly if they appear suddenly, but the pain is relieved after aspiration (removal of the fluid). The only definitive method for diagnosis of breast cancer is surgical biopsy and pathologic examination of the tumor. The earliest, least expensive method for breast cancer screening is mammography (see Table M-1 for screening guidelines). It is not foolproof, however; at least 20% of breast tumors do not show up on mammograms.

Treatment for breast cancer usually involves surgery; however, breast cancer is no longer synonymous with losing a breast. It may mean only removing the tumor itself *(lumpectomy),* and following the surgery with radiation. As many as 70% of women with early breast cancer (tumors of less than 1 centimeter and negative lymph nodes) are good candidates for lumpectomy and radiation rather than mastectomy (removal of the entire breast). However, many patients and many physicians continue to choose mastectomy, believing mistakenly that lumpectomy and radiation are a less aggressive form of treatment. The fact is that far more tissue can be treated with radiation than can be removed with surgery. Thus women need to always seek a second opinion, or even a third opinion if necessary, to feel comfortable with the decision about how much surgery is necessary. Part of that decision also relates to the size of the tumor and the size of the breast; removing a small tumor from a medium or large breast will have a much better cosmetic result than removing a large tumor from a very small breast.

For many years, surgery for suspected breast cancer meant biopsy followed by immediate radical mastectomy if cancer was found, a *one-step procedure* in which the woman consented to surgery, not knowing whether she would wake up without a breast. When studies began to suggest that survival after less radical surgery was the same as with the more extensive procedure, women began to demand a *two-step procedure*. Now, after an excisional biopsy (the first step), usually performed with local anesthetic, a woman can take time to consider which of the available surgical options (the second step) is the right choice for her. The two-step procedure is widely used today but it is not universal, so a woman needs to ask which approach the surgeon uses. We now know that there is usually plenty of time to choose a course of treatment, and that the choice should take into account not only physical factors but lifestyle factors, including a woman's relationship with her partner and how she feels about her breasts. It is also important to choose a surgeon experienced in breast surgery, rather than a general surgeon. Many major medical centers have breast health facilities with a team of surgeons, nurses, radiation oncologists, and other health professionals who specialize in breast cancer diagnosis and treatment.

After surgery for breast cancer, additional treatment may include *radiation therapy, chemotherapy* (anticancer drugs), *hormone therapy* (altering the levels of certain hormones in the body) and *immunotherapy*. The choice depends on a number of factors, including lymph node status, whether metastatic disease exists (determined by a bone scan and other laboratory tests). Tests now exist that can help predict a cancer's probable course and thus serve as a guide to the most effective treatment for each individual woman; collectively they are known as the "breast cancer risk profile." They include: *estrogen-receptor assay* (because breast cancer growth is fueled by either estrogen or progesterone); *histologic type* (based on the appearance of cancer cells); *nuclear grade* (based on size and shape of the cancer cell nucleus); *DNA flow cytometry* (based on cell activity of the genetic material); HER-2 oncogene (a controversial test useful only in a few node-negative patients); and *cathepsin D* (measurement of the cathepsin D protein which cancer cells secrete to help them spread). Women cannot take for granted that their physicians will automatically order these tests before recommending a course of treatment; however, it is important to request the risk profile so that the most effective treatment can be given. For example, the results of this profile can help determine whether chemotherapy is advisable and what drugs might be most useful in each case. A blood test, CA-15-3, is used increasingly to monitor disease states.

In the rare cases of breast cancer that occur during pregnancy, treatment depends on the woman's stage of pregnancy. During the first TRIMESTER, the woman may want to consider therapeutic ABORTION, depending on her beliefs about abortion and how important this pregnancy is to her. If she decides to continue with the pregnancy, treatment possibilities are very limited because of the danger that radiation, chemotherapy drugs, and general ANESTHESIA hold for the FETUS. During the second trimester, general anesthesia is safer, so mastectomy is possible. Chemotherapy and radiation, however, are still dangerous for the fetus and need to be delayed. During the third trimester, either lumpectomy or mastectomy is possible, with chemotherapy and/or radiation delayed until after the birth. If breast cancer is diagnosed during BREASTFEEDING, it is necessary to stop breastfeeding and start the baby on formula. It is still not known whether pregnancy and/or breastfeeding affect the course of the cancer itself.

breastfeeding   Also *lactation*. Nourishing a newborn INFANT with milk secreted by the mammary glands. Although not essential to the infant's well-being or the mother-infant relationship, breastfeeding offers many nutritional, immunologic, and psychosocial advantages to both mother and baby. Advantages and disadvantages are summarized in Table B-2 (see page 45). Deciding whether or not to breastfeed is a woman's choice, based on her feelings, beliefs, and life circumstances. Most women who choose to breastfeed find the experience pleasurable and even erotic. Those who consider breastfeeding distasteful, unclean, or embarrassing stand little chance for success in this manner of nourishing their infant. Commercially prepared formulas can meet an infant's nutritional needs, and bottle feeding can still be a time of emotional closeness between mother and baby.

See also LACTATION.

breast self-examination (BSE) A woman's examination of her own BREASTS for lumps or other indications of BREAST CANCER (see Figure B-2). BSE should be performed at the same time each month, preferably just after the menstrual period. This is particularly important for premenopausal women because their dense breast tissue limits the effectiveness of mammography screening. Learning how to do BSE from a breast health specialist, either a nurse-practitioner or a physician, and performing this examination regularly makes each woman an expert in recognizing any changes in the landscape of her

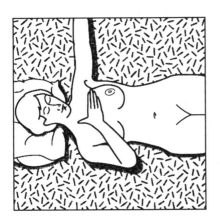
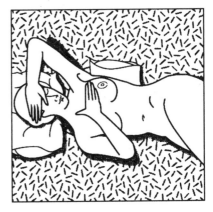

Figure B-2   Breast self-examination

(this series of illustrations, pages 55–56, courtesy of
The Informed Woman's Guide to Breast Health)

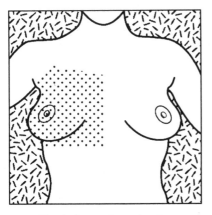
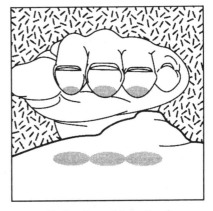

*Shaded area is perimeter
for BSE*

*Palpation with pads of
the fingers*

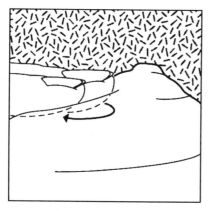

Light-pressure circles

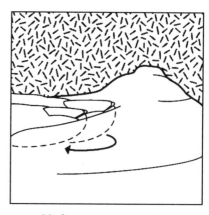

Medium-pressure circles

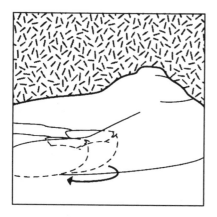

Deep-pressure circles

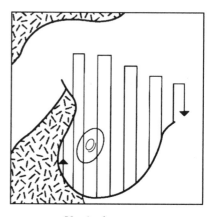

Vertical pattern

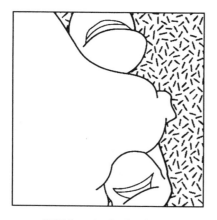

BSE for nipple discharge

breasts. Since early detection remains the best defense against breast cancer, BSE can prove to be a lifesaving skill.

Some women have been diagnosed with breast cancer during PREGNANCY and subsequently recovered sufficiently to have other children.

breech presentation Also *breech birth.* An abnormal position of the FETUS during birth in which its buttocks (breech) present (lead the way into the BIRTH CANAL) instead of the head (CEPHALIC PRESENTATION). Breech presentation occurs in 3 to 4% of all deliveries, but in one-third of premature deliveries of 28 weeks' GESTATION or less, since the fetus is small enough to turn completely around inside the UTERUS. The breech is said to be *incomplete* if a foot or knee extends below the level of the buttocks (also called a *footling* breech). Breech presentation makes vaginal delivery difficult and quadruples the risk to the baby; thus most breech babies are delivered by CESAREAN section. In normal cephalic presentation, the head—the largest part of the baby— passes through the birth canal first, and the rest of the body usually follows with little difficulty. Breech presentation forces the smallest part first, followed by successively larger structures with the head, the largest part, being last to emerge. In cephalic presentation, the flexible bones of the fetal head are molded by the CONTRACTIONS, pushing it through the birth canal, decreasing its diameter as much as half an inch. Breech presentation does not allow for this molding and consequently requires a larger pelvic diameter to permit passage of the head.

Risks to the baby include intracranial HEMORRHAGE, damage incurred in attempting to pull the head through the CERVIX, compression of the UMBILICAL CORD, and cutting off the baby's oxygen supply. To avoid these risks, most clinicians attempt external VERSION, careful maneuvering of the baby's position from outside the abdomen. Sometimes these attempts are initially successful; however, the fetus often will return to breech position. Thus most clinicians choose cesarean delivery to minimize the risk.

brow presentation An abnormal position of the FETUS during birth in which its brow (forehead) presents (leads the way into the BIRTH CANAL). Frequently a brow presentation will change into either a VERTEX (top or crown of the head) or a FACE PRESENTATION during the baby's progress through the birth canal, causing the baby to drop its chin onto its chest (see CEPHALIC PRESENTATION). If brow presentation does not change and the baby is small, vaginal delivery may still be possible; however, with a full-term baby of average size, CESAREAN DELIVERY may be the only option. Brow presentation is the rarest form of ABNORMAL PRESENTATION.

brown adipose tissue (BAT) Also *brown fat.* Fat deposits in newborns that serve as their primary source of heat, insulation, and calories in the first few days after birth before breast milk has come in. BAT begins to develop at about 26 to 30 weeks' GESTATION and continues until two to five weeks after birth unless it is depleted by COLD STRESS. It is deposited around the upper chest and throat, in the armpits, and around the kidneys.

C

calcium Nutrient essential for the formation of bones and teeth in every person. During PREGNANCY, calcium requirements increase from 800 milligrams to 1,200 milligrams per day. If a woman's DIET does not include enough calcium, the developing FETUS will take what it needs from the mother's bones and teeth. Calcium can be found in milk, cheese, and other dairy products, as well as in broccoli (also an excellent source of vitamins A and C, fiber, and potassium), spinach, kale, beans, and nuts.

calendar method
   See NATURAL FAMILY PLANNING.

caput succedaneum A swelling of the newborn head caused by collection of fluid (serum) under the scalp. This condition generally results from prolonged LABOR or use of a VACUUM EXTRACTOR during DELIVERY. Caput generally appears at birth or shortly thereafter, and disappears within 12 hours or a few days after birth. Caput succedaneum should not be confused with *cephalhematoma,* a swelling of the newborn head caused by a collection of blood between the surface of a cranial bone and the periosteum, the thick fibrous membrane covering the bones of the skull. Because of their location, cephalhematomas never cross suture lines (the spaces between the bones of the fetal/newborn skull). They may take weeks or even months to disappear.

   Neither caput nor cephalhematoma requires treatment; neither does any permanent damage.

cardiopulmonary adaptation Adaptation of the newborn's heart and lungs to life outside the WOMB. Before birth, the fetal cardiovascular system functions independently of the developing respiratory system. When the infant begins to breathe on its own, however, the two systems become interdependent.

catheter, urinary Flexible drainage tube inserted through the URE-THRA into the BLADDER. This device is used either to obtain a urine specimen free of bacteria present on the skin, or to ensure the flow of urine that might otherwise be impeded by surgery, trauma, or disease. Since inserting a catheter can carry bacteria into the bladder, sterile procedures must be used. Catheterization is often used after CESAREAN DELIVERY to ensure emptying of the bladder. Sometimes an indwelling catheter (often a *Foley catheter*) is left inserted for several days until normal bladder function resumes.

caudal anesthesia
See under ANESTHESIA.

cephalhematoma
See under CAPUT SUCCEDANEUM.

cephalic presentation Any head-first birth position of the FETUS. The ideal presentation for vaginal delivery is VERTEX, where the top or crown of the head (occiput) is the PRESENTING PART. All other positions are termed abnormal, including other cephalic presentations, each of which causes specific problems.
See also BROW PRESENTATION; FACE PRESENTATION; POSTERIOR PRESENTATION.

cephalopelvic disproportion (CPD) A condition in which the shape, size, or position of the fetal head make it impossible to pass through the mother's PELVIS.

cervical cap A cup-shaped rubber or plastic device that fits snugly over the CERVIX, blocking the entrance of SPERM. Used with spermicidal cream or jelly, it is held in place by suction and similar in effectiveness to the DIAPHRAGM (about 85% effective). Like a diaphragm, it must be fitted to the individual woman; however, it can be left in place up to 48 hours. Because menstrual flow breaks the suction that holds the cap in place, it cannot be depended on as a contraceptive during that time.
The cervical cap has been used in Europe and the United King-

dom for many years and is gaining popularity in the United States since attaining Food and Drug Administration (FDA) approval in 1988. It can be more difficult to fit due to limited size options, and more difficult than a diaphragm to insert and remove. The FDA recommends that only women with a normal PAP SMEAR use the cervical cap since it has been associated with the incidence of abnormal pap smear results; and, that they obtain another Pap smear after using the cap for three months. If irritation from the SPERMICIDE occurs, a different brand may eliminate the problem. If the cap is dislodged during intercourse, the fit should be rechecked. Authorities recommend that a CONDOM be used during the first eight times of intercourse with a cervical cap in place.

cervical dilatation   Opening of the uterine CERVIX, either naturally during the birth process or surgically using instruments. During birth, dilatation is accompanied by EFFACEMENT, a thinning of the cervix caused by the descending fetal head.

cervical eversion   The replacement of normal cells on the exterior surface of the CERVIX with cells generally found higher up in the cervical canal. Normally, the exterior surface is made up of layers of flat, shiny cells called *squamous epithelium,* while the interior surface is made up of tall, red, velvety cells called *columnar epithelium.* The columnar epithelium is richly supplied with mucous glands. Normally the squamous and columnar epithelium come together near the opening of the cervical canal. In cervical eversion, however, the columnar cells have multiplied and spread over the exterior of the cervix. The increased number of mucous glands results in a heavy mucus discharge, the most common symptom of cervical eversion. This condition is often associated with high ESTROGEN levels during PUBERTY and PREGNANCY, and while using ORAL CONTRACEPTIVES. Treatment of cervical eversion remains controversial. Some clinicians believe it should be treated by freezing (cryosurgery) or laser surgery; others maintain that it requires no treatment.

See also CERVICITIS.

cervical intraepithelial neoplasia (CIN)   Also *dysplasia.* A condition in which part of the squamous epithelium (cells on the exterior surface) of the CERVIX has been replaced by abnormal tissue. Three classifications of CIN exist: CIN I is mild dysplasia; CIN II is moderate dysplasia; and CIN III includes both severe dysplasia and carcinoma *in situ* (cancer that has not spread). CIN I may disappear without treatment; CIN II and III, however, progress to carcinoma *in situ* in at least one-third of patients. Therefore, they must be removed surgically after careful evaluation has eliminated the possibility of coexisting invasive cancer.

Usually there are no signs or symptoms of CIN; diagnosis is based on the results of a PAP SMEAR and a follow-up biopsy. This points up the importance of every woman having a Pap smear and a pelvic examination annually. For women whose Pap smears reveal CIN, follow-up evaluation and monitoring every six months are essential.

cervical mucus method   Also *ovulation* or *Billings method.* One of several FERTILITY awareness methods used to predict the time of OVULATION (fertile period) to either avoid or encourage conception, based on the amount and consistency of the cervical mucus secreted each day. Over the course of each MENSTRUAL CYCLE, cervical mucus changes gradually from a slight secretion immediately after menstruation to a heavier secretion of thick, sticky, opaque mucus. Just before ovulation, the mucus increases in volume and becomes clear and slippery, resembling raw egg white, causing a feeling of wetness around the VAGINA. The mucus becomes stringy and stretchable; this stretchability (*spinnbarkeit,* a German word meaning "able to be spun") is greatest at the time of ovulation. After ovulation, the mucus thickens again until menstruation begins, and the cycle repeats.

A woman using the cervical mucus method simply observes her mucus each day to determine if it changes according to a regular pattern. If it does, and if she becomes familiar with that pattern, this is a reasonably reliable method of avoiding or encouraging conception. If the cervical mucus method is used with the BASAL BODY TEMPERATURE METHOD, it proves even more reliable. However, foreign substances such as spermicidal creams, jellies, or foam; seminal fluid; douches; or any vaginal or cervical infection can alter or eliminate the normal mucus, making the method useless.

See also NATURAL FAMILY PLANNING.

cervical stenosis   Constriction of the cervical canal, most commonly caused by surgical manipulation such as electrocoagulation (clotting produced by a cauterizing instrument), cryotherapy (freezing), laser vaporization, or conization (cone biopsy). Symptoms include abdomi-

nal discomfort, AMENORRHEA (absence of menstruation) or cryptomenorrhea (where menstruation occurs but is retained by anatomical
obstruction), and a soft, tender midpelvic mass. Treatment includes
cautious dilation of the CERVIX and an endometrial biopsy to rule out
cancer.

cervicitis Also *cervical erosion.* Inflammation of the CERVIX, usually
caused by infection but occasionally by chemical irritants (douches)
or foreign bodies (tampons, intrauterine devices [IUDs]). In the
United States, candidiasis is the leading bacterial cause of acute cervicitis, followed by TRICHOMONAS, gardnerella, and GONORRHEA.
Chronic cervicitis affects many women of childbearing age and is
often associated with lacerations during childbirth or poor hygiene
(wiping from back to front, thereby contaminating the VAGINA with
bacteria from the anus). Mild cervicitis has no symptoms. More severe
cervicitis causes a profuse vaginal discharge, often with a disagreeable
odor, sometimes tinged with blood. Other symptoms include vulvo-
vaginal itching, pain during intercourse, spotting or bleeding after
intercourse, URINARY FREQUENCY, and INFERTILITY. Diagnostic tests are
necessary to determine the cause so that appropriate treatment can be
administered. Treatment may be topical (vaginal SUPPOSITORIES or
creams) or systemic (oral or injected antibiotics). If the condition
persists, surgical treatment using electrocauterization (burning), electrocoagulation, or cryosurgery (freezing) may be necessary to destroy
the infected tissue and promote healing and growth of new tissue.

cervix The lower, tube-like segment of the UTERUS, sometimes
called the "neck" of the uterus, extending from the EXTERNAL OS (the
opening into the VAGINA) to the INTERNAL OS (the opening into the
upper body or *corpus* of the uterus). The principal part of the cervix,
about 1 inch long (2.5 centimeters), is called the *cervical canal* or
endocervix. Before PREGNANCY, the cervix is pink; during pregnancy,
it takes on a bluish or purple hue, the result of increased blood supply.
This color change, called CHADWICK'S SIGN, is one of the earliest PRE-
SUMPTIVE SIGNS OF PREGNANCY.
 The cervix is composed of fibrous tissue, with many folds in the
cervical lining, making it highly elastic. Before childbirth, the external
os is a small, dimple-like opening, about 5 millimeters (0.2 inch) in
diameter. During labor, it expands to a diameter of 10 centimeters (4
inches) to permit passage of the baby. That expansion permanently

changes the shape of the os (opening) to a lateral slit about ½ inch long.

The cervical lining contains many small mucus-secreting glands. The secretions serve three purposes: (1) vaginal lubrication; (2) protection against bacteria; and (3) protection of SPERM from acidic vaginal secretions. During OVULATION, hormonal changes cause the cervical mucus to become thinner, clearer, and more alkaline, thus creating a more favorable environment for sperm to reach the uterus. These changes help determine when ovulation is taking place (see CERVICAL MUCUS METHOD). Many disorders can affect the cervix, including cancer, usually without symptoms but detectable by a PAP SMEAR. Other less serious but uncomfortable disorders are CERVICITIS, CERVICAL EVERSION, dysplasia, and POLYPS.

See also CERVICAL INTRAEPITHELIAL NEOPLASIA (dysplasia); INCOMPETENT CERVIX.

cesarean delivery   Also *cesarean section, C section, abdominal delivery, surgical delivery.* Delivery of the FETUS through an abdominal and uterine incision. The word *cesarean* comes from the Latin word *caedere* meaning "to cut." Cesarean delivery originated in ancient times as a way to save the life of a baby whose mother was dying or dead, and it is still used for that purpose. Modern surgical techniques have made cesarean delivery one of the safest of operations; however, many clinicians believe that it is often performed unnecessarily in the United States.

Since 1970, the cesarean rate in the United States has escalated from 5% of all births to nearly 30%. This dramatic escalation can be attributed largely to three factors: (1) increased use of ELECTRONIC FETAL MONITORING (EFM), which transmits more sounds that may be diagnosed as FETAL DISTRESS; (2) OBSTETRICIANS' belief that "once a cesarean, always a cesarean;" and (3) delivery of all BREECH births by cesarean. Contributing factors include medical insurance policies that pay more for cesarean delivery than for vaginal delivery; increase in hospital births managed by obstetricians trained in surgery; older mothers having first babies, at higher risk for complications; and an increase in malpractice suits when the newborn is imperfect.

Several recent studies have questioned the value of routine EFM, finding no relationship between routine EFM and improved fetal outcome. Some authorities believe that fetal distress is diagnosed more often than it exists, causing unnecessary cesarean deliveries.

From one-third to one-half of all cesarean births occur in women who have had prior cesarean delivery, because physicians long believed the uterine scar would rupture during LABOR. That belief is changing, however, based on European studies showing that in women with low transverse uterine scars who were allowed to labor, from 50 to 75% had successful vaginal deliveries (called vaginal birth after cesarean or VBAC). Fortunately, American physicians are beginning to accept VBAC. In 1982, the American College of Obstetrics and Gynecology reversed its policy of 75 years and declared that vaginal deliveries after cesarean were safe under many circumstances. Thus it is hoped that, eventually, this will reduce the number of cesarean deliveries performed.

The primary indication for cesarean delivery is DYSTOCIA, that is, difficult labor caused by a pelvis too small to accommodate the baby (CEPHALOPELVIC DISPROPORTION), ABNORMAL PRESENTATION (such as BREECH), inefficient uterine CONTRACTIONS, FETAL DISTRESS, or a combination of these problems. Other indications include PLACENTA PREVIA, PROLAPSED CORD, active genital HERPES, preeclampsia or ECLAMPSIA, or other serious maternal disease such as heart disease or DIABETES.

Although cesarean delivery is one of the safest of major operations, it still carries more risk than vaginal delivery. The risk of maternal death is two to four times greater than with vaginal delivery and recovery is much slower. One-fourth of maternal deaths relate to ANESTHESIA complications.

skin incisions The abdominal skin incision for cesarean birth is either transverse (Pfannenstiel) or vertical (infraumbilical midline), and does not determine the type of uterine incision. The transverse incision is made just below the pubic hair line so it remains nearly invisible when healed. Disadvantages of this type of incision are that it requires more time and does not allow for extension when needed. The vertical incision is made between the navel and the pubic area. Because it offers quicker, easier access to the fetus, it is used when time is limited, or when the mother is obese. With either type of incision, regional or general anesthesia may be administered.

uterine incisions Two types of uterine incisions are used currently: a *cervical incision,* either transverse (crosswise) or vertical; or an incision in the body (corpus) of the uterus. Cervical incisions are used most often today because repair is easier and the risk of HEMORRHAGE is reduced.

The *low transverse cervical incision* (Kerr incision) is most commonly used because it decreases blood loss and the risk of rupture during subsequent vaginal deliveries, reduces the risk of infection, and makes repair easier. Occasionally the size or position of the baby, the presence of twins, or other complication requires the use of the *low vertical cervical incision* (Selheim incision). While more likely to increase the risk of blood loss and possible rupture during subsequent vaginal deliveries, the low vertical incision is still preferred over the classic incision.

The *classic incision,* while simplest to perform, entails the greatest risk of blood loss and postoperative infection; it also increases the likelihood of rupture during subsequent pregnancies or vaginal deliveries. It involves a vertical incision in the body of the uterus, providing a larger opening and better access to the fetus. This approach is used mainly in placenta previa, where the placenta covers the lower uterine segment; or in cases of TRANSVERSE LIE, where the baby is lying horizontally instead of vertically. Today, the classic incision is reserved mainly for emergencies because it is quicker and easier to perform and offers more room for delivery of the fetus. It accounts for only about 1% of all cesarean deliveries.

The necessity for a cesarean delivery can prove very disappointing to a woman who has prepared for a vaginal birth. Thus it is important for every couple to discuss with their physician what the rate of cesarean births is in his or her practice, and what approach would be taken if a cesarean proves necessary. If the cesarean rate exceeds 15%, they might wish to talk with another physician. In the event that circumstances require cesarean delivery, couples may still have preferences about choice of anesthesia, birth partner's presence in the delivery and recovery rooms, recording the birth on audio or video tape, holding the newborn while on the delivery table or in the recovery room, and breastfeeding immediately after birth. Asking these kinds of questions helps the woman and her partner maintain a sense of control and participation in the birth process.

Women anticipating an elective or repeat cesarean birth may wish to donate their own blood ahead of time in the event that transfusion becomes necessary. Repeat cesareans are often less painful and tiring than the first.

Chadwick's sign   Color change in the CERVIX from pink to a purple or bluish hue, a PROBABLE SIGN OF PREGNANCY. As the pregnancy progresses, the color deepens and is more noticeable in second and subsequent pregnancies.

chancre A sore that is the first visible sign of SYPHILIS, occurring at the site where the organism (called a spirochete) entered the body, usually the GENITALS.

chancroid Also *soft chancre, ulcus molle.* A SEXUALLY TRANSMITTED DISEASE caused by a strain of rod-shaped bacteria, *Hemophilus ducreyi,* most commonly found in tropical climates. Cases of chancroid in North America occur largely in the southeastern United States. Like many sexually transmitted diseases, its incidence has increased in recent years. It is spread by vaginal, anal, or oral-genital intercourse, usually through an existing break in the skin or MUCOUS MEMBRANE such as a cut, scratch, or sore. Chancroid usually causes no symptoms in women, so they may unknowingly spread the disease. In men, however, it causes one or more small sores on the PENIS or in the urethra within five days after contact. The sores are raised with a thin red border and soon fill with pus. When they rupture, they become open sores with uneven edges that bleed easily and often spread. Women who do have symptoms experience similar sores on the thighs, VULVA, VAGINA, CERVIX or URETHRA and at the base of pubic hairs. While the sores may disappear in a few days, in at least half the cases, the bacteria infect the lymph glands in the groin, causing a rounded painful swelling called a bubo.

childbirth education
    See PREPARED CHILDBIRTH.

chlamydia infection The leading SEXUALLY TRANSMITTED DISEASE in the United States, caused by the bacterium *Chlamydia trachomatis.* It affects 4 million people a year in the United States. It is transmitted by vaginal, anal, or oral-genital intercourse. An infected woman can also transmit chlamydia to a female sexual partner on the fingers, a vibrator, or other sexual stimulator.

    Most women with chlamydia have no symptoms and may thus transmit the disease unknowingly. If symptoms do appear, their development is gradual, usually within three weeks after contact, and include a vaginal discharge originating in the CERVIX; irregular bleeding, especially after intercourse; pelvic pain during intercourse; and/or

URETHRITIS, resulting in itching and burning during urination. Untreated, the infection can develop into PELVIC INFLAMMATORY DISEASE (PID), causing INFERTILITY. Men with chlamydia, however, almost always develop such symptoms as a discharge from the PENIS and discomfort during urination, and may experience infection of the prostate gland or epididymis, the pathway for SPERM to exit the penis. Unless the infection is treated, male infertility may result. Chlamydia can also cause conjunctivitis (inflammation of the white portion of the eyeball) in both men and women, and pneumonia in persons with a compromised immune system. Infants born to women with chlamydia can be infected while in the BIRTH CANAL.

Chlamydia is difficult and expensive to diagnose because the organisms will not grow outside human cells. Thus many clinicians advise antibiotic therapy for any woman with GONORRHEA, pelvic inflammatory disease, or cervical discharge unidentified by other tests. Sexual partners of the infected person should also be treated to avoid repeat infection, described as the ping-pong effect.

chloasma Also *mask of pregnancy, melasma*. Irregular brownish pigmentation over the forehead, cheeks, and nose of pregnant women, usually fading or disappearing after birth. This coloration is thought to be caused by elevated levels of melanocyte-stimulating hormone or possibly by increased levels of ESTROGEN and PROGESTERONE, and thus may also happen during use of oral contraceptives. Freckles and other heavily pigmented areas of the body such as the NIPPLES, VULVA, and perianal area may also darken during PREGNANCY. The *linea alba,* the midline of the abdomen that extends from the pubic area to the umbilicus (navel), also darkens, and is then referred to as the LINEA NIGRA. Exposure to the sun can further darken the pigmented areas and decrease the likelihood of fading after DELIVERY; for this reason as well as for general health reasons, use of a sunscreen is advisable for outdoor activity.

choriocarcinoma Also *gestational trophoblastic disease*. A rare type of uterine cancer, most often caused by a HYDATIDIFORM MOLE or by normal DELIVERY or ABORTION. Heavy vaginal bleeding is the principal symptom, and can lead to fatal HEMORRHAGE. Choriocarcinoma is diagnosed by a BLOOD TEST because it is characterized by high levels of a unique tumor marker, HUMAN CHORIONIC GONADOTROPIN (HCG). This cancer demands prompt treatment to avoid rapid spread (metastases) to the lung, brain, bone, and skin. Fortunately, anticancer drugs have proven very effective in treating this condition, largely eliminating the need for HYSTERECTOMY.

chorion   The thick, outermost membrane enclosing the developing EMBRYO, the AMNION, and the yolk sac. The chorion has many finger-like projections, called *chorionic villi,* on its surface; some of these will develop into the fetal portion of the PLACENTA, through which the FETUS receives nutrients and gets rid of waste products.

chorionic villus sampling   Also *CVS.* A test used for prenatal diagnosis of BIRTH DEFECTS during the first TRIMESTER. It involves insertion of a catheter (or cannula) into the UTERUS through the VAGINA and removal of a small sample of the *chorionic villi.* ULTRASOUND imaging is used to visualize the position of the uterus, PLACENTA, and UMBILICAL CORD. By analyzing the villi, such diseases as SICKLE CELL ANEMIA, DOWN SYNDROME, PHENYLKETONURIA, and Duchenne MUSCULAR DYSTROPHY can be diagnosed. CVS is replacing AMNIOCENTESIS as a prenatal diagnostic method in some cases because it can be used earlier in PREGNANCY and thus permit therapeutic ABORTION during the first trimester if severe birth defects are indicated.

chromosome   A threadlike structure in the nucleus of body cells that carries the *genes,* the instructions that determine the cell's behavior and transmit these instructions to the cell's offspring. Each human cell normally has 46 chromosomes, 23 from each genetic parent. Chromosomal abnormalities or genetic "errors" occur in approximately one out of every 250 live births, and about three-fourths of them are problematic. Authorities estimate that about one-third of all MISCARRIAGES are the result of chromosomal abnormalities.
   See also BIRTH DEFECTS.

circumcision   Surgical removal of the foreskin, or PREPUCE, of the PENIS in males and of the CLITORIS in females. Although seldom used in females in the United States, it remains the most frequently performed surgery on males, despite the 1989 statement of the American Academy of Pediatrics that there is no longer any medical reason for male circumcision. Parents can now make an informed choice once they understand the risks and benefits of the procedure. Some studies show a lower incidence of penile cancer in circumcised males, and fewer urinary tract infections in males under one year of age. Certain religions, such as Judaism and Islam, mandate circumcision for all male INFANTS. However, it should not be performed on premature babies or newborns with bleeding problems or other serious illness.

The only valid medical reason for female circumcision (clitoridectomy) is in rare cases where uterine or vaginal cancer has spread to the external GENITALS. Yet female circumcision was practiced in 19th century Europe and some parts of the United States until the late 1930s to reduce MASTURBATION and nymphomania and ensure a woman's faithfulness to her husband. This unnecessary genital mutilation persists in some developing countries even today, often as a ceremonial rite of passage.

clitoris   A small, highly sensitive organ at the front of the female GENITALS. It is considered the center for sexual feeling and stimulation. Located between the *labia minora* (small lips of the VULVA), the clitoris is covered by a PREPUCE (hood), or foreskin. It develops from the same embryonic tissue as the male PENIS, and like the penis, has many nerve endings and becomes erect (stiff) when engorged with blood during sexual excitement. Much smaller than the penis, however, the clitoris is normally less than 1 inch long even when erect. It is the primary site of female ORGASM, particularly at the glans (tip), and has no known function other than sexual pleasure.

coach
    See PREPARED CHILDBIRTH.

coitus   Also *copulation, sexual intercourse.* Vaginal intercourse, in which the male PENIS is inside the female VAGINA. During a healthy PREGNANCY, there seems to be no valid reason to avoid coitus. However, it should be avoided if the woman is bleeding, has a history of PRETERM LABOR, or experiences strong uterine CONTRACTIONS following ORGASM. In late pregnancy, positions for intercourse other than male superior (such as female superior or vaginal rear entry) may prove more comfortable and satisfying.
    See also ORAL SEX; SEXUAL RESPONSE.

coitus interruptus   Also *French method, withdrawal method.* A Latin term meaning "interrupted intercourse," an unreliable method of CONTRACEPTION in which the male withdraws his PENIS from the VAGINA just before EJACULATION ("coming"). Because some seminal fluid may leak into the vagina or onto the external female GENITALS, depositing thousands of SPERM, this method often fails to prevent conception. In addition, many couples find that it increases the anxiety and decreases the satisfaction of the sexual experience.

cold stress   Excessive loss of heat by the newborn, causing an increase in respiratory and metabolic rate as well as muscular activity, in an attempt to maintain core body temperature. Many newborn nurseries now use tiny stocking caps on newborns to help prevent heat loss through the scalp, thus reducing the danger of cold stress.

colostrum
> See under LACTATION.

conception
> See under FERTILIZATION.

condom   Also *prophylactic, rubber, safe sex.* A BARRIER METHOD of CONTRACEPTION consisting of a thin sheath, usually made of latex rubber, placed on the erect PENIS before intercourse to capture the fluid ejaculated during male ORGASM. It is also used to reduce the risk of SEXUALLY TRANSMITTED DISEASES such as AIDS, GONORRHEA, SYPHILIS, HERPES, and CHLAMYDIA. To avoid breakage of the condom, about half-an-inch of empty space should be left at the tip to hold the seminal fluid. The condom should be held in place after EJACULATION until careful withdrawal of the penis is complete so that no seminal fluid is spilled on the woman's GENITALS. Condoms may be lubricated with water soluble jelly or saliva, or may be obtained prelubricated. Petroleum jelly (Vaseline) should not be used as a lubricant because it breaks down the rubber of the condom. Condoms are readily available without prescription in drugstores and in restroom vending machines. Vending machine purchase is not recommended, however, since the condoms may be old or outdated and thus prone to leak or break. Condoms may be stored in the original package up to two years but should not be kept in a warm place such as a wallet or pocket, because heat causes them to disintegrate.

Each act of intercourse requires a fresh condom. Should the device break or tear during withdrawal, the woman should at once insert contraceptive foam or jelly in order to avoid PREGNANCY (see

SPERMICIDE). DOUCHING should be *avoided* since it could spread the SPERM. Condom use is considered 75 to 90% effective in preventing conception; use of contraceptive foam with a condom increases the effectiveness to 95% or more. Condoms cause no harmful side effects; some couples, however, dislike the interruption of putting on a condom, and some men indicate that condoms decrease sexual sensation.

Although early condoms were made of animal (such as sheep) intestines, most modern condoms are made of latex rubber. They are available in many different colors and patterns, some with ribbing. Most are pre-rolled and prelubricated.

The AIDS epidemic has dramatically increased condom use, since they are considered the most effective protection against infection. However, even careful use of condoms during intercourse should be considered only "safer" sex, not "safe" sex, since many questions remain unanswered about transmission of the HIV virus that causes AIDS.

conduction   Loss of heat from the body surface to a cooler surface by direct skin contact. This is one of four ways that newborn INFANTS lose heat.

See also CONVECTION; EVAPORATION; and RADIATION.

conduction anesthesia
See under ANESTHESIA.

condyloma acuminata   Also *genital warts, venereal warts.* Sexually transmitted warts or small tumors that form on the VULVA and inside the VAGINA in women and on the shaft of the PENIS in men, and may appear around the anus in either sex. Caused by a human papilloma virus with a long incubation period, these tumors may not appear until one to six months after exposure. They begin as small pink or tan growths about the size of a rice grain and often itch, causing scratching, which in turn causes spread. They tend to merge or coalesce and form large, cauliflower-like masses that grow and spread rapidly during PREGNANCY and during the use of ORAL CONTRACEPTIVES. Prompt diagnosis and treatment is essential since the condition may spread to the baby during birth.

Treatment may be either medical or surgical, depending on whether the woman is pregnant. Medical treatment, suitable only for the *nonpregnant* woman, consists of repeated applications of either a podophyllum solution, or 5-fluorouracil (an anticancer drug), or injections of alpha-interferon. Surgical treatment may involve cryosurgery (freezing), cauterization (burning), excision, or laser vaporization.

Even properly treated, the warts tend to recur, necessitating further treatment. Both partners should be treated to prevent reinfection.

congenital abnormalities   Any condition transmitted from mother to baby either before or during birth. Causative organisms can be carried to the FETUS across the PLACENTA, or to the baby during passage through the BIRTH CANAL. Diseases such as RUBELLA and chicken pox can be transmitted to the baby in this way, and although not seriously affecting the mother, can be life-threatening to the infant. SEXUALLY TRANSMITTED DISEASES such as HERPES and AIDS can also infect a baby as it travels through the birth canal.

constipation   Difficult or infrequent bowel movements (elimination of dry, hard stools). Once believed essential to good health, the daily bowel movement is no longer regarded as necessary for everyone since bowel habits are very individual. Some persons may have three to four bowel movements daily while others have only one every three or four days. However, regular elimination of feces is important. Many people experience occasional constipation for a variety of reasons, such as disruption in daily habits or schedule due to travel, illness, or inactivity; change in diet; or use of medications. When constipation becomes chronic and laxatives become a way of life, however, serious disease may be present.

Constipation can be a problem during PREGNANCY, especially during the last months, as the expanding UTERUS displaces the intestines and presses on the descending colon. Oral iron supplements can also contribute to constipation. Pregnant women who have not had previous problems with constipation can usually maintain good bowel function by increasing their fluid intake to 2,000 milliliters (2 quarts) daily, eating a high-fiber diet, and getting daily exercise, such as walking. It is also important to allow adequate time after breakfast for a natural, unhurried bowel movement. Those who rush off to work or school often ignore the urge to defecate, which can lead to constipation. If the above measures do not relieve constipation, mild laxatives, stool softeners, or SUPPOSITORIES may be recommended by the caregiver.

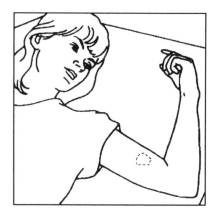

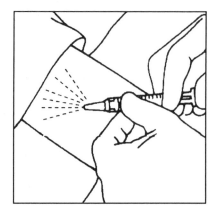

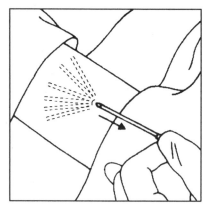

Figure C-1   Norplant®, the newest contraceptive drug

(courtesy of Wyeth-Ayerst Laboratories)

contraception Prevention of conception or PREGNANCY through behavior, devices, or medications. Contraceptive behaviors include abstinence, BREASTFEEDING, DOUCHING, FERTILITY awareness methods, withdrawal (COITUS INTERRUPTUS), and surgical STERILIZATION. Devices include the CONDOM, DIAPHRAGM, CERVICAL CAP, CONTRACEPTIVE SPONGE, and INTRAUTERINE DEVICES (IUD). Medications include SPERMICIDES (foam or jelly that kills *sperm)*, ORAL CONTRACEPTIVES, Norplant® (implantable levonorgestrel) and Depo-Provera (injectable contraceptive approved for use in the United States in late 1992). These methods vary in effectiveness and in possible side effects. Douching is the least effective method and surgical sterilization the most effective. The various devices such as condoms and diaphragms involve the smallest number of side effects, while the medications involve the greatest number. See Table C-1 for comparison of the various methods.

contraceptive sponge A soft, pillow-shaped polyurethane foam device with a cup-like depression in the center of one side to fit over the

(text continued on page 76)

***Table C-1   Comparison of the Effectiveness
of Contraceptive Methods***

Method	Percentage of women experiencing accidental pregnancy in the first year of use
Female sterilization	0%
Male sterilization	.15
Norplant	.04
Spermicide only (jelly, foam, vaginal suppository)	21.
Diaphragm with spermicide	18.
Cervical cap with spermicide	18.
Contraceptive sponge	
Women with previous childbirth	18.
Women without previous childbirth	28.
Condom	12.
IUD	
Progestasert	2.0
Copper T	0.8
Pill	
Combination	0.1
Progestogen only	0.5
Withdrawal (coitus interruptus)	18.
Fertility awareness	
Calendar	14.4
Ovulation	10.5

CERVIX. Marketed in the United States under the name Today™, it is available without a prescription. The sponge is presoaked with the SPERMICIDE nonoxyl 9, which is activated when the sponge is moistened with tap water before insertion. The sponge entraps and kills the sperm, while blocking the cervix. Although theoretically as effective as the DIAPHRAGM, in practice the sponge is much less effective for women who have borne children, most likely because only one size of sponge is available and childbearing enlarges the cervix. The sponge is more convenient than the diaphragm since it may be left in place for as long as 24 hours without reapplying more spermicide for each act of intercourse within that period. It must be left in place for at least six hours after intercourse. A variety of problems have been reported, including difficulty in removal, disintegration of the sponge with the risk of fragments being retained in the VAGINA, vaginal tenderness, inflammation of the cervix, and a higher-than-admitted failure rate. Occasionally it can cause an allergic reaction, and should not be used by women who have experienced TOXIC SHOCK SYNDROME.

contraction, uterine   Also *labor pain.* Involuntary shortening of the outer layer of uterine muscle fiber that helps expel the baby from the UTERUS and through the BIRTH CANAL. Periodic contractions begin in early pregnancy but are painless and not noticeable until the ninth month (see BRAXTON HICKS CONTRACTIONS). When LABOR begins, contractions occur at regular intervals, becoming closer together and more intense as labor progresses. During the first stage of labor, they are brief, mild, and intermittent, first sensed as discomfort in the small of the back but soon felt in the lower ABDOMEN as well. During this phase, contractions alternate with 10- to 20-minute periods of relaxation. These periods allow the laboring woman and her uterine muscles to rest. As labor progresses, contractions become longer, stronger, and more intense, and the periods of relaxation briefer. When the cervix is dilated to about 4 to 7 centimeters, contractions last about one full minute, with four to eight minutes between contractions. When the cervix is dilated to 7 to 10 centimeters, contractions may last one and one-half minutes with as little as 30 seconds between contractions. With full dilation, during the second stage of labor (when the baby is born) contractions last between 50 to 100 seconds and occur at two- to three-minute intervals. Abdominal muscles then begin to play a role; the woman feels an urge to bear down (unless ANESTHESIA numbs this sensation) and help push the baby out. A few minutes after

DELIVERY, regular uterine contractions begin again, continuing until the PLACENTA is expelled. Following delivery of the placenta, the BIRTH ATTENDANT massages the woman's abdomen to be sure that contractions are continuing. Unless contractions continue, HEMORRHAGE may result (see POSTPARTAL HEMORRHAGE). These periodic contractions can be painful and are called AFTERPAINS; however, they serve two useful purposes: helping the uterus return to its pre-pregnant size and reducing the risk of hemorrhage. Afterpains can be especially painful during BREASTFEEDING due to the release of OXYTOCIN, and some women may require mild ANALGESICS for several days. For most women, however, these contractions diminish in intensity during the first 48 hours after birth.

Uterine contractions occur whether they can be felt or not. Regional anesthesia such as *caudal* or *epidural,* does not stop them, nor does lack of control over other pelvic muscles, as in women with paraplegia. They also occur during menstruation (see DYSMENORRHEA) and occasionally, in a milder form, during ORGASM. Opinions vary as to the cause of the pain associated with contractions of labor. Some authorities believe it originates in the stretching of the CERVIX and perineal tissues; others that it is due to hypoxia (lack of oxygen) in the muscles, and still others from the compression of nerves in the PELVIS.

See also ANESTHESIA.

contraction stress test (CST)   Also *OCT, NSCST.* A technique to assess fetal respiratory function. During uterine CONTRACTIONS, blood flow to the PLACENTA is reduced momentarily, decreasing delivery of oxygen to the FETUS. A healthy fetus can tolerate this temporary reduction of oxygen, showing little change in the FETAL HEART RATE (FHR). The test can identify a fetus at risk by the degree of changes in the FHR during a contraction. The test requires uterine contractions that occur three times in ten minutes. These contractions may be spontaneous or induced, either by intravenous OXYTOCIN (PITOCIN) or by NIPPLE stimulation. Until recently, intravenous oxytocin was used for the CST, also called the oxytocin challenge test (OCT). Many clinicians now use the nipple stimulation contraction stress test (NSCST), based on the fact that stimulation of the nipple or the breast causes the release of natural oxytocin. This kind of CST is also called breast self-stimulation test (BSST) or breast stimulation test (BST).

Prior to inducing contractions, the clinician places an electronic fetal monitor on the mother's abdomen and monitors blood pressure, heart rate, fetal activity, and spontaneous contractions for 15 minutes. This is called a baseline recording. The monitoring continues as contractions are induced; if three contractions lasting 40 to 60 seconds each occur within a 10-minute period, the results are evaluated and the test is concluded. Nipple stimulation usually is sufficient to produce satisfactory contractions within 15 to 30 minutes.

Indications for CST include maternal DIABETES mellitus, suspected INTRAUTERINE GROWTH RETARDATION (IUGR), POSTMATURITY (42 or more weeks' GESTATION), and other problems. However, CST should not be performed in the presence of bleeding during the third TRIMESTER, previous CESAREAN birth with classical incision, premature RUPTURE OF THE MEMBRANES, INCOMPETENT CERVIX, or MULTIPLE PREGNANCY (twins, triplets, and so on).

contragestive Also *contragestant*. A birth control drug known as RU-486, developed by Dr. Etienne Baulieu and the French pharmaceutical company Roussel-Uclaf as an alternative to surgical ABORTION. Marketed under the name Mifepristone, this contragestive blocks PROGESTERONE receptors in the uterine lining (ENDOMETRIUM), preventing the progesterone-induced buildup of the uterine lining that enables it to sustain a PREGNANCY. Because it does not prevent FERTILIZATION or IMPLANTATION, RU-486 is an abortifacient rather than a CONTRACEPTIVE. The efforts of antiabortion forces in the United States resulted in an import ban on the drug, a ban lifted in 1993 by President Clinton. However, Roussel-Uclaf has not applied for approval of the drug in the United States because of the political climate. It is only marketed in countries with legalized abortion, universal health care, and controllable distribution, to avoid a black market.

If RU-486 is taken monthly near the time of an expected menstrual period, it can be used for birth control. During the first two months of pregnancy, it causes abortion in about 85% of women, and is more effective when administered with PROSTAGLANDINS.

Because it acts to block progesterone, RU-486 is also being studied as a treatment for other hormonally related diseases such as BREAST CANCER, uterine cancer, ENDOMETRIOSIS, and Cushing's syndrome. However, it remains controversial in the United States because of its use as an abortifacient, which has had a chilling effect on research. In 1992, a small Canadian study was initiated to study RU-486 as a breast cancer therapy.

contraindication   Any condition that makes a particular drug or procedure inadvisable. An *absolute contraindication* means that the procedure is dangerous to the patient and should not be used; a *relative contraindication* means that both the risks and the benefits of the procedure must be considered before a decision is made. For example, allergy to the anesthetic is an absolute contraindication for *epidural anesthesia;* mild-to-moderate bleeding is a relative contraindication since the use of *general anesthesia* may pose even greater risk.

convection   Loss of heat from the body surface into the cooler air. Convection is one of four ways that newborn INFANTS lose heat (see CONDUCTION, EVAPORATION, and RADIATION). Air-conditioning, oxygen by mask, and procedures such as weighing, done outside an incubator without an overhead warmer, contribute to convective heat loss in the newborn.

Coombs' test   A test to detect Rh incompatibility of mother and FE-TUS. It may be either direct or indirect. A direct Coombs' test indicates sensitized Rh-positive red cells (cells that cause antibodies to form in the mother's blood) in the newborn's blood. The indirect Coombs' test measures the Rh-positive red cells in the mother's blood. A newborn with a positive direct Coombs' test will need treatment for jaundice and perhaps *hyperbilirubinemia* (elevated levels of bilirubin, a reddish yellow bile pigment, in the blood). Treatment may include PHO-TOTHERAPY, drug therapy, and/or transfusion.
    See also NEONATAL JAUNDICE.

corpus luteum   See OVARY.

couvade syndrome   The involuntary or sympathetic development of physical symptoms by the partner of a pregnant woman. These symptoms can include increased appetite, anxiety, insomnia, fatigue, upset stomach, or other problems similar to those experienced by the woman. Studies suggest that men who experience couvade syndrome tend to be more involved in preparation for their role as fathers. Originally, the term "couvade" referred to certain cultural rituals and taboos observed by men to mark the transition to fatherhood.

crabs
    See PUBIC LICE.

crack cocaine
> See DRUG USE AND PREGNANCY.

cramp   Involuntary, painful CONTRACTION (shortening) or spasm of a muscle or group of muscles. *Menstrual cramps* are uterine contractions similar to LABOR pains but less intense and more irregular. *Leg* or *foot cramps* often occur during PREGNANCY, particularly at night, and during the second stage of labor when the baby's head presses on the pelvic nerves leading to the legs. Massaging the muscles until they relax is usually effective in relieving the pain; sometimes standing on the affected foot is helpful as well.

cravings
> See FOOD CRAVINGS, AVERSIONS.

crowning   Appearance of the fetal head at the external opening of the VAGINA, signaling that birth is imminent. In many facilities, a mirror is positioned so the woman can see the baby's head crowning; often this gives her renewed energy and impetus for the final push needed to give birth.

cryptorchidism   Also *undescended testicles*. The failure of one or both testicles to descend into the SCROTUM of male INFANTS at birth. This condition occurs in less than 4% of full-term infants, but in nearly 30% of PREMATURE INFANTS. In about half these cases, the affected testicle descends spontaneously during the first month of life. In others, descent may not occur until PUBERTY; however, most authorities recommend surgical correction by one year of age if descent has not occurred. If this condition is not corrected by age five or six, INFERTILITY may eventually result.

culdocentesis   A diagnostic procedure involving withdrawal of fluid from the *cul-de-sac* portion of the ABDOMEN (the section behind the UTERUS and beneath the intestines) by inserting a needle through the VAGINA. Bloody fluid can indicate a ruptured ECTOPIC PREGNANCY, necessitating additional procedures, such as CULDOSCOPY or LAPAROSCOPY, for accurate diagnosis of the problem. Fluid containing pus indicates acute SALPINGITIS (infection of the FALLOPIAN TUBES). Atypical cells indicate cancer.

culdoscopy   Examination of the pelvic organs by means of a culdoscope, an instrument inserted through a small vaginal incision into the *cul-de-sac* area of the ABDOMEN. This procedure is usually performed to assess the function of the FALLOPIAN TUBES or to detect tubal pregnancy. It requires that the woman be positioned on her knees, with her buttocks elevated toward the examiner. After administering local ANESTHESIA, the clinician injects indigo, carmine, or other dyes through a cannula inserted into the CERVIX to detect any blockage in the tube.

cunnilingus   Also *eating* (slang). Stimulation of the female GENITALS (VULVA, CLITORIS) using the mouth or tongue. The term comes from the Latin words *cunnus* meaning "vulva" and *lingere,* meaning "lick." Authorities believe cunnilingus should be avoided during late PREGNANCY, at least any practice that might include blowing air into the woman's VAGINA, since this could cause an air embolism, which is potentially fatal.
    See also EMBOLUS; FELLATIO; ORAL SEX.

curettage   A scraping of the uterine lining, or the inner lining of another organ, to remove tissue for diagnostic examination, using an instrument called a curette.
    See also DILATATION AND CURETTAGE (D & C).

cycle
    See CERVICAL MUCUS METHOD; MENSTRUAL CYCLE; OVULATION.

cyst   An abnormal sac of tissue, filled with liquid, gaseous, or semisolid substance. A cyst can develop in various areas of the body such as the BREASTS, OVARIES, and skin.

Bartholin cyst   A cyst that results from blockage of the ducts of the Bartholin's glands, vulvovaginal glands that secrete mucus during sexual excitement. A small cyst requires no treatment. Large or infected cysts, however, must be surgically drained and the cyst wall removed to prevent recurrence. Infectious organisms include gonococcus, so a GONORRHEA culture is required.

chocolate cyst   Also *endometrial cyst*. See under ENDOMETRIOSIS.

Nabothian cyst   Also *cervical cyst*. A cyst that develops around a blockage of one of the many mucus-producing glands that line the CERVIX. They can occur as a single cyst or as clusters of cysts, usually on the surface of the cervix. Nabothian cysts look like small white pimples, no bigger than a small pea. They require no treatment unless they are accompanied by CERVICITIS, in which case they are removed by surgical cauterization (burning) or cryosurgery (freezing).

ovarian cyst   A cyst that forms on the OVARY. These cysts can develop at any age, but most commonly occur between PUBERTY and MENO- PAUSE. They may be as small as a pea or as large as a grapefruit, and usually do not cause symptoms but are discovered on GYNECOLOGIC EXAMINATION. Although many ovarian cysts are benign (noncancer- ous), it is important to rule out the presence of ovarian cancer, also a "silent" malignancy, seldom giving rise to symptoms. This is particu- larly important in women who have a history of ovarian cancer in their family, since this does seem to have a genetic link.

More than half of ovarian cysts are *functional*, meaning that they result from normal ovarian function during the MENSTRUAL CYCLE. Two types of functional cysts occur: *follicle cysts* and *corpus luteum cysts*. *Follicle cysts* form when an ovarian FOLLICLE develops incompletely and fails to release an egg. They range from microscopic size to 4 centimeters (1.6 inches) in diameter, generally cause no symptoms, and disappear without treatment within 60 days. Large cysts, however, may cause pelvic pain, a notable variation in the menstrual cycle, pain during intercourse, and occasionally, abnormal uterine bleeding. Cor- pus luteum cysts arise from the *corpus luteum,* the structure formed by the ovarian follicle after OVULATION, when it fails to shrink. If these cysts do not disappear spontaneously, the physician may prescribe ORAL CONTRACEPTIVES as treatment.

dermoid cysts   The most common kind of *nonfunctional* ovarian cyst. They are benign and contain fragments of skin, bone, teeth, cartilage, and even hair, thought to originate from undeveloped em- bryonic tissue. These cysts can twist (torsion), rupture, and bleed, causing severe pain; then they must be surgically removed. If the cyst is very large, the affected ovary may also need to be removed.

In women under age 30, physicians usually wait 60 days to see whether a cyst disappears spontaneously. If it does not, and the woman is not pregnant, ULTRASOUND or X-ray examination of the abdomen will reveal the difference between a cyst and a solid tumor. In women over 40, ultrasound or X-ray examination may be ordered at once and, if questions remain, the physician may perform a LAPAROSCOPY to view the ovaries through a small incision, or he or she may perform a larger incision and a biopsy.

cystitis   Also *bladder infection, urinary tract infection.* Inflammation of the urinary BLADDER, most commonly caused by bacterial infection. It can also result from injury, mechanical irritation, or a foreign body such as a CATHETER. Frequent sexual intercourse can cause cystitis, because the movement of the PENIS irritates the floor of the URETHRA and bladder, and may introduce bacteria from the VULVA into the urethra. Cystitis stemming from frequent sexual intercourse has been termed *honeymoon cystitis.* To avoid this condition, women should urinate before and immediately after intercourse and increase their intake of water. This dilutes the urine, decreasing the likelihood of bacterial growth. A too-large DIAPHRAGM can irritate the urethra during intercourse. The chlorinated water in swimming pools can also irritate the urethra.

The bacterial organism most likely to cause cystitis is *Escherichia coli,* normally found in the intestinal tract. Thus it is important for women always to wipe from front to back after urinating or having a bowel movement. A CYSTOCELE (fallen bladder) can lead to infection by preventing complete emptying of the bladder, making the urine more concentrated and thus more conducive to bacterial growth. During PREGNANCY, the expanding UTERUS has a similar effect as it presses on the bladder, making cystitis a common problem for expectant women.

Symptoms include urgency, FREQUENCY (feeling the need to void often but producing little urine at one time), a burning sensation during urination, and often a sensation of pressure above the pubic area. Sometimes the urine contains blood or pus. Diagnosis includes a urinalysis and culture to identify the infecting organisms and determine the most effective drug. In addition to drug therapy, treatment includes drinking six to eight glasses of water daily. Drinking cranberry juice is also recommended since it makes the urine more acidic and less conducive to bacterial growth. It is important to take all of the medication prescribed, even after symptoms disappear, to ensure that the infection is eliminated.

cystocele   Also *dropped bladder, fallen bladder.* Protrusion of the urinary BLADDER into the VAGINA, owing to relaxation of the pelvic muscles that normally support the bladder. This condition often results from childbirth, particularly in women who have had very large babies or many pregnancies, and may be accompanied by PROLAPSED UTERUS. The major symptom of cystocele is leakage of urine, especially when coughing, sneezing, or laughing (see STRESS INCONTINENCE). It can mean repeated urinary tract infections, signaled by urgency and frequency of urination and a burning pain during urination (see also CYSTITIS). Cystocele can be easily diagnosed during a pelvic examination. Minor cases can be treated with KEGEL EXERCISES to strengthen pelvic muscles, or by insertion of a plastic or rubber pessary, a device used to support the bladder. Severe cystocele must be surgically repaired.

cytology   Study of the formation, structure, function, and pathology (diseases and disorders) of cells. One of the most common cytologic studies is the PAP SMEAR.

D

deceleration   Periodic decrease in the baseline FETAL HEART RATE as measured by electronic FETAL MONITORING. These patterns of decrease are classified as *early, late,* and *variable,* depending on when they occur in relation to uterine CONTRACTIONS. *Early* decelerations are usually caused by pressure on the fetal head as it descends through the BIRTH CANAL, with the nadir (lowest point) occurring at the peak of the contraction; generally these do not indicate FETAL DISTRESS. *Late* decelerations, on the other hand, signal decreased blood flow and oxygen transfer to the FETUS, the nadir occurring near the end of the contraction. Late decelerations sometimes may be alleviated by the mother's assuming a semi-upright position. *Variable* decelerations are so named because they vary in onset, occurrence, and pattern, and are thought to be due to compression of the UMBILICAL CORD.
See also NUCHAL CORD.

decidua   The MUCOUS MEMBRANE lining of the pregnant UTERUS that is expelled after DELIVERY.

decrement   Decrease or decline, as in a uterine CONTRACTION.

delivery   Birth of a baby; childbirth.
See also LABOR.

demand feeding   Feeding schedule based on the infant's desire to nurse rather than on a regular pattern.

Demerol   Brand name for meperidine, a narcotic ANALGESIC (pain-relieving drug) often used in childbirth and other severe pain. For many years it was used in LABOR with SCOPOLAMINE ("twilight sleep") to induce a light ANESTHESIA. Although effective in relieving pain, it depresses the baby's respiratory system and makes the newborn drowsy, unresponsive, and less able to nurse.

dental hygiene   Regular brushing and flossing of teeth, plus periodic checkups by a professional dentist and professional cleaning of teeth by a dental hygienist. Ideally, a thorough dental examination and any necessary repairs should be completed prior to conception. During pregnancy, it is important to maintain good oral hygiene at home and to continue with regular dental checkups. Any dental repairs or extractions should be done only with local anesthetic, and the woman should let her dentist know that she is pregnant to avoid exposure to any TERATOGENS, including dental X-ray examinations. Extensive dental work, such as oral surgery, should be delayed until after DELIVERY.

Depo-Provera
See under PROGESTERONE; CONTRACEPTION.

depression, postpartum   Also *baby blues*. A type of depression, usually short-lived, that affects more than half of all women within the first few days after giving birth, thought to be related to sudden hormonal changes. ESTROGEN levels return to their pre-pregnant state within 24 hours after PREGNANCY and total blood volume is reduced by one-third. Symptoms vary from brief feelings of sadness to immobilizing fear, anxiety, and withdrawal. If the symptoms last longer than two weeks, a support group may help alleviate the depression. If a woman's symptoms also include sleeplessness, loss of appetite, extreme MOOD SWINGS, or thoughts of harming herself or her infant, prompt professional counseling is needed. This severe form of depression is termed *postpartum psychosis* and is rare, affecting an estimated 1 in 1,000 women. Often these women are found to have serious hormonal imbalance, including very high levels of ESTROGEN and low levels of PROGESTERONE. In these cases, medication and/or hospitalization may be required.

DES
See DIETHYLSTILBESTROL.

diabetes   Also *diabetes mellitus, sugar diabetes*. A common, chronic disorder resulting from inadequate production or utilization of insulin, a powerful HORMONE that enables glucose (sugar) to move from the blood into muscle and fat cells, or into the liver for storage. It affects about 10% of the United States population, and twice as many women as men. Diabetes is characterized by the presence of high levels of glucose in the blood *(hyperglycemia)* and in the urine *(glycosuria)*. Symptoms include frequency of urination, excessive hunger and thirst, and sudden weight loss (most diabetics are overweight). Female diabetics often experience vaginal YEAST INFECTIONS and vaginal itching. The cause of diabetes is unknown; however, it does seem to be related to age, OBESITY, hereditary factors, and possibly an autoimmune response. Because the cause is unknown, diabetes cannot be cured but only controlled, sometimes by DIET alone, other times by oral medication or by administration of insulin. Uncontrolled diabetes can have severe complications, largely because it impairs the circulatory system, which can result in gangrene necessitating amputation, and/or in blindness.

Diabetes is classified in three categories: *Types I, II,* and *III.* Type I, also called *insulin-dependent diabetes mellitus (IDDM)* or *juvenile onset diabetes,* begins in childhood or early adulthood, and generally requires insulin therapy for life. Type I accounts for only about 8% of persons with diabetes. Type II, also known as *non-insulin-dependent diabetes mellitus (NDDM)* or *mature onset diabetes,* begins after age 30. This type accounts for more than 90% of persons with diabetes in the United States. Type II diabetes can often be controlled by carefully following a high-fiber, high-carbohydrate diet and exercising to control weight. Type III, also called *gestational diabetes,* occurs during PREGNANCY and, in about half the cases, disappears after DELIVERY. Some clinicians believe gestational diabetes is not a different type of the disease but, instead, that pregnancy simply reveals existing Type II diabetes.

Any type of diabetes during pregnancy increases the risk of complications for both mother and FETUS. Careful monitoring by both an internist (or an endocrinologist) and an obstetrician who specializes in HIGH-RISK PREGNANCY, plus strict adherence to diet, EXERCISE, and rest in order to maintain normal blood sugar levels *(euglycemia)*, can increase the likelihood of a successful pregnancy and a healthy baby.

If blood sugar levels are not controlled during pregnancy, the woman may be subject to shock (severe HYPOGLYCEMIA), signaled by sweating, tremors, anxiety, double vision, progressing to delirium, convulsions, and collapse, or ketoacidosis *(hyperglycemia)*, a medical emergency that must be immediately corrected to prevent fetal and/or maternal death. She is also at risk for high blood pressure, preeclampsia and ECLAMPSIA, various infections, difficult delivery, and possibly STILLBIRTH. HYDRAMNIOS (too much amniotic fluid, associated with abnormality of mother or fetus in about 50% of cases) is often a problem, as is POSTPARTAL HEMORRHAGE. The baby is likely to be very large, with abnormally large but immature or malformed organs, born prematurely and with RESPIRATORY DISTRESS. Thus it is important that women with known diabetes have normal blood sugar levels *before* pregnancy begins, and that all other women be screened for diabetes at the beginning of pregnancy. Women with Type II diabetes often need insulin therapy during pregnancy, since oral medications for diabetes are not considered safe for the fetus. In the event of any type of diabetes, medical followup and self-care must be thorough and continuous.

Babies of diabetic mothers have a high PERINATAL mortality rate (10 to 15%); those who survive often have serious BIRTH DEFECTS. Therefore, many physicians recommend an ALPHA-FETOPROTEIN test between 16 and 18 weeks' GESTATION and a sonogram (ULTRASOUND test) between 18 and 22 weeks to detect any major problems. To monitor the baby's well-being, weekly NONSTRESS TESTS begin at about 28 weeks, increasing to twice weekly at 34 weeks.

During the third TRIMESTER, the woman's condition must be monitored more closely than ever. She should be alert for symptoms of either hypoglycemia or hyperglycemia (see Table D-1). Blood sugar levels should be checked several times a day and recorded. Although CESAREAN DELIVERY at 38 weeks' gestation is no longer automatic for all women with diabetes, close monitoring should begin at 35 weeks, often with ultrasound examination and AMNIOCENTESIS at 37 or 38 weeks. Women with carefully controlled Type III diabetes can often have a full-term (42 weeks) vaginal birth, unless the baby is too large for the BIRTH CANAL, in which case a cesarean delivery will be performed. LABOR may be induced if DELIVERY has not occurred by 42 weeks since the risk to the baby is greatly increased. Women with Types I and II may also have a vaginal delivery; labor may be induced at 38 weeks, however, provided the fetal lungs are sufficiently mature.

After birth, the diabetic mother's insulin requirements drop dramatically, and she may not need insulin for several days. BREASTFEEDING is encouraged as it benefits both infant and mother. Daily nutritional requirements increase during lactation from 500 to 800 calories above pre-pregnant levels. Insulin dosage must be carefully

(text continued on page 90)

Table D-1   **Symptoms of Hypoglycemia and Hyperglycemia**

	Hypoglycemia	*Hyperglycemia*
Causes	Too much insulin	Too little insulin
	Too little food	Too much food (especially carbohydrate)
	Increased exercise without increased food	Emotional stress
		Infection
Onset	Usually sudden (minutes to half-hour)	Slow (days)
Symptoms in general order of appearance	Nervousness	Polyuria
	Shakiness	Polydypsia
	Weakness	Dry mouth
	Hunger	Increased appetite
	Sweatiness	Tiredness
	Cool, clammy skin	Nausea
	Pallor	Hot, flushed skin
	Blurred or double vision	Abdominal cramps
	Headache	Abdominal rigidity
	Disorientation	Rapid deep breathing
	Shallow respirations	Acetone breath
	Irritability	Paralysis
	Convulsions	Headache
	Coma	Soft eyeballs
		Drowsiness
		Oliguria or anuria
		Depressed reflexes
		Stupor
		Coma

Source: Adapted from Guthrie, D.W.; Guthrie R.A., *Nursing Management of Diabetes Mellitus,* 2nd ed. St. Louis: Mosby, 1982. Used with permission.

monitored and adjusted to individual needs. Women with Type I diabetes will need to continue blood glucose monitoring at home. Women with Type II diabetes can resume oral medications only after they have stopped breastfeeding. Some women with Type III diabetes will go on to develop Type II after pregnancy; in others, however, the symptoms will disappear after delivery.

In an ideal situation, all pregnancies would be planned. For the woman with diabetes, however, it is essential to plan each pregnancy. BARRIER METHODS of CONTRACEPTION (DIAPHRAGM, CONDOM, and so on) used with SPERMICIDE are recommended for diabetic women, since ORAL CONTRACEPTIVES are believed to increase the risk of cardiovascular disease. Couples who have completed their families may consider elective STERILIZATION to prevent the risk of future pregnancies.

diaphragm   A muscular organ stretched across the bottom of the rib cage, separating the chest cavity from the abdominal cavity. During the latter part of PREGNANCY, the expanding UTERUS can push the diaphragm up as much as an inch, causing shortness of breath, particularly when lying down. Turning to the side and using pillows to prop up the abdomen will help relieve pressure on the diaphragm.

Also, a barrier form of contraception, consisting of a flexible (springy) metal ring covered with a soft rubber dome that fits over the CERVIX, behind the pubic bone. To be effective as a contraceptive, the diaphragm must always be used with spermicidal cream or jelly; otherwise SPERM may slip in around the edges of the diaphragm. It must be inserted no more than two hours before intercourse and left in place at least eight hours after intercourse; additional SPERMICIDE should be added with an applicator for each act of intercourse within the eight-hour period. A diaphragm should not be left in the VAGINA longer than 24 hours. Available only with a doctor's prescription, a diaphragm must be properly fitted, large enough to allow for expansion during sexual arousal, small enough to prevent slipping out during intercourse, but not tight enough to cause discomfort. Proper fit should be checked annually, and after childbirth, ABORTION, or a weight change of 10 to 15 pounds or more. Theoretically, proper use of a diaphragm with spermicide is about 98% effective as a contraceptive. Some researchers, however, judge the actual effectiveness to be only about 85%. A diaphragm does help protect against some SEXUALLY TRANSMITTED DISEASES.

See CONTRACEPTION.

Dick-Read method Preparation for childbirth based on eliminating the fear-tension-pain syndrome; named for the British OBSTETRICIAN, Grantly Dick-Read, who developed the method in the 1930s. He believed that teaching women how their bodies function during LABOR and how they can relax their voluntary muscles during CONTRACTIONS would help reduce their fear and avoid the tension that intensifies pain.

See also NATURAL CHILDBIRTH.

diet A pattern of food intake. A normal, healthful diet contains a variety of foods that provide a balance of carbohydrates, proteins, and fats with sufficient quantities of essential vitamins, minerals, and trace elements. During PREGNANCY, a healthful diet is particularly important both for mother and baby (Table D-2). Proper nutrition helps the woman's body meet the increased demands that pregnancy places on it, and protects her against such problems as ANEMIA, infections, and TOXEMIA. A balanced diet also helps prevent prematurity, low BIRTH WEIGHT, STILLBIRTH, and developmental delays in the baby.

The average pregnant woman requires 300 or more extra calories each day, 65% more protein (about 54 grams), and calcium equal to one quart of milk. Many clinicians believe that iron and FOLIC ACID supplements also are needed; recent studies show that folic acid supplements can help prevent NEURAL TUBE DEFECTS such as spina bifida (see ANEMIA). ALCOHOL should be eliminated from a pregnant woman's diet since no safe level of alcohol consumption has been established. Caffeine should also be minimized, as should all nonessential medications.

A woman who breastfeeds may need 500 calories a day more than her pre-pregnant intake, chiefly in the form of protein. Her diet should also include plenty of calcium and B vitamins, plus increased fluid intake. What the nursing mother eats may affect her baby's digestion; however, this is highly individual. Some babies seem more prone to colic and gas pains, particularly when mother has eaten cruciferous vegetables (cabbage and its relatives, such as cauliflower, brussel sprouts, broccoli), onions, garlic, and chocolate. Any alcohol consumption should follow rather than precede nursing; otherwise, it may depress the baby's central nervous system.

(text continued on page 94)

Table D-2   Healthful Diet for Pregnancy

Food group	Nutrients	Food source	Recommended daily
Fruits and vegetables	Vitamins A and C; minerals; fiber	Citrus fruits and juices; berries, melon, apple, bannana, grapefruit; leafy green vegetables; yellow or orange vegetables such as carrots, sweet potatoes, squash; green vegetables such as broccoli, green beans, peas; also beets, cabbage, potatoes, corn, lima beans	4 or more servings (1 serving = 1 medium apple, orange, banana; 4 oz juice; ½–1 cup cooked fruits; ½–1 cup cooked or raw vegetables; two tomatoes; one medium potato)
Whole grain breads and cereals	B vitamins; iron; minerals; fiber	Breads: including corn muffins, waffles, pancakes, biscuits, dumplings; cereals: including rice, oatmeal, corn meal (or grits); pasta: noodles, spaghetti, macaroni	4 or more servings (1 serving = 1 slice bread; ¾ cup cereal; ½ cup rice)

Table D-2   Healthful Diet for Pregnancy (continued)

Food group	Nutrients	Food source	Recommended daily
Milk and milk products	Calcium; protein; riboflavin; vitamins A, D, and others; zinc; phosphorus; magnesium	Milk, buttermilk, cottage cheese, yogurt, soy bean milk	4 servings (1 serving = 8 oz. or 1 cup)
Meat, poultry, fish, eggs, nuts, and beans	Protein; iron; thiamine, niacin, and other vitamins; minerals	Beef, pork, veal, lamb, poultry, fish, dry beans, peas, lentils, peanut butter, eggs	3 to 4 servings (1 serving = 2 oz.)
Sweets, desserts		Sugar, brown sugar, honey, molasses, custards, puddings	Occasionally, if desired

The pregnant woman should eat three nutritious meals each day, supplemented by healthful snacks such as fruit, carrots, or yogurt. Smaller, more frequent meals will help avoid heartburn and indigestion. She should drink four to six 8-ounce glasses of water and a total of 60 to 80 ounces of fluid each day. Caffeinated beverages such as coffee, tea, and cola drinks should be avoided, as should those sweetened with NutraSweet® (ASPARTAME). Vegetarians should consult their clinician or a nutritionist to be sure that their diet includes sufficient protein. Women with lactose intolerance need to seek nondairy alternatives for calcium, such as tofu, broccoli, or other dark green leafy vegetables, pinto beans, and canned salmon.

diethylstilbestrol (DES)   A potent synthetic ESTROGEN prescribed for 3 to 6 million women between 1941 and 1971 to prevent MISCARRIAGE, later discovered to cause vaginal cancer (clear-cell adenocarcinoma) and other abnormalities of the reproductive system in the daughters of women who took the drug during PREGNANCY. A high incidence of GENITAL and urinary abnormalities have also been shown in sons of DES mothers; these include CYSTS, CRYPTORCHIDISM (unde-scended TESTES), low SPERM count, abnormally shaped sperm, or absence of sperm. In addition, studies suggest that the mothers who took DES have a higher incidence of BREAST CANCER and uterine cancer. Despite its tragic long-term effects, DES is still approved for use in treating advanced breast and prostate cancers, in estrogen replacement therapy in postmenopausal women, for premenopausal women with low levels of estrogen, to suppress lactation in women who do not wish to BREASTFEED, and sometimes as a morning-after pill for birth control. It is also used to stimulate growth of cattle and sheep, even although the Food and Drug Administration prohibited the use of DES in animal feed in 1979.

DES daughters may have many difficulties with pregnancy related to abnormalities of the UTERUS and/or CERVIX (many have a small T-shaped uterus and a malformed cervix), including spontaneous ABORTION, premature birth, or ECTOPIC PREGNANCY (occurring in the FALLOPIAN TUBE rather than the uterus). Both mothers and daughters exposed to DES should avoid the use of estrogens, such as ORAL CONTRACEPTIVES or postmenopausal estrogen replacement therapy.

dilatation of the cervix   Enlargement of the EXTERNAL OS (opening) from a few millimeters to approximately 10 centimeters, large enough to permit passage of the baby's head during childbirth.

dilatation and curettage (D & C)   Dilation of the EXTERNAL OS to permit insertion and manipulation of a curette, a small instrument used in scraping (CURETTAGE) part of the uterine lining (ENDOMETRIUM). The most frequently performed minor gynecologic surgery in the United States, D & C may be either diagnostic or therapeutic. It is used in diagnosing uterine cancer, causes of dysfunctional bleeding, or INFERTILITY. Therapeutically, D & C is used to stop heavy bleeding, remove uterine POLYPS, and remove fragments of PLACENTA or other tissue that remain in the UTERUS after childbirth, MISCARRIAGE, or therapeutic ABORTION. Any tissue removed from the uterus should be examined by a pathologist to rule out unsuspected cancer.

For many years, D & C was the principal method used for first TRIMESTER abortion; however, since the early 1960s, VACUUM ASPIRATION has replaced it in most cases. Many physicians also prefer vacuum aspiration for biopsy and treatment of dysfunctional bleeding. Depending on the purpose of the D & C, some physicians prefer to hospitalize the patient and use general ANESTHESIA because it allows for a more thorough pelvic examination. However, increasing emphasis on cost-containment often means that the procedure is performed on an outpatient basis using regional or local anesthesia, reducing both expense and risk to the patient. With the woman in the LITHOTOMY position (lying on her back with feet in the stirrups), the surgeon inserts a SPECULUM into the VAGINA and dilates the CERVIX by inserting a series of progressively larger rods, the largest about 11 millimeters ($\frac{1}{2}$ inch) in diameter. An alternate method of dilation uses LAMINARIA (long stems of kelp, a seaweed) inserted about 24 hours before the procedure; this gradual, painless procedure is becoming increasingly popular with many practitioners. After dilatation, the surgeon inserts a long, spoon-shaped curet and scrapes shreds of tissue from the endometrium and often from the cervical canal. When the instruments are removed, the procedure is completed, usually taking no more than 15 to 20 minutes.

Most women experience some bleeding or staining, CRAMPS or backache, for a day or two. Any heavy bleeding or foul-smelling discharge, fever, or severe pain can mean infection and should be reported at once to the clinician. Infection is the most common complication of a D&C, and is generally controlled by antibiotics; untreated, however, infection can become life-threatening. Most physicians recommend that women avoid vaginal intercourse, DOUCHING, and use of tampons for two weeks after D&C to reduce the risk of infection. If intercourse is desired, the partner should wear a CONDOM. Most women are asked to return for a postoperative checkup two weeks after the surgery.

Although complications after D&C are rare, they can include uterine perforation, excessive scarring of the uterus (ASHERMAN'S SYNDROME; see AMENORRHEA), HEMORRHAGE, or damage to nearby organs (bladder and bowel). It is essential that the clinician rule out pregnancy before doing D&C, if the woman wishes to continue the pregnancy. Any infection or inflammation of the uterus, FALLOPIAN TUBES, or cervix should be alleviated before surgery.

dilatation and evacuation (D & E)   Also *dilatation and extraction*. A procedure used to terminate mid-TRIMESTER pregnancies (from 16 to 24 weeks' gestation), combining VACUUM ASPIRATION, surgical curettage (D&C), and usually the use of FORCEPS. It is performed on an OUTPATIENT basis using local ANESTHESIA. To dilate the CERVIX, the clinician inserts LAMINARIA in the INTERNAL OS 6 to 12 hours before the procedure. The procedure takes from 10 to 30 minutes, and the woman usually remains in the hospital several hours for observation.

diuretic   Also *water pill*. A drug that acts on the kidneys to eliminate fluids from body tissues. These drugs should *not* be used during PREG-NANCY; they endanger both the FETUS and the mother. At one time, doctors believed that diuretics should be used to reduce the fluid reten-tion and swelling (EDEMA) of pregnancy and prevent toxemia (pree-clampsia); however, research has shown that diuretics can mask the symptoms of toxemia and also cause HYPERTENSION. Because some physicians cling to outdated ideas, it is important for pregnant women to know when to question or disregard advice from a physician, or better still, find a more up-to-date caregiver.

dizziness
    See FAINTING.

donor egg   An egg from the OVARY of a donor, fertilized by a male's SPERM *in vitro* (outside the UTERUS; *in vitro* means "in glass") and placed in his partner's uterus so that PREGNANCY can occur. Just one of several methods of assisted reproduction, donor egg IVF (IN VITRO FERTILIZATION) is used in women who experience early MENOPAUSE (premature ovarian failure) but can still sustain a pregnancy once a fertilized egg is implanted in their uterus. It can also be used for women who have a genetic disorder that might otherwise be transmit-ted to the child. Either the woman wishing to become pregnant or her infertility clinic selects the female donor, who must then undergo physical and psychological screening, including BLOOD TESTS and UL-TRASOUND. The procedure is timed according to the donor's OVULATION cycle. A week before egg retrieval she is given HORMONES to increase the number of eggs produced from one to four or more (see FERTILITY PILL). The eggs are harvested from her ovarian follicles using needle aspiration, guided by ultrasound. The eggs are then mixed with sperm in a laboratory container. If FERTILIZATION occurs, the EMBRYOS are transferred to the uterus of the woman desiring pregnancy. To increase the chance for successful IMPLANTATION, the woman receiving the eggs is given PROGESTERONE injections. To further ensure pregnancy, some clinicians put not one embryo but two or more into the woman's uterus. Additional fertilized embryos can be frozen for later use. About half the embryos survive the freezing and thawing process; 10% of these result in pregnancy.

Within two weeks after the EMBRYO TRANSFER, the woman is given a pregnancy test. If the results are positive, the progesterone shots are continued up to 12 weeks. Women with early menopause using this method have a 30 to 40% pregnancy rate. The overall success rate for all types of IVF is only 16 to 20%. One in four pregnancies resulting from IVF ends in MISCARRIAGE.

Donor egg IVF is a costly procedure (about $5,000 for each attempt if there is a reputable clinic nearby; otherwise, it will involve travel and other expenses as well), and is not always reimbursed by health insurance. The woman choosing this approach also risks potential complications from the various hormones and other drugs involved; some authorities speculate that the hormonal manipulation may greatly increase the risk of ovarian, endometrial, cervical, and BREAST CANCER for 20 to 30 years after treatment. Legal and ethical questions are also involved in donor egg IVF, similar to those of SURROGATE MOTHERHOOD or ARTIFICIAL INSEMINATION: whose baby is it?

See also INFERTILITY.

dorsal lithotomy   The position used for pelvic examination and other gynecologic procedures, with the woman lying on her back (supine), her feet in the stirrups, knees drawn up, and legs spread and raised. While less than comfortable or dignified for the woman, this position offers the clinician the best visibility and access to the reproductive organs. From the time of Louis XIV, who enjoyed watching the birth process, this position was also used for childbirth, especially in hospitals. However, it is not the most physiologically effective position for LABOR and birth because it denies the mother and the emerging infant the force of gravity. Unlike the upright positions—sitting, standing, or squatting—that hundreds of generations of women used for labor and birth (see BIRTHING STOOL, BIRTHING CHAIR), the dorsal lithotomy position puts the weight of the pregnant uterus on the vena cava, the body's largest vein, reducing the supply of oxygen to the baby during CONTRACTIONS. It also tightens the PERINEUM, increasing the need for EPISIOTOMY. Women with such disabilities as scoliosis may find the lithotomy position difficult or impossible, even for a brief time. In these cases, a side-lying position with the upper leg elevated (resting on the clinician's shoulder or supported by an assistant) may prove more comfortable and effective.

douching   Cleansing the VAGINA with water or other liquid. Unless a clinician has prescribed a medicated douche for a specific vaginal infection, there is no reason to douche. It is useless as a form of birth control, and unnecessary as a hygienic measure. In fact, studies have shown that douching can promote the growth of bacteria by changing the relative acidity of the vagina, and actually force an infection up into the UTERUS. Douching can be dangerous during PREGNANCY, after an abortion or dilatation and curettage (D&C), and after childbirth. It should not be done before a GYNECOLOGIC EXAMINATION because it may remove organisms that should be detected by the examiner.

Down syndrome   Also *Down's syndrome, mongolism.* The most common serious BIRTH DEFECT, characterized by mental retardation; stunted growth; poor muscle tone; a small, flat nose and slanted eyes, (from which came the earlier name, mongoloid); protruding tongue; and short, wide feet and hands. Many Down syndrome children have serious congenital heart defects and blood disorders; until recently, few survived to adulthood, and those who did were institutionalized. Thanks to research, advances in pediatric heart surgery, and a more humane approach to children with disabilities, many Down syndrome children can be helped to live useful lives, either with their families or in sheltered communities. Their intelligence levels vary widely, and they often benefit from early development and education programs designed to help make maximum use of their abilities.

Down syndrome occurs in about 1 of every 600 births in the general population; however, the risk is much higher in adolescents and mothers over 35. In women age 40, the incidence is 1 in 100. At age 45, the incidence is about 1 in 40 deliveries.

Down syndrome is generally due to the presence of an extra CHROMOSOME 21 (trisomy 21); however, about 3% of cases are caused by translocation (see BIRTH DEFECTS). Fortunately, this condition can be detected by AMNIOCENTESIS and CHORIONIC VILLUS SAMPLING, so that women can choose whether to continue the pregnancy and give birth to a child with this defect.

dreams
   See SLEEP.

dropping
   See LIGHTENING.

drug use and pregnancy   Nearly everything a pregnant woman eats, drinks, or inhales finds its way to the baby, sometimes with tragic results. Substances that cause BIRTH DEFECTS are called TERATOGENS. One example is Thalidomide, the tranquilizer prescribed during the 1960s that caused hundreds of INFANTS to be born with "flippers" rather than arms or legs; another is DIETHYLSTILBESTROL (DES), the drug prescribed between 1941 and 1971 to prevent MISCARRIAGE, which has since caused thousands of young women to die of vaginal cancer and hundreds of thousands more to suffer from various malformations. Prescription drugs are only one category of substances that can harm the FETUS. Everyday products such as coffee, tea, aspirin, and other over-the-counter medications are also drugs that may endanger the fetus. So are beer, wine, and liquor (see ALCOHOL USE). Thus the pregnant (and BREASTFEEDING) woman should avoid *all* unnecessary drugs, prescription or otherwise. Any addictive (habit-forming) drug such as crack, cocaine, heroin, morphine, opium, and methadone can cause addiction in the baby, plus congenital malformations, retarded growth, poor feeding, irregular sleep patterns, and diarrhea; at birth, the drug-addicted INFANT immediately experiences withdrawal symptoms. Long-term effects on the child of maternal use of illegal drugs include hyperactivity and learning disabilities.

Aspirin should be avoided throughout pregnancy, but particularly in late pregnancy because it may interfere with the blood-clotting mechanism of both mother and baby, increasing the risk of HEMORRHAGE. Antibiotics such as tetracycline can permanently stain the baby's teeth and can retard limb growth in premature infants. Caffeine, found in coffee, tea, cola drinks, chocolate, and some pain-relieving drugs, has not been shown to cause birth defects; however, it can increase the FETAL HEART RATE just as it does the mother's heart rate; therefore, its use should be minimized during pregnancy. Vitamins can also have toxic effects on the fetus and the mother, particularly in large quantities. Pregnant women should avoid the following: Vitamin A (possible eye damage), B6 (possible maternal nerve damage), C (daily dosage should not exceed 1,000 milligrams), D (can cause HYPERCALCEMIA, E (possible elevation of mother's blood pressure), and K (possible NEONATAL JAUNDICE).

The Food and Drug Administration has developed a classification system for medications administered during pregnancy, based on risks and benefits (Table D-3). Any drug that is necessary for the health of the mother should be given in the smallest possible dosage

Table D-3 *Teratogenicity Drug Labeling Now Required by U.S. Food and Drug Administration (FDA)**

Category A	Well-controlled human studies have not disclosed any fetal risk.
Category B	Animal studies have not disclosed any fetal risk; or have suggested some risk not confirmed in controlled studies in women; or there are not adequate studies in women.
Category C	Animal studies have revealed adverse fetal effects; there are no adequate controlled studies in women.
Category D	Some fetal risk, but benefits may outweigh risk (e.g., life-threatening illness, no safer effective drug). Patient should be warned.
Category X	Fetal abnormalities in animal and human studies; risk not outweighed by benefit. *Contraindicated in pregnancy.*

*The FDA has established five categories of drugs based on their potential for causing birth defects in infants born to women who use the drugs during pregnancy. By law, the label must set forth all available information on teratogenicity.

and for the shortest possible time. The greatest danger to the fetus occurs during the first TRIMESTER of pregnancy when major organs are developing; thus any woman planning a pregnancy or learning that she is pregnant should consult her caregiver about any medications she is taking or might take. She should also remind other health-care providers, such as dentists, that she is pregnant.

To get up-to-date information on specific drugs and chemicals that may be harmful to the fetus, call the California Teratogen Registry at the University of California/San Diego Medical Center at 800-532-3749.

dry labor   LABOR that occurs after the breaking of the AMNIOTIC SAC (bag of waters) and release of the amniotic fluid. Generally the sac does not rupture until late in the first stage of labor, but occasionally it breaks very early in labor or before labor begins. Sometimes the clinician ruptures the sac (AMNIOTOMY) as part of INDUCTION OF LABOR or to strengthen the CONTRACTIONS. The labor that ensues is not actually dry because the cells that line the amniotic sac continue to secrete large quantities of fluid.

ductus arteriosus   A vessel in the fetal circulatory system that connects the main pulmonary artery (the artery that will carry deoxygenated blood from the right side of the heart into the lungs after birth) and the aorta (the major vessel that carries oxygenated blood from the left side of the heart to the organs of the body). Because the baby's lungs do not function until the moment of birth, the oxygenated blood bypasses the fetal lungs by way of the ductus arteriosus. Normally this vessel closes after birth when the INFANT begins to breathe on its own; the ductus then becomes a nonfunctional fibrous cord. In some infants, however, the vessel remains open, a condition termed patent ductus arteriosus, limiting the infants' supply of oxygen. These infants are sometimes called "blue babies" because inadequate oxygen gives their skin a bluish tinge. Although some cases of patent ductus arteriosus resolve spontaneously, most require surgical correction.

ductus venosus   A fetal vessel that carries oxygenated blood between the umbilical vein through the liver to the inferior VENA CAVA, the major vessel that brings deoxygenated blood from the lower body back to the heart. It normally closes after birth and becomes a nonfunctional fibrous cord; its closure forces an additional blood supply to the liver.

due date
See ESTIMATED DATE OF CONFINEMENT (EDC).

Duke's test   A BLOOD TEST used to determine whether a woman has developed ANTIBODIES that destroy or inactivate her partner's SPERM, thus preventing PREGNANCY.
See also SPERM.

duration   The length of time a uterine CONTRACTION lasts, from the beginning of the INCREMENT to the completion of the DECREMENT.

dysmenorrhea   Physical or emotional problems related to menstrual periods, including CRAMPS, HEADACHE, bloating, MOOD SWINGS.
See also PREMENSTRUAL SYNDROME.

dyspareunia   Pain during vaginal intercourse.

dystocia   Difficult LABOR, usually caused by one of three factors, or some combination of them: ABNORMAL PRESENTATION (position) of the baby; a PELVIS too small for the baby to pass through (see PELVIMETRY); and uterine dysfunction.

See also PROLONGED LABOR.

dysuria   Pain when urinating, usually related to a BLADDER or kidney infection.

See also CYSTITIS; PYELONEPHRITIS.

early pregnancy test
See PREGNANCY TEST.

eclampsia Also *metabolic toxemia of pregnancy, toxemia*. A major, sometimes fatal complication of PREGNANCY occurring after 20 weeks' GESTATION, during LABOR, or after DELIVERY, and characterized by seizures (convulsions), unconsciousness, and coma. About half the postpartum seizures occur in the first 48 hours after delivery, but they may occur as long as six weeks after birth. Eclampsia occurs in less than 1% of all deliveries because it can usually be prevented by controlling *preeclampsia,* also called *pregnancy-induced hypertension* (PIH), a condition that usually precedes eclampsia. Eclampsia is the leading cause of maternal death in the United States; many of these deaths could be prevented through good PRENATAL CARE. See HYPERTENSION.

The cause of eclampsia and preeclampsia is not known; however, it is much more common among women having their first baby, particularly women over age 35; teenagers in lower socioeconomic groups; women with MULTIPLE PREGNANCIES; and women with a family history of PIH. It is also associated with HYDATIDIFORM MOLE, Rh incompatibility, DIABETES, chronic hypertension (high blood pressure), and kidney disease.

Eclampsia may begin with a single seizure or many seizures, that can occur at any time, even during sleep, and are followed by coma. Other signs include oliguria (decreased urine output), proteinuria (protein in the urine), fast pulse rate, elevated blood pressure and fever, EDEMA (swelling due to retention of fluids), and hyperreflexia (exaggerated reflexes). When seizures begin before delivery, labor begins soon thereafter. CONTRACTIONS quickly increase in frequency and duration, and progress rapidly to completion, sometimes before the clinician is even aware of the contractions. The condition usually improves within a day or two, although sometimes the seizures resume, in which case they may be more severe or even fatal.

When eclampsia cannot be prevented, the treatment is aimed at stopping the seizures through sedation. The woman must be hospitalized and given anti-hypertensive drugs (to lower blood pressure) and DIURETICS to increase urinary output.

Babies of mothers with eclampsia are at high risk from the disease and from its treatment. Sedation to control the seizures reduces the flow of oxygen to the baby; rapid delivery may injure the infant. Frequently the baby is premature, with all the attendant risks of being born too soon. Any woman who has had eclampsia is more likely to develop it in subsequent pregnancies. It may also predispose her to develop hypertension later in life. Thus she may wish to consider STERILIZATION to avoid the dangers inherent in future pregnancies.

ectoderm   The outer layer of cells in the EMBRYO that develop into skin, hair, and nails.

ectopic pregnancy   Also *tubal pregnancy*. The implantation of a fertilized egg (ZYGOTE) outside the UTERUS, most commonly in or near the FALLOPIAN TUBES, but occasionally in the OVARIES, ABDOMEN, or CERVIX. The incidence of ectopic pregnancy has quadrupled since 1970, probably due to the dramatic increase in PELVIC INFLAMMATORY DISEASE (PID). If the growing EMBRYO causes the tube to rupture, severe HEMORRHAGE can result. Ectopic pregnancy is now the leading cause of maternal death during the first TRIMESTER of pregnancy.

Ectopic pregnancy occurs when the fallopian tubes have been damaged or blocked, generally from PID but sometimes from tubal surgery, ENDOMETRIOSIS, previous ectopic pregnancy, CONGENITAL ABNORMALITIES of the tube, or hormonal factors that impede the movement of the egg through the tube down to the uterus. Other less common factors include chromosomal defects or other abnormalities in the ZYGOTE, or the presence of an INTRAUTERINE DEVICE (IUD) to prevent conception. Women who have one ectopic pregnancy are more likely to have another.

Diagnosis of ectopic pregnancy can sometimes be difficult unless ULTRASOUND is performed. Symptoms may include abdominal pain and tenderness, and at least one missed menstrual period followed by irregular vaginal BLEEDING. PREGNANCY TESTS may be inconclusive. Some women may continue to have periods and show no other signs of early pregnancy. Warning signals of tubal rupture include sudden sharp pain or continuing one-sided pain in the lower abdomen, fainting, shoulder pain (called referred pain, caused when the abdomen fills with blood), and vaginal bleeding. These symptoms merit immediate emergency treatment.

Surgery is the usual treatment for ectopic pregnancy; its extent depends on how much the tube is damaged, whether infection is present, and whether the woman wishes to attempt another pregnancy. Generally the affected tube must be removed, but if the woman desires future pregnancy, the adjacent OVARY is spared. However, if both tubes are damaged, HYSTERECTOMY should be considered because pregnancy is no longer possible.

EDD   Estimated date of delivery.
See also NAGELE'S RULE.

edema   Also *bloating, fluid retention, water retention.* An excessive accumulation of fluid in body cells and tissues, outside the vessels of the circulatory system. The primary symptoms are swelling, especially in the feet and ankles, and weight gain. Mild edema is normal before menstruation and during the last half of PREGNANCY. The high levels of ESTROGEN produced in the PLACENTA cause the body's connective tissue to retain fluid. This additional fluid contributes to the increased blood volume necessary to nourish the placenta, protects the mother from shock if HEMORRHAGE occurs, and helps ensure an adequate flow of breast milk after delivery. Elevating the feet and legs can relieve some of the swelling and any discomfort.

Normal edema of pregnancy *(gestational edema)* affects primarily the lower body. Any edema of the face and hands suggests *preeclampsia* and should be reported to the clinician at once. Under no circumstances should a pregnant woman take a DIURETIC (water pill); these drugs endanger her and her baby.

effacement   A gradual thinning and shortening of the cervical canal, beginning in the final month of PREGNANCY and continuing through the first stage of LABOR. It changes the shape of the cervical canal from tubular to funnel-shaped. BRAXTON HICKS CONTRACTIONS initiate the effacement process before labor begins; during labor, dilatation (dilation) also occurs, expanding the opening of the cervical os into the VAGINA. Clinicians measure effacement in percentages, with complete

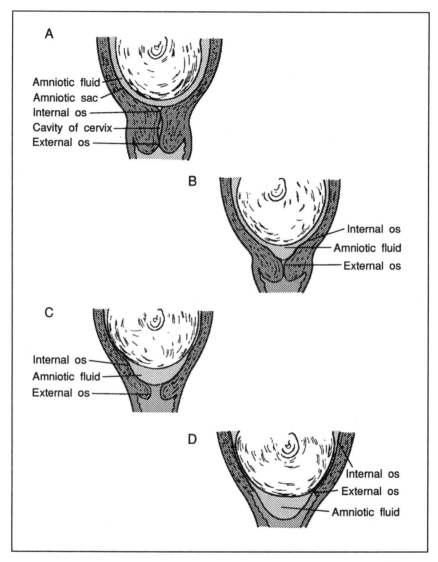

Figure E-1 Effacement of the cervix in the PRIMAGRAVIDA. *A. At the beginning of labor there is no cervical* EFFACEMENT *or* DILATATION. *The fetal head is cushioned by amniotic fluid. B. Beginning cervical effacement. As the cervix begins to efface, more amniotic fluid collects below the fetal head. C. Cervix is about one-half effaced and slightly dilatated. The increasing amount of amniotic fluid exerts hydrostatic pressure. D. Complete effacement and dilatation.*

(From Maternal Newborn Nursing, *Fourth Edition, by S. Olds, M. London, and P. Ladewig. © 1992 by Addison-Wesley Nursing. Reprinted by permission.)*

effacement being 100%. In many women, 80% effacement has been achieved before labor starts.

ejaculation Also *coming* (slang). The expulsion of SEMEN (ejaculate) from the PENIS at ORGASM.

premature ejaculation A man's inability to delay ejaculation until his partner has become fully aroused. This ability varies widely among men.

retarded ejaculation Also *ejaculatory incompetence.* Inability to ejaculate with the penis in the VAGINA. Usually resulting from psychological factors, this condition can cause INFERTILITY unless resolved through sex therapy or other counseling.

retrograde ejaculation A disorder in which the ejaculate surges back into the BLADDER instead of out through the penis because the bladder SPHINCTER fails to close at ejaculation. Since the ejaculate is eventually eliminated in the urine, there is little or no opportunity for impregnation of the partner. Retrograde ejaculation can occur after prostate surgery or in association with DIABETES, paraplegia, or anti-hypertensive medications. In some cases, medication can correct the problem; in others, surgery may be necessary.

See also SEXUAL RESPONSE, SPERM.

embolus Any foreign matter blocking a blood vessel; it may be solid, liquid, or gaseous. The blockage itself is called an *embolism.* An *air embolus* (air bubble) can enter the bloodstream during intravenous infusion or injection, or by exposure to increased air pressure, as in deep-sea diving. A *fat embolus* can result from fracture of the hip or other large bone. One of the most serious, potentially fatal types of embolism is a *pulmonary embolism* (also called *thromboembolism),* in which a blood clot (THROMBUS), generally formed in the deep veins of the leg or PELVIS, travels upward and blocks the blood flow to the lungs. Symptoms include sweating, pallor (looking pale), lightheadedness, cough, rapid heart beat, shortness of breath, chest pain, a feeling of pressure in the bowel and rectum. Thromboembolism can occur during the POSTPARTUM period; treatment involves heparin infusion to dissolve the thrombus, pain-relieving drugs such as DEMEROL, lidocaine to regulate the heartbeat, and oxygen. Surgery may be necessary in severe cases.

embryo   A fertilized egg, or ZYGOTE, during the first eight weeks of development. Throughout the rest of the PREGNANCY, it is referred to as a FETUS. The embryo develops through the process of cell division, based on the genetic material inherited from both parents and influenced by the mother's DIET, medications, and lifestyle.

The single-celled zygote moves through the FALLOPIAN TUBES down into the UTERUS, where it divides in two. Cells continue to divide and differentiate, one cluster becoming a sphere and the other the embryo itself. On the sixth or seventh day, the sphere of cells implants itself in the lining of the uterus, ultimately developing into the PLACENTA. Other cells develop into the AMNIOTIC SAC that surrounds the growing embryo. By the fourth week of GESTATION, the embryo is about one-quarter inch long but recognizable as a mammal. This is the most vulnerable period for the embryo, a time when genetic abnormalities or external influences (TERATOGENS) can damage or interfere with normal growth and development. By the eighth week, the embryonic heart begins to beat, facial features are recognizably human, most internal organs are formed. The embryo is about 2.5 centimeters (1 inch) long.

See also FERTILIZATION; FALLOPIAN TUBES; FETUS; PLACENTA; PREGNANCY; UTERUS.

embryo transfer   Also *embryo transplant*. A method of assisted reproductive technology that involves placing a live EMBRYO into a woman's UTERUS. The embryo may have resulted from IN VITRO FERTILIZATION (IVF) of the woman's egg and her partner's SPERM or a DONOR EGG and her partner's sperm. Women who have been unsuccessful with ARTIFICIAL INSEMINATION or IVF may wish to consider embryo or ZYGOTE transfer.

See also GAMETE INTRAFALLOPIAN TRANSFER [GIFT], INFERTILITY.

emmenagogue   A substance used to induce a delayed menstrual period. This may be a drug, herb, or other chemical. Physicians may suggest HORMONE injections or pills to bring on a delayed period; however, this is not an accurate test for PREGNANCY and may be dangerous. If the woman is pregnant, these drugs may cause uterine CONTRACTIONS and eventual ABORTION; if she continues the pregnancy, BIRTH DEFECTS may result from the drugs.

endocervical   Within the cervical canal.

endocrine glands   Also *ductless glands*. Glands that secrete HOR-
MONES and other chemicals directly into the bloodstream rather than
through ducts (as sweat glands do, for example). The major endocrine
glands are the PITUITARY; the pancreas; the THYROID; parathyroid, and
ADRENAL GLANDS; the hypothalamus and the PINEAL BODY; the gonads
(or sex glands—OVARIES and TESTES) and the PLACENTA. These glands
interact in various complex ways to influence many body functions,
including the reproductive cycle, from PUBERTY to CONCEPTION, to
PREGNANCY, childbirth, and MENOPAUSE. All together they comprise the
endocrine system.
     See also HORMONE.

endoderm   The inner layer of cells in the EMBRYO that develops into
such internal organs as the intestines.

endometriosis   A common chronic condition in which endometrial
tissue (glandular tissue from the lining of the UTERUS) is present on
other organs outside the uterus, usually within the pelvic area. Researchers estimate that endometriosis affects 10 to 20% of women in
their reproductive years (ages 15 to 50). It is the single most common
gynecologic diagnosis responsible for hospitalization of women ages
15 to 44. Like many women's health problems, however, it has been
inadequately studied, so the cause is unknown and the only real "cure"
remains total HYSTERECTOMY (removal of the uterus) and OOPHOREC-
TOMY (removal of the OVARIES).
     Endometriosis can cause severe pain, periodic pain, break-
through bleeding, or no symptoms except INFERTILITY. Prior to menstruation, ESTROGEN and PROGESTERONE secretion causes the ENDO-
METRIUM to thicken, expand, and form additional arteries and veins to
increase the uterine blood supply in preparation for PREGNANCY. If
pregnancy does not occur, the hormone levels drop, the newly formed
arteries and veins close off, and the endometrium is shed through
menstruation. In endometriosis, the endometrial tissue outside the
uterus goes through the same process, except the blood collects in the
pelvic cavity because it has no outlet. Eventually this old, dark blood
forms an *endometrial cyst* or *chocolate cyst*.
     In early endometriosis, the woman experiences severe menstrual
CRAMPS. As the disease advances, scar tissue and adhesions build up
and crowd the reproductive organs, causing pain before menstruation.
Adhesions can block eggs in the ovary, causing INFERTILITY. In addi-

tion, it can cause pain during sexual intercourse, lower back pain, diarrhea and/or constipation, and increased risk of ECTOPIC PREGNANCY and/or spontaneous ABORTION.

Symptoms of endometriosis mimic those of PELVIC INFLAMMATORY DISEASE (PID); thus the only definitive diagnosis is by LAPAROSCOPY or exploratory surgery. Treatment is either hormonal or surgical, depending on the woman's age, location and severity of the endometriosis, plans for bearing children, family and medical history. One of the HORMONES used is danazol, a weak male hormone whose side effects include weight gain, acne, deepening of the voice, and growth of facial hair. Another hormone, PROGESTIN, is helpful to some women; however, if a woman becomes pregnant while taking progestin, the drug can cause BIRTH DEFECTS.

The hormonal agents only provide temporary remission of endometriosis, as does pregnancy. Nearly half of all women with endometriosis cannot conceive, however, and those who do are three times as likely to have MISCARRIAGES as women without endometriosis.

Women who want to get pregnant may consider surgery to remove endometrial tissue, either by cauterization (burning), CURETTAGE (scraping), or laser surgery. This approach corrects infertility in 30 to 50% of women with this problem. To relieve the pain of endometriosis, some surgeons will sever the major nerve networks that send pain impulses from the pelvic area to the brain. This procedure, called *presacral* and *uterosacral neurectomy,* is often performed using laser surgery.

In severe endometriosis, when adhesions are heavy and the tubes are damaged, if the woman wants to bear children, major surgery (LAPAROTOMY) is required to remove or clean out the CYSTS and repair the tubes. For the woman with severe endometriosis that has proved unresponsive to hormone therapy, and who does not desire children, hysterectomy may be performed.

After MENOPAUSE, endometriosis usually subsides without further treatment. Many women seek information and emotional support from the Endometriosis Association, an international self-help organization based in Milwaukee, Wisconsin, with chapters throughout the world. This organization has literature, cassette tapes, and crisis telephone services available. Further information is available by calling 800-992-3636 in the United States and 800-426-2363 in Canada, or by writing The Endometriosis Association, 8585 North 76th Place, Milwaukee WI 53223.

endometritis   Inflammation or infection of the uterine lining (EN-DOMETRIUM) that can occur in the POSTPARTUM period. Symptoms may include fever, chills, pain in the pelvic or abdominal area, and a bloody or yellowish vaginal discharge. Depending on the infectious organism, discharge may be either foul-smelling or odorless. Postpartum endometritis may be caused by bacteria introduced during vaginal examination; endometritis unrelated to PREGNANCY can result from irritation by an INTRAUTERINE DEVICE or complications from an early ABORTION. Antibiotic therapy is usually effective.

endometrium   The innermost layer of MUCOUS MEMBRANE lining the UTERUS. It varies in thickness from 0.5 to 5 millimeters in response to the female hormonal cycle and, unless a woman becomes pregnant, the lining is shed each month as menstrual flow. After MENOPAUSE, the endometrium atrophies.

The endometrium is subject to several disorders, the most common of which is endometrial POLYPS. When endometrial tissue develops outside the uterus, menstrual pain can become severe (see ENDOMETRIOSIS). The most serious endometrial disorder is cancer, for which the initial treatment is complete HYSTERECTOMY.

en face   A face-to-face position, often used to describe early mother-baby interactions in which the mother arranges herself and the infant to face each other and maintain eye-to-eye contact.

engagement   The beginning of the baby's descent through the BIRTH CANAL, wherein the widest part of the baby's head has passed through the *pelvic inlet* (see PELVIMETRY). Engagement may occur during the last few weeks of PREGNANCY or as late as the second stage of LABOR when the CERVIX is completely dilated.

engorgement, breast
See under LACTATION.

engrossment   A father's sense of absorption, preoccupation, and intense interest in his newborn child.

epidural anesthesia
See under ANESTHESIA.

episiotomy   A surgical incision in the PERINEUM, the skin and muscle tissue between the VAGINA and the rectum. This is the most frequently performed surgery related to childbirth, used in more than 62% of all births, and in 90% of first births. Physicians are taught to perform episiotomy to decrease the risk of lacerations (tearing) during DELIVERY, relieve compression of the fetal head, and shorten the second stage of LABOR; however, many authorities believe that it accomplishes none of these goals and, in fact, increases the risk of more serious lacerations, blood loss, and pain. One study showed that 27% of women who had episiotomy and used stirrups during birth had serious lacerations (third- and fourth-degree) compared with less than 1% of women who gave birth without episiotomy or stirrups. Women who give birth in a semi-upright position (sitting, standing, or squatting) experience little if any tearing. Massage of the perineum by the BIRTH ATTENDANT using warm oils and wet compresses also helps the perineum expand without tearing, and allows much quicker healing and recovery. Women have the right to refuse episiotomy.

epispadias   A congenital malformation of the PENIS characterized by an opening on the dorsal (top) surface and exposure of the urinary BLADDER.

Epstein-Barr virus   Human herpes virus IV, the agent that causes infectious mononucleosis (sometimes called "kissing disease" because it is believed to be spread primarily through saliva) and HEPATITIS. Named for the two British virologists who identified it, Michael A. Epstein and Y. M. Barr, this virus is also associated with some cancers. Women infected with this virus are at higher risk of MISCARRIAGE or STILLBIRTH.

   See also HEPATITIS.

Epstein's pearls   Small, shiny white specks on the gum margin and hard palate of the newborn. These feel hard to the touch but are of no significance and disappear in a few weeks.

Erb's Duchenne palsy   Paralysis of the upper arm and chest wall resulting from birth injury to the brachial plexus (network of nerves and blood vessels that control arm function), usually occurring when the baby's shoulder lodges behind the mother's pubic bone during DELIVERY.

erection A stiffened, hard, elevated condition of body tissue caused by stimulation, most commonly referring to the PENIS. Tissue that responds in this way is called *erectile tissue;* it contains many small blood vessels that expand in response to stimulation (usually sexual), causing engorgement (swelling). With engorgement, the tissue darkens, swells, and stiffens. Women have erectile tissue in the NIPPLES, CLITORIS, inner LABIA and vaginal opening. In addition to the penis, men's erectile tissue includes the nipples. Erection is necessary for vaginal intercourse; inability to have or sustain an erection is called *impotence.*

See also SEXUAL RESPONSE.

erythema toxicum Also *erythema neonatorum toxicum.* A rash that appears suddenly over the trunk and diaper area of the newborn, usually between 24 and 48 hours after birth. It may spread; however, the LESIONS do not appear on the palms of the hands or on the soles of the feet. The lesions are pink at the base with a white or yellowish papule or pustule on the top. The cause of the rash is unknown and it disappears in a few days without treatment.

erythroblastosis fetalis A blood disease of the newborn whose blood type is incompatible with the mother's blood type (usually the RH FACTOR). This condition is characterized by ANEMIA, JAUNDICE, generalized EDEMA, and enlargement of the liver and spleen.

estimated date of delivery (EDD) Also *estimated date of confinement (EDC).*

See NAGELE'S RULE.

estrogen The principal female sex hormone, produced in women primarily by the OVARIES and (during PREGNANCY) by the PLACENTA, but also by the ADRENAL GLANDS. In men, small amounts of estrogen are produced by the TESTES. There are three major types of estrogen, *estrone, estradiol,* and *estriol,* and more than a dozen minor types. In premenopausal women, *estradiol,* produced by the ovaries, is the most potent estrogen; in postmenopausal women, the most influential estrogen is *estrone,* produced in the adrenal glands, skin, and fatty tissue. This may explain why larger, heavier women often experience fewer menopausal symptoms than do small, thin women. Estrone is metabolized to *estriol,* probably in the liver, making it the least potent of the three major estrogens.

Most of the characteristics associated with "femaleness" such as development of the BREASTS, UTERUS, FALLOPIAN TUBES, and VAGINA, broadening of the hips, fat deposits in the buttocks and above the pubic bone, and the growth of body hair are regulated by estrogen. Estrogen also helps regulate OVULATION, menstruation, and sexual function. It strengthens the vaginal tissues and stimulates the mucus-secreting glands that lubricate the vagina during sexual arousal. During pregnancy, the placenta produces even higher levels of estrogen, increasing the blood supply to the FETUS; these levels drop dramatically after birth.

Estrogen production decreases after MENOPAUSE, sometimes resulting in vaginal dryness, discomfort during intercourse, and possible loss of LIBIDO. This is highly individual, however, since many women enjoy a satisfying sex life after menopause. Other common, although not universal, symptoms of menopause related to estrogen decrease include drying and wrinkling of the skin, weight increase with "spare tire" around midriff, thinning of hair, hot flashes, and MOOD SWINGS. Although these symptoms can be relieved or alleviated with estrogen replacement therapy, this hormonal manipulation carries certain risks and remains controversial.

Estrogen was discovered in the early 1900s and synthesized shortly thereafter; both its natural and synthetic forms have found many uses. Estrogen is used for FAMILY PLANNING, regulation of menstrual periods, suppression of LACTATION, relief of menopausal symptoms, and for treatment of some forms of cancer. Side effects include breast tenderness and enlargement, HEADACHE, nausea and vomiting, fluid retention, and irregular vaginal BLEEDING. In addition, estrogen is considered a contributing factor in such disorders as blood clots, high blood pressure, and certain cancers. Estrogen therapy is CONTRAINDICATED for any woman with a personal or family history of breast or pelvic cancer, thromboembolic disease, severe kidney or liver disease, SICKLE CELL ANEMIA, HYPERTENSION (high blood pressure), or cerebral vascular diseases. In women who are obese or have gallbladder disease, epilepsy, migraine headaches, or DIABETES, the use of estrogens holds high potential for harmful side effects.

evaporation   One type of heat loss, occurring when water on the skin changes to a vapor.

exchange transfusion   Replacement of 70 to 80% of a newborn's blood with donor blood to avoid destruction of the baby's red blood cells by maternal ANTIBODIES. The most common reason for exchange transfusion is Rh incompatibility.

excise   To cut out or remove surgically.

exercise during pregnancy   Physical activity to promote good health for mother and baby. Most women can continue much of their normal physical activity throughout PREGNANCY; however, all women should consult their physician or other clinician before launching into any new exercise program. Walking, swimming, and cycling on a stationary bike are good basic exercises for most women with normal pregnancies. Athletic women who regularly work out, jog, cross-country ski, or cycle may be able to continue those activities with caution, particularly to avoid falls. Books and videotapes are available with calisthenics developed especially for pregnant women; pelvic exercises (KEGEL EXERCISES, PELVIC TILT, and relaxation exercises) all help to improve muscle tone and heart function. It is important to exercise regularly and in moderation, with gradual warm-up and cool-down movements, and to replace fluid and calories consumed with plenty of liquids (at least one 8-ounce glass of liquid every half hour of strenuous activity). Pregnant women need to avoid HYPERTHERMIA (overheating) by exercising too long in hot weather; hot tubs and saunas should be avoided for the same reason. Any symptoms of dizziness, shortness of breath, tingling, numbness, PALPITATIONS, abdominal pain, or vaginal BLEEDING should be reported to the physician or other caregiving clinician at once.

external os   The opening between the CERVIX (the "neck" of the UTERUS) and the VAGINA.

face presentation   A rare, chin-first position of the baby as it moves down into the BIRTH CANAL. In this position, the baby's neck is so greatly extended that the back of the head touches the back. Normally the top of the baby's head is the presenting or leading part; however, face presentation happens once in every 400 to 500 deliveries. Depending on the size of the mother's PELVIS and whether the chin is anterior (facing the mother's pubic bone) or posterior (facing the mother's tailbone), vaginal delivery, perhaps assisted with FORCEPS, may be possible. If the chin is posterior or severely extended, or if the mother's pelvis is small, CESAREAN DELIVERY may be necessary.

faintness   Also *syncope*. A feeling of dizziness, lightheadedness, as although the surroundings were swirling, sometimes leading to a temporary loss of consciousness (fainting). This sensation is not uncommon during PREGNANCY, particularly when standing for long periods of time or just being in crowded or overheated areas. Faintness is caused by changes in the volume of circulating blood and by postural hypotension (low blood pressure resulting from pooling of blood in the veins). To avoid fainting (and the possible injury to the woman or her FETUS that could result), the pregnant woman should sit down and put her head between her legs. If this does not relieve the symptoms, she should be helped to a place where she can lie down with her feet elevated and breathe fresh air. When getting up from a resting position, it is important for her to move slowly.

fallopian tubes   Also *oviducts, uterine tubes*. A pair of narrow tubes, one attached to each side of the UTERUS, leading to a flared opening *(fimbria)* near each OVARY. Eggs released by the ovary travel through the fallopian tubes to the uterus where they are either implanted (if fertilized by union with a male SPERM) or shed as part of the monthly menstrual flow. The fimbria contains many fingerlike projections (*fimbriae ovarica*) that reach out toward the ovary to help capture the egg as it is released. The tube is lined with *cilia* (moving, hairlike projections) to propel the egg through the tube toward the uterus. The lining also contains nonciliated cells that produce a protein-rich fluid to nourish the egg.

Normally, the egg takes three or four days to move from ovary to uterus. However, FERTILIZATION is only possible within the first 24 hours of the egg's release from the ovary since the egg is not viable after that. Thus fertilization usually occurs when the egg is about one-third of the way down the tube. Occasionally, the fertilized egg fails to move into the uterus and is implanted in the tube itself, a critical condition termed tubal or ECTOPIC PREGNANCY. Unless the fallopian tubes function properly, conception is impossible. INFERTILITY in young women most often results from scar tissue blocking the tubes, caused by either PELVIC INFLAMMATORY DISEASE, a previous ectopic pregnancy, ruptured appendix, gynecologic or abdominal surgery, or postoperative infection. Blocked tubes can sometimes be repaired by microsurgery or laser surgery.

Women who wish to avoid all further pregnancies may choose to have a TUBAL LIGATION, a surgical closing or interruption of the tubes (having one's tubes "tied") to avoid conception. This surgery can be completed through a very small incision using LAPAROSCOPY, sometimes called Band-Aid surgery.

SALPINGITIS (inflammation and infection of the tubes) is the primary disease that affects the fallopian tubes and may result from GONORRHEA, pelvic inflammatory disease, pelvic tuberculosis, an ABORTION, childbirth, or an INTRAUTERINE DEVICE. Cancer rarely begins in the fallopian tubes but can spread from there to the uterus or ovaries. Surgical removal of the tubes is termed SALPINGECTOMY, and may be done at the time of HYSTERECTOMY or excision of an ectopic pregnancy.

false labor   Uterine CONTRACTIONS, both regular and irregular, that occur throughout PREGNANCY and may be mistaken for true LABOR during the last TRIMESTER, but do not dilate the CERVIX. Relatively painless, often irregular, these contractions do not increase in duration, frequency, or intensity.

See also BRAXTON HICKS CONTRACTIONS.

false pregnancy Also *pseudocyesis*. Symptoms of PREGNANCY appearing in a woman who is not pregnant. She may stop menstruating, gain weight, feel nauseated in the morning, and experience BREAST tenderness and occasional sensations of fetal movement. When examined, however, her pelvic organs are normal and the UTERUS a normal nonpregnant size. Sometimes these symptoms signal ECTOPIC PREGNANCY, a *corpus luteum* CYST, or a missed ABORTION, all of which need to be ruled out by the clinician. Most often, however, false pregnancy is caused by a woman's overwhelming wish to have a child, and indicates the need for counseling on and perhaps treatment of INFERTILITY.

family planning Determining if, when, and how a family's children will be born. In a perfect world, every baby would be a wanted child, born to parents who were in optimum physical, emotional, and financial readiness to receive the new life. Although such perfection remains impossible, many women and couples can determine the number and spacing of their children by using one or more methods of CONTRACEPTION. Family planning began in America with Margaret Sanger, a public health nurse in New York City, who recognized women's needs for education about birth control in the early 1900s. In many communities, information about family planning services and clinics is available from the Department of Public Health, Planned Parenthood, or other agencies. These services may include contraception counseling and care (including surgical STERILIZATION), PREGNANCY TESTING and counseling, ABORTION and post-abortion counseling, as well as treatment for SEXUALLY TRANSMITTED DISEASES and counseling for survivors of RAPE. Family planning clinics may be freestanding facilities or part of a public or private hospital.

See also ABORTION; CONTRACEPTION; GENETIC COUNSELING; NATURAL FAMILY PLANNING; PREGNANCY COUNSELING; RAPE.

fatigue A feeling of extreme tiredness, not uncommon during pregnancy, particularly during the first and third TRIMESTERS. In the first trimester, the woman's body is working hard to produce the PLACENTA, the complex connection through which the FETUS receives nutrients and expels waste materials. In the third trimester, fatigue can result from the additional weight of the expanding UTERUS, the mental and emotional weight of planning for all the events and responsibilities to come, and the possible loss of sleep that these factors cause. Fatigue is a signal that the body needs rest, perhaps a nap (or at least a rest period with feet elevated) in the afternoon, an earlier bedtime, and help with household chores. Eating a healthful DIET is important as is getting plenty of exercise (such as walking). During the third trimester, ANEMIA sometimes occurs, causing extreme fatigue, breathlessness, PALPITATIONS, FAINTNESS, and/or pallor (very pale skin tones).

fellatio Also *fellation, penilingus, oral coitus* or *buccal onanism; blowing, blow job, going down* (slang). Using the mouth to stimulate the PENIS, including kissing, licking, or sucking. See also CUNNILINGUS; ORAL SEX.

female reproductive cycle (FRC) The pattern of monthly changes in sexually mature females, including OVULATION and MENSTRUATION, and the hormonal changes that regulate them.

fertility For women, the biological ability to become pregnant and carry the PREGNANCY to TERM; for men, the biological ability to impregnate a woman. Women attain peak fertility around age 25, after which begins a gradual descent until age 40, when fertility declines rapidly; at MENOPAUSE, fertility ceases. Men attain peak fertility around age 21 or 22, and although their fertility begins a very slow decline after age 25, many men remain fertile after age 70.

About 50% of couples will conceive during the first three months of unprotected sex; 80 to 90% will conceive within a year. Between 10 and 15% of American couples have difficulty achieving conception.

See also INFERTILITY; STERILITY.

fertility pill A synthetic HORMONE or other substance prescribed to force OVULATION or replace hormones in women who are unable to become pregnant. Now that treatment of INFERTILITY has become a growth industry, these drugs are also used to cause multiple ovulation (release of more than one egg), helping to ensure the success of IN VITRO FERTILIZATION. One of the most commonly used drugs is *clomiphene citrate*, sold under the brand names Clomid and Serophene. About 70% of women taking this drug begin to ovulate, achieving about the same pregnancy rate as the general population. Clomiphene citrate has also been used to treat irregular MENSTRUAL CYCLES and anovulatory bleeding, and, in men, to stimulate SPERM production. It can also make the cervical mucus too thick for sperm to penetrate, unless a low-dose ESTROGEN is given with it. Side effects can include ovarian CYSTS and enlargement of the OVARIES.

Other potent drugs used to stimulate ovulation are HUMAN CHORIONIC GONADOTROPIN (HCG), extracted from the human PLACENTA; human menopausal gonadotropin (HMG), extracted from the urine of menopausal women, sold under the brand name Pergonal. Both these drugs require close monitoring by the clinician since they can over-stimulate the OVARIES, causing large ovarian cysts and/or MULTIPLE PREGNANCIES—twins, triplets, even quadruplets and quintuplets, all of whom face much higher risks than single births. Clinicians can detect multiple births or potentially life-threatening complications through estrogen assays and ULTRASOUND. This has led to a practice called "selective reduction" of pregnancy, in which the clinician, with per-mission of the couple, removes and discards some of the EMBRYOS so that the remaining embryos will have a better chance for survival. This practice raises ethical questions, particularly with those persons whose beliefs forbid ABORTION.

Treatment with these drugs is time-consuming and expensive: daily injections and periodic BLOOD TESTS and ultrasound are required. Each attempt at pregnancy costs $5,000 to $10,000. In addition to ovarian cysts, the side effects can include ovarian HEMORRHAGE, rup-ture, or torsion (twisting), sometimes necessitating surgical removal of an ovary. Most women who take Pergonal will ovulate and about two-thirds will conceive, usually within three cycles—and $15,000 to $30,000! Of those who conceive, about half will have a single birth, one-fourth will have multiple births, and one-fourth will miscarry.

Sometimes clinicians prescribe other drugs to enhance the ef-fects of Pergonal; these include FOLLICLE STIMULATING HORMONE (FSH) and gonadotropin-releasing hormone (GnRH) agonists (drugs that ac-tivate these hormones). Available as nasal sprays or injections, the GnRH drugs reduce all hormone levels temporarily, making the body more responsive to Pergonal and sometimes inducing menopause-like symptoms (hot flashes and vaginal dryness). Generally these drugs are used from 5 to 14 days.

Some authorities believe that women treated with fertility drugs face a high risk of cancer of the BREAST, ovary, ENDOMETRIUM, and CERVIX for 20 to 30 years after treatment.

See also INFERTILITY.

fertilization Also *conception.* The union of SPERM and egg, causing the fusion of their two nuclei, resulting in a fertilized egg, or ZYGOTE. Normally, FERTILIZATION occurs in the FALLOPIAN TUBES. After EJACULATION, sperm swim up through the CERVIX, UTERUS, and tubes during a 24- to 48-hour period. If the OVARIES release an egg during that time, a sperm may penetrate it, after which the CHROMOSOMES unite and cell division begins. Once fertilized, the egg moves through the fallopian tube and becomes implanted in the uterus. The fertilization process takes about one week, and most PREGNANCY TESTS will show positive results within a few days after IMPLANTATION, or within two weeks after conception.

See also EJACULATION; FALLOPIAN TUBES; FERTILITY; IMPLANTATION; INFERTILITY; OVUM; SPERM; UTERUS.

fetal alcohol syndrome (FAS)
See ALCOHOL USE.

fetal blood sampling   Drawing a blood sample from the fetal scalp, or from the fetal body if in a BREECH (rump as PRESENTING PART) position, to evaluate acid-base balance of the FETUS.

fetal bradycardia   A FETAL HEART RATE of less than 120 beats per minute measured during a 10-minute cycle of continuous monitoring.

fetal death   Also *fetal demise*. Death of the FETUS after the 20th week of PREGNANCY.

fetal distress   Indications that the FETUS is in danger, particularly a change in heart rate or activity.

fetal heart rate (FHR)   Number of fetal heartbeats per minute, normally ranging from 120 to 160 beats per minute.

fetal monitoring   Evaluating the physical condition of the baby during PREGNANCY, LABOR, and birth. There are several methods of fetal monitoring, both external and internal, ranging from simple to complex. The simplest form is daily monitoring of fetal activity by the mother, beginning in the 27th week of pregnancy. The mother keeps a daily record of how many times the baby moves or kicks within 30 or 60 minutes. Although babies vary widely in how often they move, fewer than 10 movements in 10 hours for two days in a row should be reported to the clinician.

Another method of external fetal monitoring is listening to the baby's heartbeat, either with the ear (something fathers like to do) or with a stethoscope, usually discernible between 16 and 20 weeks' GESTATION. A special obstetrical stethoscope with a metal headband transmits the sound even more clearly. The fetal heartbeat can be heard as early as 11 to 14 weeks by using an ultrasonic device called a Dopptone. The normal FETAL HEART RATE is 120 to 160 beats per minute. Any marked slowing or irregularity of the heart rate indicates potential danger for the baby.

AMNIOCENTESIS (examination of amniotic fluid) is yet another means of monitoring fetal well-being, when used just before the onset of labor. The fluid is normally clear; brownish-green amniotic fluid indicates the presence of MECONIUM (the baby's stool), passed only when the FETUS is in distress. By inserting a fiberoptic instrument through the CERVIX, the clinician can see whether the fluid is clear or cloudy.

Fetal monitoring generally refers to electronic fetal monitoring (EFM) used during labor and DELIVERY to measure and record the baby's heart rate and the mother's CONTRACTIONS. This type of monitoring, developed during the 1950s for use in HIGH-RISK PREGNANCIES, has become almost routine for all hospital births. Several long-range studies indicate that EFM has not reduced the newborn mortality rate or the number of brain-injured children; nonetheless, it continues to be widely used.

External EFM involves placing two belts around the mother's abdomen, one to hold the tocodynamometer, the device that monitors and records uterine contractions, and the other to hold an ultrasonic transducer, which monitors and records the fetal heartbeat.

Internal EFM, used almost routinely in hospital births, involves inserting two electronic catheters (wires inside a plastic tube connected to external electrodes) into the VAGINA and through the cervix. One is attached to the presenting part of the baby, most often the scalp, with metal clips or screws, to monitor the heart rate. The other remains between the fetus and the uterine lining, monitoring the duration, frequency, and intensity of contractions.

Internal EFM is essential if the woman receives epidural ANESTHESIA since FETAL DISTRESS increases with the length of time the anesthesia is used. It is also mandatory if labor is induced. Although internal EFM may be valuable in very high-risk situations, it can mean discomfort and risk for mother and baby. In fact, some fetal distress

detected by the monitor may be the result of invasive hospital procedures, including the monitor itself. If not properly maintained, monitors can produce inaccurate or misleading information. Women
attached to a monitor are not permitted to walk or change positions
frequently to relieve labor pain, thus diminishing the effectiveness of
contractions and prolonging labor. Some clinicians believe that keeping the mother in bed, lying on her back, may compress the VENA CAVA,
a major vein, and thus interrupt uterine blood flow, depriving the baby
of oxygen. This invasive form of monitoring increases the risk of
infection and injury to the baby's scalp (see VENA CAVAL SYNDROME).

Fetal monitoring remains a controversial practice, one that has
contributed to the increased number of CESAREAN DELIVERIES performed. Most authorities suggest that internal EFM be limited to truly
high-risk births or those in which complications develop during labor,
and that EFM not be used simply as routine. However, it behooves the
expectant woman to be informed about the risks and benefits of EFM
and what effects it could have on her and her baby.

fetal movement
See FETAL MONITORING.

fetal presentation   The presenting part of the fetal body that enters
the mother's PELVIS first. Normally the head presents first, called CE-
PHALIC PRESENTATION. The other types are BREECH (rump first) and
SHOULDER presentation.

fetoscopy   A microsurgical procedure that permits direct observation
of the FETUS and withdrawal of blood or skin samples to detect possible BIRTH DEFECTS. Developed in the early 1970s, it remains an experimental, high-risk procedure, performed in only a few medical centers
throughout the world. It is used only when there is strong probability
of serious birth defects, or when intrauterine therapy is necessary to
treat a disease before the baby is born. Fetoscopy allows the clinician
to see any gross defects in the fetal body and to diagnose blood disorders such as HEMOPHILIA, thalassemia, and SICKLE CELL ANEMIA. Risks
associated with fetoscopy include spontaneous ABORTION, preterm
birth, ABRUPTIO PLACENTAE, amniotic fluid leakage, and intrauterine
FETAL DEATH. Performed at about 18 weeks' gestation, fetoscopy uses
an instrument called an endoscope inserted inside the AMNIOTIC SAC.

ULTRASOUND is used before and during the procedure to determine gestational age, fetal position, placental location and thickness, location of UMBILICAL CORD insertion into the PLACENTA, pockets of amniotic fluid, and the position of the part of the fetus or tissue to be observed or sampled. After intravenous sedation and use of a local ANESTHETIC, the endoscope is inserted into the amniotic sac through a small incision in the abdomen and UTERUS. The tube containing the endoscope is no larger than a pencil lead. A tiny needle or FORCEPS can be inserted through the endoscope to obtain tissue or blood samples from the placenta.

Fetoscopy carries much greater risk for the fetus than AMNIOCEN-TESIS; in about 5% of cases, it causes spontaneous ABORTION. As other diagnostic techniques such as MAGNETIC RESONANCE IMAGING (MRI), CHORIONIC VILLUS SAMPLING (CVS), and PERCUTANEOUS UMBILICAL BLOOD SAMPLING (PUBS) become more sophisticated and widely used, the need for fetoscopy will be greatly reduced.

fetus   The baby in utero, from about the seventh or ninth week of GESTATION until birth.

fever   Also *pyrexia, hyperthermia.* Body temperature that exceeds 98.6 degrees Fahrenheit (37 degrees Celsius), often a sign of infection or inflammation. When fever occurs during PREGNANCY, the woman should consult her clinician about methods to bring her temperature back to normal. She should *not* take aspirin without consulting her clinician. Sometimes a cool bath is sufficient to reduce the fever. A fever of 102 degrees Fahrenheit sustained for more than two days can harm the FETUS, as can a single day or more of a fever of 104 degrees.

fibrocystic breasts   Also *fibrocystic breast disease.* A catch-all term to describe lumpy BREASTS or any breast irregularity that is benign (not cancerous).
See also BREAST; BREAST CANCER.

fibroid   Also *fibromyoma, leiomyoma, myoma.* A benign (noncancerous) ESTROGEN-dependent tumor that can develop inside, outside, or within the uterine wall. Fibroids can be found in nearly one-third of all women by age 35, and occur more frequently in black women than in white. Because their growth is stimulated by estrogen, fibroids shrink and sometimes disappear after MENOPAUSE. Unless they become painful or grow large enough to obstruct other organs, fibroids require no treatment. Nonetheless, many HYSTERECTOMIES are performed for no other reason than to remove fibroids. Problem fibroids can be surgically removed without hysterectomy; the procedure is called a myomectomy.

If a woman with fibroids becomes pregnant, the tumors are likely to grow very rapidly during PREGNANCY due to the high levels of estrogen. Even although the tumors can be very large, they seldom interfere with the pregnancy because they generally move up into the abdomen. If they remain in the PELVIS, however, CESAREAN DELIVERY may be necessary. Fibroids can interfere with placental function, sometimes causing BLEEDING during the pregnancy. Women with fibroids should not use an INTRAUTERINE DEVICE, since the tumors may have changed the shape of the uterus, increasing the risk of uterine bleeding.

See also POLYP.

fimbria
> See FALLOPIAN TUBES.

fistula   An abnormal passage from one body cavity into another, or to the outside of the body. A *rectovaginal fistula* connects the VAGINA and rectum, as indicated by leakage of gas and/or feces from the vagina. A *vaginal fistula* connects the vagina and the BLADDER (also call a *vesicovaginal fistula),* signaled by leaking of urine from the vagina. Vaginal fistulas usually result from injury inflicted during surgery, such as HYSTERECTOMY or CESAREAN DELIVERY. Small vaginal fistulas may heal without treatment; if not, they require surgical correction.

An *anal fistula* generally leads from the anal canal to an opening in the skin near the anus, from which fecal matter may leak. These fistulas seldom heal spontaneously, and almost always must be surgically corrected.

folic acid   One of the B complex vitamins, found in green, leafy vegetables. Folic acid is essential to maternal and fetal health, contributing to the formation of blood and new cells. Taking folic acid supplements before and during PREGNANCY can greatly reduce the risk of such NEURAL TUBE DEFECTS as spina bifida.

follicle, ovarian   A cluster of cells in the OVARY that encircle an egg.

Every month the PITUITARY GLAND secretes FOLLICLE-STIMULATING HOR-MONE (FSH), causing several follicles to grow and produce ESTROGEN. This process is called the proliferative or follicular stage of the MEN-STRUAL CYCLE. During the next phase, all but one of the follicles atrophy and deteriorate. The remaining follicle, termed the GRAAFIAN FOLLICLE, matures and, influenced by another HORMONE, LUTEINIZING HORMONE (LH), travels to the surface of the ovary, ruptures, and releases an egg. This process is called OVULATION. Following ovulation, the cells of the ruptured follicle merge and fill with a yellow pigment called lutein. At this stage, the follicle, now called a corpus luteum, continues producing estrogen and begins to also produce PROGESTER-ONE. If FERTILIZATION of the egg does not occur, the corpus luteum disintegrates. Occasionally a follicle fails to disintegrate and remains a fluid-filled CYST.

See also CYST, OVARIAN.

follicle-stimulating hormone (FSH)   A HORMONE secreted by the PITUITARY GLAND in both women and men. In women, FSH promotes growth of the ovarian FOLLICLES, release of a mature egg, and production of ESTROGEN by the OVARIES. In men, FSH helps SPERM cells mature.

See also MENSTRUAL CYCLE; OVULATION.

fontanelle   A "soft spot" in a newborn baby's head where the bones of the skull have not fused. The bones of the baby's skull are joined only by connective tissue to allow for overlapping during passage through the BIRTH CANAL, a process called MOLDING.

food cravings, food aversions   Changes in appetite that occur often during PREGNANCY, creating a strong desire for certain foods (cravings) and a strong distaste for others (aversions). This is more of a problem for some women than others; however, most pregnant women are affected with this problem, especially during the first TRIMESTER. Although food cravings and aversions are not completely understood, they are believed to result in part from hormonal changes, and in part from the body's need for a particular nutrient (such as citrus fruit) or rejection of a harmful food or beverage (such as coffee). Sudden cravings for healthful foods (such as fruits, vegetables, cereal, or pasta) should be indulged, as should aversions to unhealthful foods (such as coffee or brownies). When the cravings are for sugary or high-fat foods (such as chocolate chip cookies), the pregnant woman needs to find a satisfactory substitute. In some cultures, women may crave nonfood items such as clay or laundry starch; called PICA, this kind of craving is often a sign of nutritional deficiency.

forceps   Also *obstetrical forceps*. An instrument that resembles a pair of large salad tongs, used to help pull a baby from the BIRTH CANAL or to turn a baby who is in POSTERIOR PRESENTATION. The clinician inserts one blade at a time into the VAGINA, placing them on the sides of the baby's head. Once the blades are in position, the clinician attaches them and pulls gently to pull the baby out. Forceps generally have been replaced by the VACUUM EXTRACTOR or CESAREAN DELIVERY; some older physicians, however, may still use forceps to shorten the pushing phase of LABOR. Unless there is evidence that the baby is having difficulty in emerging, there is no medical reason to use forceps because they can seriously injure the baby.

See also VACUUM EXTRACTOR.

foreskin

See PREPUCE.

frequency, urinary   Urgent need to void often, but without an increase in the amount of urine released. PREGNANCY often triggers urinary frequency, particularly in the first three months, and again in the final weeks, often interrupting sleep as often as two or three times each night (nocturia). Frequency during early pregnancy is most often related to anteversion of the UTERUS (a tilting forward that irritates the BLADDER). In the late stages it results from pressure of the expanding uterus and the presenting part of the baby on the bladder.

Urinary frequency also may signal infection, perhaps intensified by a fallen bladder. Pressure from a FIBROID can also result in urinary frequency.

See also CYSTITIS; CYSTOCELE; STRESS INCONTINENCE; URETHRITIS.

FSH

See FOLLICLE-STIMULATING HORMONE.

fundus

See under UTERUS.

G

galactocele Also *milk cyst*. A CYST that forms in the BREAST when one of the lactiferous (milk-secreting) glands is blocked.

galactorrhea Secretion of breast milk by a woman who has not recently given birth.
See also AMENORRHEA-GALACTORRHEA SYNDROME.

gamete Also *germ cell*. A reproductive cell containing 23 CHROMOSOMES, half the number of other types of cells. SPERM and egg cells are gametes; CONCEPTION occurs when two gametes unite to form a single cell.
See also FERTILIZATION; OVUM; SPERM.

gamete intrafallopian transfer (GIFT) A method of ARTIFICIAL INSEMINATION developed for women who have normal FALLOPIAN TUBES but remain infertile due to one or more of several factors such as ENDOMETRIOSIS, problems with cervical or uterine secretions, low SPERM count or low sperm MOTILITY. The procedure is similar to IN VITRO FERTILIZATION, with OVULATION induced by fertility drugs, and eggs retrieved using LAPAROSCOPY. Rather than mixing the eggs and sperm in a laboratory container, however, the clinician places the eggs in a catheter with sperm obtained earlier and inserts them through the laparoscope into the FIMBRIA of the fallopian tube. Thus FERTILIZATION occurs in the fallopian tube, similar to normal conception, and is achieved in about 25% of couples.
See also ARTIFICIAL INSEMINATION; FERTILITY; INFERTILITY; LAPAROSCOPY; OVUM; SPERM.

Gaucher's disease An incurable genetic disorder characterized by the lack of an enzyme that enables the body to metabolize certain fats, resulting in accumulation of fats in the liver, spleen, and bone marrow. These organs become enlarged, joints become painful, and bones brittle. Like TAY-SACHS DISEASE, it is a single-gene disorder (see under BIRTH DEFECTS) and occurs most often in Jews of European ethnic origin, of whom an estimated 4% are carriers. If both parents are carriers, detectable by a skin biopsy, there is a 25% chance that any child of theirs will have the disease. The presence of Gaucher's disease can be detected by AMNIOCENTESIS.

Gaucher's disease is named for its discoverer, Philippe Gaucher, a French physician. Unlike Tay-Sachs, it is not always fatal, but varies from patient to patient, depending on the age of onset. Infants affected seldom survive more than a year or two. When the disease appears in adult life, it is usually less severe and patients may survive for many years. No treatment is known; however, enzyme replacement therapy produces signs of remission in some adults.

gender identity   A person's sense of being male or female, and an acceptance and awareness of his or her biologic sex. Several factors influence the development of gender identity, including: (1) biologic factors originating in fetal life; (2) sex assignment at birth by parents and clinicians; (3) parental attitudes; (4) conditioning; and (5) development of body image and body ego. Although many children show some evidence of gender confusion, by the age of two years most develop a core gender identity consistent with their biologic sex.

gene
    See under GENETICS.

genetic counseling   Professional advice concerning the risk of occurrence or recurrence of a hereditary disease within a family, and the options available for prevention and/or treatment. Many young couples seek genetic counseling prior to conception, particularly if they anticipate problems based on their knowledge of their families' history. Women who delay childbearing until after age 35 may also seek counseling about the probability of having a child with a chromosomal disorder. Other women may have a history of spontaneous ABORTION or exposure to environmental hazards. Some couples may wait until early PREGNANCY to seek counseling; others may have given birth to a child with a genetic disorder. Fortunately, prenatal testing can now detect many serious genetic disorders so that couples can make informed choices about whether to continue a pregnancy.

Genetic counseling generally uses a team approach, with a medical geneticist, a genetics associate and/or a nurse-geneticist, and perhaps a social worker. The genetics team works with the primary physician to provide the woman or couple with complete and accurate information that will enable them to make informed choices about reproduction. The ultimate goal is to decrease the incidence and impact of genetic disease.

The key element in genetic counseling is a complete family history and personal medical history for both parents. Specific diagnostic tests may be performed, including metabolic screening, urinary screening, and chromosome analysis. See also KARYOTYPING.

After gathering and analyzing all the relevant information, the counselor reviews the results with the woman or couple and explains the available options.

See also AMNIOCENTESIS; ARTIFICIAL INSEMINATION.

genetic disorders
See under BIRTH DEFECTS.

genetics   The science of heredity, named for the basic unit of heredity, the gene. Each of the 50,000 to 100,000 human genes is a blueprint for producing a particular protein.

genitals   Also *genitalia*. The external reproductive organs. In women, the primary external organs are called the VULVA or pudendum; in men, they include the PENIS and SCROTUM.

genital warts
See CONDYLOMA ACUMINATA.

genotype   The genetic makeup of an individual (the pattern of the genes on the CHROMOSOMES).

German measles
See RUBELLA.

gestation   Also *term*. The period of intrauterine development from conception to birth; PREGNANCY. Gestation normally lasts $9\frac{1}{3}$ months (40 weeks); an INFANT born near the end of 40 weeks is called full-

term. A baby born before 36 weeks' gestation is described as PREMA-
TURE, and one born after 42 weeks is described as POSTMATURE.

Since it is usually impossible to tell which act of intercourse
resulted in pregnancy, gestation is calculated from a woman's LAST
MENSTRUAL PERIOD (LMP), even though that may have occurred two
weeks prior to conception. The date of DELIVERY is determined to be
nine months and seven days from the first day of the LMP.

The precise timing of each stage of development varies among
individuals and ethnic groups, as does the size of a FETUS; however, the
process is the same. Milestones in development are illustrated in the
fold-out chart of Maternal and Fetal Development.

gestational age   The number of complete weeks of fetal development, calculated from the first day of the LAST MENSTRUAL PERIOD
(LMP).

gestational trophoblastic disease (GTD)
   See CHORIOCARCINOMA; HYDATIDIFORM MOLE.

gonad   Sex gland. The female gonads are the OVARIES; the male gonads are the TESTES.
   See also OVARY; TESTES.

gonorrhea   Also *GC, clap, dose, drip, strain* (slang). The second
most commonly reported SEXUALLY TRANSMITTED DISEASE in the United
States, usually transmitted by sexual intercourse, either vaginal, anal,
or oral. CHLAMYDIA is the most common. The causative organism in
gonorrhea is the gram-negative gonococcus, *Neisseria gonorrhoeae.*
This organism cannot live outside the body; it thrives on the mucosal
lining of the mouth, throat, URETHRA, and CERVIX. Symptoms appear in
men within 1 to 14 days after sexual contact, and include painful
urination and a urethral discharge that may be white, yellow, or yellow-green. In 80% of infected women (and 20% of infected men),
however, there are no symptoms, increasing the possibility for un-
knowing transmission to other sexual partners. The only symptoms
that do appear in women are pelvic pain, a yellow-green vaginal discharge, and irritation of the VULVA. When infection occurs through
ORAL SEX, it can cause sore throat and enlarged, tender lymph nodes in
the groin. Anal transmission usually causes no symptoms.

Gonorrhea in pregnant women can result in spontaneous ABOR-

TION or tubal infection in the first TRIMESTER. At birth, the baby can contract gonococcal conjunctivitis (inflammation of the eyes) during passage through the BIRTH CANAL. If not treated, it can cause severe infection, STERILITY, and arthritis. See PELVIC INFLAMMATORY DISEASE.

Injectable penicillin is the drug of choice for treating gonorrhea, accompanied by an anti-gout medication called probenecid, given orally to prevent quick excretion of the penicillin by the kidneys. Oral ampicillin with probenecid is also effective, as is oral tetracycline; however, oral tetracycline should not be taken by pregnant women.

Goodell's sign   A softening of the CERVIX, one of the PROBABLE SIGNS OF PREGNANCY, usually discernible by the second month.

Graafian follicle   The single ovarian FOLLICLE that matures during each OVULATION and breaks through the ovarian wall to release a mature egg. Named for the 17th century physician, Reinier de Graaf, who discovered it, this follicle is made up of three principal layers of cells, the *granulosa,* which enclose the mature egg in the center, the *thecae interna,* which surround the granulosa and produce and store ESTROGEN, and the *theca externa,* an avasculer (without vessels) layer of connective tissue. After the egg breaks through the ovarian wall, the Graafian follicle collapses inward. The cavity formerly occupied by the egg fills with blood, forming a new structure, the corpus luteum.

gram stain   One method of staining samples of body tissue to help identify microscopic organisms. Gram staining is used to detect fungus and bacterial infections, including GONORRHEA and TRICHOMONAS.

granuloma inguinale   Also *lymphogranuloma venerum.* A SEXUALLY TRANSMITTED DISEASE occurring primarily in tropical climates; few cases are found in North America, except in the southern United States. More common among men than women, it is caused by an organism called *Donovania granulomatis,* named after Charles Donovan, its discoverer, and is also called Donovanosis. Granuloma inguinale is believed to be transmitted by sexual intercourse but, unlike many STDs, is not highly contagious; many persons exposed to the infection do not contract it. Symptoms may appear as soon as three days or as long as four months after contact. They include swelling, generally in the groin but sometimes on the GENITALS or near the anus, followed by formation of painful, foul-smelling ulcers. The ulcers bleed easily and, unless treated with antibiotics, will spread to the thighs, lower abdomen, and buttocks, increasing the risk of further infection. It can cause massive swelling of the genitals (elephantiasis).

Granuloma is most often treated with three or more weeks of tetracycline; in PREGNANCY, however, erythromycin is used since tetracycline can permanently stain the teeth of the developing FETUS. Recurrence of the disease is common.

gravida   Medical term meaning a pregnant woman.

grief   An emotional reaction to loss, such as the death of a loved one. Although PREGNANCY and childbirth are joyous events for most women and families, unusual circumstances can change them into times of grief and sadness. MISCARRIAGE, STILLBIRTH, or the death of a baby at or soon after birth all represent major losses to the woman and family involved, and grief is the normal reaction. A HIGH-RISK PREGNANCY holds the possibility of loss: the baby may be born prematurely or with a defect; or the mother's health or life may be threatened. Fear of such losses can evoke *anticipatory grief,* a psychological preparation for the possibility of losing the baby and/or the mother. Mothers who, for whatever reason, choose to relinquish their babies for adoption often mourn the loss of that INFANT. Infertile couples also experience grief at the loss of the hoped-for child. See INFERTILITY.

It is important to realize that grief is a normal human response to loss, universal and yet individual in its intensity and duration. *Mourning* is the behavioral process that helps to resolve or "work through" grief, so that the survivor can continue to live without the person who has died. Grief and mourning may disrupt the survivor's life for six months to two years or longer. Clinicians believe that arbitrary timetables should not be assigned to grieving. Studies of grief related to loss of a pregnancy show no correlation between the length of time a FETUS or infant survives and the intensity of the mother's grief. Those who experience stillbirth may mourn as intensely as mothers whose infants survived for several months.

Miscarriage triggers grief for the loss of a baby who is very real to the parents, the baby of their dreams and fantasies. Miscarriage often occurs before the woman has begun to think of the fetus as separate from herself; thus she experiences the loss as losing part of herself. Most cultures have developed rituals for mourning death; however, there are no rituals for the death of the unborn—no casket, no funeral—and so parents are isolated in their mourning. Well-meaning friends and family members sometimes say insensitive things in their wish to comfort parents; others say nothing, fearing they will say the wrong thing.

A family whose baby dies near the time of birth may find it helpful to touch and hold the baby, name the baby, and hold a memorial service appropriate to their religious beliefs and values. Hospital staff are often willing to provide photographs and a lock of the baby's hair. If there are other children, it is important to talk with them about the baby's death and let them know that they are not responsible. Often siblings resent the idea of a new baby and then feel guilty if the baby dies. The mother often feels guilty too, wondering whether her emotions or behaviors were responsible for the baby's death. Until the grief and the guilt are resolved, another pregnancy can be traumatic. Couples are advised to talk with their clinician about possible causes for the baby's death and what implications that might have for future pregnancies. Fortunately, support groups for grieving parents are available in many communities; in these groups parents can share their feelings with other parents who have had the same experience. One such organization is Compassionate Friends, P.O. Box 1347, Oak Brook IL 60521; 312-990-0010.

gynecologic examination   A physical examination that focuses on the BREASTS and pelvic area, performed to detect any abnormalities, to obtain diagnostic specimens, and/or to treat an existing problem. This examination may be performed by a GYNECOLOGIST, family physician (general practitioner, family practitioner, or internist), or a nurse-practitioner. All women need to have this examination at regular intervals to detect any disorders requiring treatment, but some disagreement exists on the length of the intervals. Ideally, the first gynecologic examination should take place before a girl becomes sexually active, or by age 16 or 17 if she has not begun to menstruate. It is essential to have this examination if PREGNANCY is suspected, whatever the age of the patient.

A complete gynecologic examination includes: (1) taking the family and medical history; (2) the physical examination; (3) tests; and (4) discussion of the findings with the clinician. The history will include questions related to the woman's health history: age; number of pregnancies and their outcomes; primary complaint or problem; menstrual history; contraceptives used; hospitalizations and surgeries;

medications; use of drugs, alcohol, or tobacco; allergies or drug reactions; and use of DIETHYLSTILBESTROL (DES) by the woman or by her mother.

The *physical examination* includes measurement of height, weight, temperature, pulse, and blood pressure. Most clinicians also assess the heart and lungs using a stethoscope, inspect the mouth and throat, and palpate (feel) the neck to detect lymph node tenderness and THYROID enlargement. Heart and lung examinations are essential for any woman planning to use ORAL CONTRACEPTIVES. Breasts are examined to detect any sign of a CYST or tumor: lumps, tenderness, NIPPLE discharge, dimpled or puckered skin. See BREAST SELF-EXAMINATION.

The *pelvic examination* is conducted with the woman in the DORSAL LITHOTOMY position for maximum visibility of external and internal pelvic organs. The clinician first inspects the external GENITALS: LABIA, pubic area, CLITORIS, anus, and URETHRA. Both Bartholin's glands and Skene's glands are palpated to detect any lumps. The internal examination begins with insertion of a metal or plastic SPECULUM into the VAGINA. This affords visibility of the vaginal walls and CERVIX so that any irritation, inflammation, swelling, or abnormal discharge can be detected. If specimens are needed for diagnostic tests, they are obtained by inserting a swab or spatula through the speculum.

The other part of the internal examination is a *bimanual examination,* in which the clinician inserts two fingers of one hand into the VAGINA and places the other hand on the woman's abdomen. Using both internal and external palpation, the clinician can assess the position, size, firmness, and mobility of the UTERUS, the location and size of the FALLOPIAN TUBES and OVARIES, and can detect any abdominal tenderness or masses. The clinician may ask the woman to bear down as though she were having a bowel movement to check for uterine relaxation or prolapse.

Next the clinician performs a *rectovaginal examination,* inserting one finger into the VAGINA and another into the rectum, to check the wall between the rectum and vagina and to assess the pelvic organs from this position. The last step of an exam is the *rectal examination,* insertion of one finger into the rectum to detect any growths or other abnormalities.

Although the pelvic examination normally is not painful, it can be uncomfortable, and, for some women, embarrassing. Emptying the bladder just before such an examination helps minimize the discomfort. DOUCHING should be avoided, however, so as not to mask any symptoms of disorders that might be present. Women who are concerned or embarrassed about this procedure might find it helpful to have a friend accompany them.

Laboratory tests performed in conjunction with a gynecologic examination include: *urinalysis,* recommended annually to screen for DIABETES; PAP SMEAR, recommended every year; a GONORRHEA culture, done routinely by some clinicians, and by others only when infection is suspected; a blood count for ANEMIA. Other tests are performed only when a specific problem is suspected; these include a SYPHILIS test; urine or stool culture; BLOOD TESTS for cholesterol, triglycerides, and other substances; and a MAMMOGRAM, recommended annually for women over 50, much less often for younger women.

At the end of the physical examination, most clinicians discuss the findings with the woman, prescribe any necessary medications, and answer questions.

See also PRENATAL CARE.

gynecologist A physician specializing in female reproductive health. For many years, this medical specialty was combined with obstetrics, which includes PREGNANCY, DELIVERY, and POSTPARTUM care; and the clinician was called an obstetrician-gynecologist (ob-gyn). The threat of malpractice litigation and the increasing number of women who choose to remain childless have combined to cause many physicians to discontinue the obstetrics portion of their practice, or to charge higher fees and practice in a subspeciality such as INFERTILITY or HIGH-RISK PREGNANCY. As a result, some communities do not have a physician willing to assist in childbirth.

Although family physicians and internists are capable of performing routine gynecologic care, they are less experienced in the areas of obstetrics and gynecology. Thus, if no obstetrician is readily available in the community, a pregnant woman may want to seek the services of a certified nurse-MIDWIFE for prenatal care.

habitual miscarriage Also *habitual abortion*. Spontaneous loss of three consecutive pregnancies by MISCARRIAGE. Inability to carry a PREGNANCY to TERM may be due to genetic defects in the FETUS, or problems with the mother or father. Maternal factors include infection, hormonal imbalance, or structural defects in the UTERUS. (See DIABE-TES, DIETHYLSTILBESTROL (DES), HERPES VIRUS). Use of ALCOHOL and other DRUGS, tobacco, and caffeine may also be related to miscarriage; environmental factors such as exposure to copper, lead, sulfur, or video display terminals may also play a role.

Women who miscarry repeatedly, particularly during the first TRIMESTER, may benefit from tests to determine the cause. These include an endometrial biopsy, THYROID function test, and CHROMOSOME studies of both parents. Depending on the results of these tests, X-RAY evaluation of the UTERUS and FALLOPIAN TUBES may be performed.

hair loss Also *alopecia*. Thinning of scalp hair, possibly related to hormonal changes not completely understood. Hypothyroidism (abnormally low production of thyroid) and ANEMIA are common causes of hair loss and should be ruled out by BLOOD TESTS. ORAL CONTRACEP-TIVES can trigger hair loss in some women; in others, hair loss occurs after discontinuing oral contraceptives. PREGNANCY can affect hair growth and texture; generally hair grows faster and thicker during pregnancy, sometimes thinning temporarily after DELIVERY.

Halsted radical mastectomy
    See MASTECTOMY.

Harlequin sign A rare skin change in the newborn in which one side of the body becomes deep red while the other side remains pale when the infant is lying on its side. This effect generally lasts from 1 to 20 minutes, but is insignificant and requires no treatment.

headache   Moderate to severe pain in the head that can indicate a variety of disorders but does not require medical treatment unless it becomes chronic or so severe that it interferes with normal activity. Most headaches respond to ANALGESICS; however, pregnant women should consult their caregiver before taking any medications to relieve headache. Relaxation techniques, biofeedback, and massage can prove highly effective in relieving tension headaches. Some clinicians recommend eating foods rich in calcium and the B vitamins. Another noninvasive treatment is acupressure: pressing the index finger on certain pressure points of the body and rotating the finger slowly for 20 or 30 seconds.

Severe and/or chronic headache can indicate a brain tumor; serious infection of the brain, spinal cord, eye, ear, nose, mouth, teeth, or sinuses; or allergy. *Migraine* headaches are caused by disturbances in the external carotid artery which carries oxygenated blood to the brain. ORAL CONTRACEPTIVES can also cause headaches.

heartburn   Also *pyrosis, indigestion.* A burning sensation near the heart (but totally unrelated to it) caused when food and gastric juices in the stomach back up into the esophagus, irritating the tender lining of the esophagus and sometimes leaving an unpleasant taste in the mouth. Heartburn is a fairly common problem in PREGNANCY, caused mainly by the upward pressure of the expanding UTERUS on the stomach. It can be relieved or prevented by avoiding overeating and excessive weight gain; eating small, frequent meals; avoiding fatty, fried, or highly spiced foods; drinking six to eight glasses of water each day; and sleeping with one's head elevated. Antacids such as Maalox® can help relieve heartburn; however, Alka-Seltzer® and other products containing sodium or sodium bicarbonate should not be used.

Hegar's sign   A PRESUMPTIVE SIGN OF PREGNANCY involving the softening of the isthmus of the UTERUS, an area just above the CERVIX at the bottom of the corpus (the body of the uterus). The clinician detects this softening during bimanual examination of the PELVIS.

hematuria   Blood in the urine, generally indicating an infection of the urinary tract, but occasionally a more serious problem such as kidney stones, CYSTS, BLADDER or kidney tumor, or SICKLE CELL ANE-

MIA. The urine appears brownish or reddish, depending on the acidity of the urine. Hematuria always requires medical attention because it can signal serious disorders.

hemolytic disease of the newborn   Also *erythroblastosis fetalis.* A neonatal blood disorder which destroys the baby's red blood cells. It results from Rh incompatibility with the mother. The best treatment is prevention by treating the mother during PREGNANCY. The most severe form of the disorder, *hydrops fetalis,* causes life-threatening ANEMIA; HEMORRHAGE in fetal lung and other tissue; and enlargement of the heart, liver, and spleen due to EDEMA. It is a frequent cause of intrauterine death and can cause uterine rupture.

hemophilia   An incurable, sex-linked (transmitted from mother to son) chromosomal disorder characterized by serious bleeding that is difficult to stop. It is related to the absence of one or more chemical factors that cause blood to clot. There are several types of hemophilia, classified by which clotting factor is defective or missing. The most common types are hemophilia A (Abnormal Factor VIII) and hemophilia B (Abnormal Factor IX). Symptoms appear early in life and include HEMATURIA (bloody urine) and hematoma (a collection of blood in an organ or body space resulting from rupture of a blood vessel), cuts and wounds that heal slowly, and severe bleeding after minor injuries or exercise. The only treatment for this condition is administration of the missing clotting factor, available from blood banks in frozen form. Severe bleeding may require transfusions; less severe conditions may be treated at home with injections by the patient or a family member. Since the advent of AIDS, and before donated blood was screened, some hemophiliacs have been infected with the HIV virus through transfusions.

hemophilus vaginalis   Also *HV, Corynebacterium vaginale, Gardnerella vaginalis.* An organism causing VAGINITIS, a SEXUALLY TRANSMITTED DISEASE characterized by white or grayish, foul-smelling vaginal discharge, itching, and burning. The treatment of choice is oral metronidazole for five to seven days; this drug is CONTRAINDICATED during early PREGNANCY and LACTATION. Oral cephradine for six days is an effective alternative treatment. DOUCHING temporarily removes secretions but does not cure the infection. Sexual partners should be treated at the same time to reduce recurrence.

hemorrhage, vaginal Uncontrollable flow of blood from the VA-GINA, usually originating in the UTERUS. Hemorrhage in adult women most often results from MISCARRIAGE or ECTOPIC PREGNANCY. During the third TRIMESTER of pregnancy, hemorrhage usually indicates placental abnormalities such as PLACENTA PREVIA or premature separation of the PLACENTA, abnormalities of blood-clotting factors, or uterine rupture. POSTPARTAL HEMORRHAGE, the third leading cause of maternal death in the United States, is related to uterine relaxation (failure to contract after DELIVERY), or fragments of placental or fetal tissue retained in the uterus.

Vaginal hemorrhage is a life-threatening emergency requiring immediate treatment: stopping the bleeding, transfusion to restore blood volume, and treatment for shock.

hemorrhoid Also *piles*. A VARICOSE VEIN (distended vein) in the anus or lower rectum, most commonly caused by PREGNANCY as the expanding UTERUS compresses major blood vessels. Other causes include CONSTIPATION (resulting in straining to defecate), OBESITY, prolonged coughing or sneezing, and abdominal tumors. Bleeding after a bowel movement is the primary symptom.

Hemorrhoids may be either *external* or *internal*. An *external* hemorrhoid is a small, bluish or purplish skin-covered mass, usually occurring in clusters, that becomes more pronounced with straining during bowel movements. This condition is seldom painful unless the hemorrhoids thrombose (form a clot); when that happens, they may become inflamed and tender, bleeding profusely. In a few days, the clot is absorbed and the swelling reduced. *Internal hemorrhoids* also occur in clusters and are covered by MUCOUS MEMBRANE. They often ulcerate and bleed during passage of a hard stool, and can cause itching and mucus drainage from the anus.

Hemorrhoids resulting from pregnancy generally disappear without treatment after DELIVERY. A DIET high in fiber and liquid intake helps relieve CONSTIPATION; occasional use of a stool softener can make defecation easier. SITZ BATHS help relieve discomfort.

hepatitis Inflammation of the liver caused by viruses, drugs, or toxic chemicals, and a complication of 0.2% of all pregnancies. The most common viral agents causing hepatitis in PREGNANCY are hepatitis A virus; hepatitis B virus; non-A, non-B hepatitis virus; and EPSTEIN-BARR VIRUS.

Hepatitis A is caused by fecal/oral contamination due to poor hygiene or contamination of food and water. Disease may take from two to six weeks after contact to appear. It causes mild to severe liver inflammation but recovery is usually complete.

Hepatitis B is transmitted by sexual intercourse or exchange of blood or other body fluids (transfusion, sharing needles, maternal-fetal transmission during birth). Symptoms appear one to three months after contact and can lead to cirrhosis (degeneration of the liver) or liver cancer. About 5 to 10% of persons infected with Type B become permanent carriers of the disease.

Type non-A, non-B hepatitis is spread primarily by blood, but also by sexual intercourse and passage through the BIRTH CANAL. Although it usually causes only mild disease initially, it can cause cirrhosis as well. Infected persons sometimes become lifetime carriers.

Hepatitis B can be prevented by administration of a vaccine, given in three doses over a six-month period. Prevention is essential because no treatment can completely eliminate an entrenched infection or control liver damage from chronic infection. The United States Centers for Disease Control recommend that all pregnant women be tested for hepatitis B so that any infected babies can be treated within the first 12 hours after birth. Unless they are treated quickly, they will become lifetime carriers of the infection. Additional vaccine is administered at one month and six months of age. Untreated, these individuals are subject to hepatitis, cirrhosis, and liver cancer in later life.

hermaphroditism   A form of intersexuality in which both ovarian and testicular tissue are present in the same individual. This disorder can occur in both men and women, affecting those characteristics that determine sex: chromosomal arrangement (see CHROMOSOME), external and internal GENITALS, and GONADS (sex glands). *A female hermaphrodite* may have OVARIES but the chromosomal arrangement of a male. A *male hermaphrodite* may have TESTES but external genitals resembling a female VULVA.

Hermaphroditism stems from defects in fetal development, sometimes related to HORMONES given to the mother to prevent MISCARRIAGE. Correction of the problem often involves hormonal therapy and surgery.

hernia, umbilical   Protrusion of the navel resulting from a weakness in the abdominal wall. When this condition is present in newborns, no treatment is needed, even though it may take several months or years to retract. Adults are also subject to umbilical hernias, particularly women who have had several pregnancies or are obese.

herpes virus Also *herpes virus hominis (HVH), genital herpes, herpes genitalis, herpes simplex Types I* and *II.* A chronic disease of the GENITALS caused by one of a family of viruses. Genital herpes is one of the most common SEXUALLY TRANSMITTED DISEASES in the United States, thought to affect at least 10% of adult women. Most such infections are related to Type II herpes virus, although about 15% are caused by Type I, the virus responsible for "cold sores" around the mouth and nose. This same virus occasionally infects the eyes (herpes simplex keratitis), brain, or stomach. Genital herpes is more common in women than men.

Symptoms of genital herpes usually appear within two to seven days of exposure and include itching, followed by the eruption of painful vesicles (blister-like sores) that break, developing into small patches of painful ulcers. These LESIONS may last up to six weeks, healing spontaneously unless they become infected with bacteria. Urinary symptoms may develop, including painful urination or even urinary retention and fever. Despite the disappearance of symptoms, however, infected persons can continue to transmit the virus to sexual partners, to a FETUS in utero, or to an INFANT during birth. At least half of patients will experience a recurrence within six months of the primary infection. Babies born vaginally to an infected mother face a 50% chance of becoming infected; 60% of infected newborns die. If the clinician is aware of the infection, CESAREAN DELIVERY may be recommended. Infection can be transmitted even before birth either through the PLACENTA or through premature RUPTURE OF THE AMNIOTIC MEMBRANES. Genital herpes also seems to predispose women to cervical cancer; precisely how or why this happens is unknown.

When herpes lesions are active, it is especially important to practice good genital hygiene and wear loose-fitting cotton undergarments. Cool compresses, SITZ BATHS, and oral ANALGESICS help reduce the discomfort until lesions have healed.

Although herpes cannot be cured, it can be treated successfully with Acyclovir, either topically (on the skin) or orally. This drug helps reduce the frequency and severity of recurrence; however, it has not been approved for use during PREGNANCY.

heterosexual   Also *straight*. A term denoting male-female sexual relationship or a person who is sexually attracted to individuals of the opposite sex.

high-risk pregnancy   Also *pregnancy at risk*. A description of a pregnant woman whose health problems put her and/or the FETUS in jeopardy. Chronic diseases such as asthma, epilepsy, DIABETES, HYPERTENSION (high blood pressure), kidney or heart disease, cancer, liver disease, SICKLE CELL ANEMIA, or other blood disorders can all have severe effects on the health of the fetus.

Genetic diseases or anatomical abnormalities such as uterine malformations caused by exposure to DIETHYLSTILBESTROL (DES) increase the risk of complications in pregnancy. Socioeconomic and lifestyle factors may put a pregnancy at risk. Women who live in poverty may not have access to good PRENATAL CARE or adequate nutrition. Use of ALCOHOL or other DRUGS can increase the risk to the fetus, often resulting in multiple BIRTH DEFECTS. Women who smoke are more likely to have smaller, premature babies, than women who do not smoke; they also have a higher risk of MISCARRIAGE, PLACENTA PREVIA, and ABRUPTIO PLACENTAE. Infections in the mother can also threaten the baby's health, particularly RUBELLA, HERPES VIRUS, AIDS, GONORRHEA, and SYPHILIS. Mothers over age 35 or under age 16 are considered to be at higher risk, as are obese women, those who have had problems in previous pregnancies, and those who are carrying more than one fetus (MULTIPLE PREGNANCY).

PRENATAL CARE is important for every pregnant woman, but for the high-risk pregnant woman, it is essential. She and her clinician must carefully and frequently monitor her health and the health of the fetus throughout the pregnancy. Measures to help prevent PRETERM LABOR are listed in Table H-1. During the last TRIMESTER, the woman needs to have convenient access to a medical center with special staff and facilities devoted to high-risk obstetrics and intensive care of the newborn.

hirsutism   Excessive growth of body hair on the face, chest, and lower abdomen of women. Although sometimes a hereditary trait, hirsutism is more commonly caused by high levels of ANDROGENS (male hormones) produced by the ADRENAL GLANDS (ADRENOGENITAL SYNDROME), by an adrenal tumor (Cushing's Syndrome), or an ovarian abnormality such as the STEIN-LEVENTHAL SYNDROME. Treatment varies

Table H-1   Measures to Prevent Pre-term Labor

Rest two or three times a day lying on your left side.

Drink 2 or 3 quarts of water or fruit juice each day. Avoid caffeine drinks. Filling a quart container and drinking from it will eliminate the need to keep track of numerous glasses of fluid.

Empty your bladder at least every two hours during waking hours.

Avoid lifting heavy objects. If other small children are in the home, work out alternatives for picking them up, such as sitting on a chair and having them climb on your lap.

Avoid prenatal breast preparation such as nipple rolling or rubbing nipples with a towel. This is not meant to discourage breastfeeding but to avoid the potential increase in uterine irritability.

Pace necessary activities to avoid overexertion.

Sexual activities may need to be curtailed or eliminated.

Find pleasurable ways to help compensate for limitations of activities and to boost the spirits.

Try to focus on one day or one week at a time rather than on longer periods of time.

If on bed rest, get dressed each day and rest on a couch rather than becoming isolated in the bedroom.

Source: Prepared in consultation with Susan Bennett, RN, ACCE, Coordinator of the Prematurity Prevention Program. From *Maternal Newborn Nursing,* Fourth Edition, by S. Olds, M. London, and P. Ladewig. © 1992 by Addison-Wesley Nursing. Reprinted by permission.

according to the cause of the disorder and may include surgery (to remove an adrenal tumor), hormone replacement, and/or electrolysis (for permanent hair removal). ORAL CONTRACEPTIVES can sometimes cause hirsutism; changing to a different brand of oral contraceptives normally corrects the problem.

See also HAIR LOSS.

home birth   Also *home delivery.* Giving birth at home rather than in a BIRTH CENTER, clinic, or hospital. Until the early 1900s, most babies were born at home, attended by a family member, lay MIDWIFE, or general practitioner. As the industrial revolution brought people into the cities, families lost their traditional support systems and, of necessity, began going to the hospital for childbirth. As an infection control measure, physicians set up LABOR and DELIVERY areas like surgical suites and treated childbirth as an illness rather than a normal life process. This practice continued until the consumer movement of the late 1960s and early 1970s raised objections to the high-tech environment and the attendant high costs. Home birth began to have more appeal for couples who wanted a voice in how and where their children were born.

Home birth involves both risks and benefits for mother and baby. Risks are related to the complications that occur in 5% of all births: ABNORMAL PRESENTATION, a baby too large to pass through the mother's PELVIS, prolonged or difficult labor, FETAL DISTRESS caused by PROLAPSED CORD or other problems that might have been detected with FETAL MONITORING, and maternal HEMORRHAGE resulting from PLACENTA PREVIA or ABRUPTIO PLACENTAE. These complications can be life-threatening even in the hospital; at home, medical backup is unlikely to be available. Most OBSTETRICIANS oppose home birth. Many physicians refuse to provide PRENATAL CARE for couples planning home birth, and many refuse to act as back-up caregivers for home birth. Despite this opposition, however, home births seem to be gaining in popularity.

In some states, home births may be attended by a certified nurse-MIDWIFE (CNM), but more often a lay midwife serves as birth attendant. Although many lay midwives have years of experience attending births, they may have limited formal education and be ill-equipped to deal with complications. Certified nurse-midwives are well-educated, skilled practitioners; their participation in home births remains controversial, however, even within their profession.

Benefits of home birth include the close, loving, family-centered atmosphere in which the woman can labor and give birth, the ongoing contact between the parents and the newborn, and the ability to have siblings and/or friends present. Home birth is much less expensive than hospital or birth center birth, and gives the family a sense of control. In addition, the rate of complications is very low since clinicians screen women very carefully beforehand.

Despite the disagreement between those who favor home birth and those who oppose it, most agree that women experiencing a HIGH-RISK PREGNANCY (10 to 15% of all women) should *not* choose birth at home. Critics of home birth point out that even "normal" pregnancies can quickly become high-risk once labor begins since this is the period of greatest stress for the baby.

Ideally the woman giving birth at home will be attended by a qualified professional, either a CNM or a physician. Minimal precautions should include an emergency backup for recognizing signs of FETAL DISTRESS, resuscitating the infant, recognizing and controlling excessive maternal bleeding, and accurately assessing the condition of mother and baby immediately after birth. Oxygen should be available, plus transportation to a nearby hospital if needed, preferably one where emergency arrangements have been worked out beforehand to ensure prompt admission and treatment.

See also BIRTHING ROOM; MIDWIFE; PREPARED CHILDBIRTH.

homosexual   Also *gay* (slang). A term denoting a sexual relationship between persons of the same sex or a person who is sexually attracted to persons of the same sex.

See also HETEROSEXUAL; LESBIAN.

hormones   Potent chemicals produced primarily by the ENDOCRINE glands that regulate the function of various body organs and tissues. Hormones are secreted into the bloodstream which transports them throughout the body. The principal hormones control growth, development of sexual organs, the reproductive cycle, composition of the blood, METABOLISM of nutrients, transmittal of messages in the nervous system, and production of other hormones.

Endocrinology (the study of hormones) is a comparatively new science and so not all hormone functions are clearly understood. Some hormones, such as insulin, are essential to life. When the body fails to produce adequate amounts of insulin, the resulting disorder is DIABETES, and the treatment is synthetic insulin. Other types of hormonal treatment include estrogen replacement therapy for postmenopausal women, and ORAL CONTRACEPTIVES to prevent PREGNANCY.

Hormones may be classified according to where they are produced—for example, ovarian hormones, pituitary hormones—or the functions they affect—sex hormones, metabolic hormones, and so on. Important hormones are discussed under separate entries.

See also HYPOTHALAMUS; PITUITARY GLAND.

hormone therapy   Also *endocrine therapy*. Use of natural or synthetic HORMONES or the removal of hormone-producing organs to treat a disease or disorder. Treating DIABETES with insulin is a kind of hormone therapy; however, the term hormone therapy more commonly refers to the use of hormones to treat various cancers. Women with BREAST CANCER sometimes have their OVARIES removed to decrease the production of ESTROGEN. If their tumors are estrogen-dependent, they also may be given tamoxifen, an estrogen antagonist. Women with PROGESTERONE-dependent tumors are given progesterone antagonists, drugs that block the action of progesterone.

See also CONTRAGESTIVE.

human chorionic gonadotropin (HCG)   A HORMONE secreted by the *chorionic villi* (fingerlike projections on the surface of the embryonic membrane) during PREGNANCY. It is also present in the urine, providing the basis for most types of PREGNANCY TEST. Although more remains to be learned about the function of HCG, it has characteristics similar to LUTEINIZING HORMONE (LH) and FOLLICLE-STIMULATING HORMONE (FSH), and is thought to sustain the corpus luteum in the first weeks of pregnancy. HCG is used to treat INFERTILITY, since it induces OVULATION when injected into an OVARY stimulated by FSH.

human immunodeficiency virus (HIV)
See AIDS.

human menopausal gonadotropin (HMG)   A synthetic HORMONE used to treat INFERTILITY in women who do not ovulate. It replaces the natural PITUITARY hormones, LUTEINIZING HORMONE (LH) and FOLLICLE STIMULATING HORMONE (FSH), which normally trigger OVULATION. HMG is also used to stimulate ESTROGEN production in women with pituitary or hypothalamic dysfunction, as well as to stimulate SPERM production in men. It is marketed under the name Pergonal.

See also FERTILITY PILL.

human placental lactogen (HPL)   Also *human chorionic somatomammotropin* or *HCS*. A HORMONE produced by the PLACENTA, similar to human pituitary growth hormone. It stimulates changes in the mother's METABOLISM that make more protein, glucose, and minerals available for the FETUS. By measuring levels of HPL, clinicians can determine whether the fetus is growing at a normal rate.

husband-coached birth
 See BRADLEY METHOD.

hyaline membrane disease Also *respiratory distress syndrome, RDS*. A life-threatening condition primarily affecting PREMATURE INFANTS whose lungs lack a substance called *surfactant* that helps keep the air sacs (alveoli) open. Without surfactant, the alveoli collapse each time the baby exhales, depriving the baby of oxygen. Babies with this condition breathe rapidly and deeply, grunting with each breath in an attempt to get more air. Their skin is cyanotic (bluish), and their nostrils flared. This is a leading cause of infant mortality; death generally occurs within 72 hours after birth. Treatment includes warming (premature infants are subject to rapid heat loss), administration of oxygen under positive pressure, and intravenous antibiotics to prevent pneumonia. Clinicians sometimes perform AMNIOCENTESIS to determine fetal lung maturity so that CESAREAN DELIVERY can be properly timed.

hydatidiform mole Also *hydatid mole, molar pregnancy*. A tumor that results from abnormal development of embryonic tissue, characterized by multiple grapelike vesicles that fill and distend the UTERUS more rapidly than a normal PREGNANCY. It is the most common gestational trophoblastic neoplasm (tumor), occurring in 1 of every 1,500 deliveries in the United States and 1 in every 125 in Mexico. It is found more often in women under age 20 and over age 40, and in those whose DIETS are deficient in protein, beta carotene, and FOLIC ACID.
 Abnormal uterine bleeding is the most frequent symptom, often with severe NAUSEA and vomiting. The condition is diagnosed with ULTRASOUND and blood or urine tests, which reveal abnormally high levels of HUMAN CHORIONIC GONADOTROPIN (HCG) that has been secreted by the tumor. Unless the tumor is expelled spontaneously by the end of 12 weeks, suction CURETTAGE is performed, followed by sharp curettage (scraping of the uterine lining using a curette) to obtain tissue samples for pathologic study. Most hydatidiform moles are noncancerous, but can give rise to a cancer called CHORIOCARCINOMA. Following curettage, chemotherapy is given, usually methotrexate or dactinomycin, until blood levels of HCG have returned to normal and remained there through two cycles of chemotherapy. The woman is then monitored for a full year to ensure that HCG levels remain normal. Unless CONTRAINDICATED, ORAL CONTRACEPTIVES are prescribed

during that year to prevent another pregnancy. At the end of that year, it is safe for her to attempt another pregnancy, provided there are no signs of tumor recurrence.

hydramnios   Also *polyhydramnios*. An excessive amount of amniotic fluid, usually more than 2,000 milliliters of fluid at TERM (see also AMNIOTIC SAC). Normally, the amniotic sac contains about 1,000 milliliters at the end of nine months. Hydramnios may be either *acute* (a sudden buildup of fluid, distending the UTERUS in a matter of days) or *chronic* (fluid increases gradually throughout the PREGNANCY).

Although the cause of hydramnios is not known, it is often associated with BIRTH DEFECTS, particularly NEURAL TUBE DEFECTS and gastrointestinal abnormalities, or MULTIPLE PREGNANCIES. It also occurs in diabetic mothers. Symptoms are related to the pressure of the distended uterus on nearby organs: difficulty in breathing and swelling of the legs, VULVA, and ABDOMEN due to fluid retention. ULTRASOUND is used to confirm the diagnosis. Extreme hydramnios points to a poor prognosis for the baby. The high probability of life-threatening abnormalities may be further complicated by difficult LABOR and premature birth, leading to a perinatal (before and after birth) death rate of 50% or greater.

There is no treatment for hydramnios, other than comfort measures for the mother such as bed rest and sedation. Fluid continues to build up, relieved only by AMNIOCENTESIS, which itself frequently induces labor.

hydrops fetalis
    See HEMOLYTIC DISEASE OF THE NEWBORN.

hydrosalpinx   A FALLOPIAN TUBE that has filled with fluid and become obstructed near the *fimbria* (the end closest to the OVARY), preventing the egg from entering the tube. It most often follows GONORRHEA or PELVIC INFLAMMATORY DISEASE, which give rise to *pyosalpinx* (pus in the tube). As the body absorbs the pus from the infection, the cavity fills with fluid. If both tubes are affected, the woman is INFERTILE. If the condition is detected early, it can be surgically corrected.

hyperbilirubinemia
    See NEONATAL JAUNDICE.

hypercalcemia Abnormally high levels of calcium in the blood which can result in fetal cardiac defects and even death.

hyperemesis gravidarum
See MORNING SICKNESS.

hypertension Also *high blood pressure*. Elevated blood pressure, occurring as a single symptom *(primary or essential hypertension)* or in association with another condition such as PREGNANCY or kidney disease *(secondary hypertension)*. It occurs twice as often in African Americans as in whites; overall, it affects about 15% of American adults. High blood pressure tends to occur in middle age, but is increasingly diagnosed in young people.

Hypertension that occurs in pregnancy is termed *pregnancy-induced hypertension* (PIH), usually occurring after 24 weeks' gestation. This condition poses serious risk to both mother and baby if it develops into preeclampsia, a combination of hypertension, edema, and proteinuria (protein in the urine). Preeclampsia has been known to occur without edema, making hypertension the most important criterion in diagnosis.

Preeclampsia is found in about 8% of pregnancies, depending on geographic location. It is most common with first babies in women under 20 years of age or over 35 years, in multiple pregnancies, and in women with diabetes, chronic hypertension, and underlying kidney disease. It occurs most often in black women, and in women of low socioeconomic status. Its cause is unknown; however, prenatal care has been shown to reduce the incidence of preeclampsia by one-half.

There are two categories of preeclampsia: mild and severe. Women with mild preeclampsia are usually confined to bed at home until the baby is sufficiently mature to be delivered. Urine is measured daily using a dipstick strip to determine protein content; blood pressure is monitored regularly. If the woman experiences severe headaches, visual disturbances, or stomach pain, she should call her caregiver at once and will likely be hospitalized. Women with severe preeclampsia are hospitalized in order to prevent convulsions, control blood pressure, and proceed with delivery, the only treatment measure possible. Untreated, preeclampsia becomes ECLAMPSIA, medical toxemia of pregnancy, a life-threatening condition that can include severe seizures, coma, and death.

If the pregnancy has advanced less than 28 weeks, the prognosis for the infant is poor. In pregnancies of 28 or more weeks, the outlook is more hopeful but the infant will need the special care available in a newborn intensive care unit (NICU).

Primary hypertension is a "silent" disease; generally no symptoms appear until the affected person has a stroke (cerebral vascular accident), or heart attack, or develops kidney disease. Measurement of blood pressure, however, is part of almost every adult's visit to any physician, so the problem frequently can be detected and treated before more serious illness strikes.

Clinicians use an instrument called a *sphygmomanometer* to measure blood pressure, which is the pressure exerted by the blood against the walls of the arteries. This pressure varies according to the strength of heart action, the elasticity of the arterial walls (which decreases in later adulthood), and the volume and thickness (viscosity) of the blood. Blood pressure is measured in two steps: first, the *systolic pressure,* measured when the left ventricle of the heart contracts, and second, the *diastolic pressure,* measured when the heart is at rest and the ventricle refills with blood. Systolic pressure in a healthy adult may be about 120 and diastolic pressure about 80; such a reading would be stated as blood pressure of 120/80. In hypertension, the diastolic pressure rises, so that a diastolic reading between 90 and 104 would be considered mild hypertension, between 105 and 114 moderate hypertension, and 115 and higher, severe hypertension. Adult blood pressure readings that consistently exceed 140/90 are considered hypertensive; however, some clinicians regard higher levels as normal in elderly patients.

hyperthermia Elevated body temperature caused by FEVER or external factors such as use of a sauna or hot tub. Studies indicate that maternal hyperthermia is associated with NEURAL TUBE DEFECTS in the FETUS and other central nervous system problems.

hypocalcemia Abnormally low levels of calcium in the blood.

hypoglycemia Abnormally low blood sugar (glucose).

hypothalamus A part of the brain near the posterior PITUITARY GLAND that secretes several HORMONES and regulates the secretion of other hormones by the anterior pituitary gland. The hypothalamus secretes OXYTOCIN (which influences uterine CONTRACTIONS) and vasopressin, which constricts blood vessels, elevates blood pressure, and affects the UTERUS and kidneys. It also releases prolactin-inhibiting factor, which as its name suggests, prevents the release of PROLACTIN, the hormone that triggers and maintains LACTATION. Hypothalamic function is incompletely understood.

hysterectomy   Surgical removal of the UTERUS. *Total hysterectomy* consists of removing the entire uterine corpus (body) and the CERVIX; *subtotal* or *partial hysterectomy* leaves the cervix intact. This latter procedure is seldom performed since the cervix has no function and remains subject to cancer. Hysterectomy does not include removal of the OVARIES or FALLOPIAN TUBES; thus it does not induce MENOPAUSE but it does prevent PREGNANCY and end menstruation. Surgical removal of the ovaries (OOPHORECTOMY) and of the fallopian tubes (SALPINGEC-TOMY) is frequently performed at the time of hysterectomy, in which case the operation is termed a *complete hysterectomy*. This operation is performed by means of an abdominal incision and requires longer recovery time than a vaginal hysterectomy, which involves removal of the uterus and cervix through an incision inside the VAGINA.

hysterosalpingography   A radiologic (X-RAY) study of the uterine cavity and FALLOPIAN TUBES, generally used to detect uterine abnormalities or tubal blockage or constriction. Usually an outpatient procedure, it involves injecting radiopaque dye into the CERVIX so that the uterine and tubal structures become visible on a screen. Many clinicians consider hysterosalpingography dangerous because of the high dose of radiation to the OVARIES, preferring the minor surgical procedure of LAPAROSCOPY.

hysterotomy   Termination of a second-TRIMESTER PREGNANCY by removing the FETUS and PLACENTA through a small incision in the UTERUS. Similar in technique to a CESAREAN DELIVERY, this operation sometimes produces a live fetus who dies almost immediately because its organs are too immature to sustain life. This is a high-risk procedure with potential for major complications; most clinicians now prefer AM-NIOINFUSION for second-trimester ABORTION whenever possible.

I

iatrogenic disorder   A disorder caused by medical treatment, such as urinary tract infection caused by catheterization.

identical twins
> See under MULTIPLE PREGNANCY.

idiopathic   Description of a health problem with no known cause. INFERTILITY is sometimes idiopathic.

immunoglobulins   Proteins that act as ANTIBODIES in the immune system when ANTIGENS (such as bacteria, foreign blood cells, or the cells of transplanted organs or tissues) are introduced.
> See also ACTIVE ACQUIRED IMMUNITY; PASSIVE ACQUIRED IMMUNITY; RH FACTOR.

implantation   Also *nidation*. Attachment of the fertilized OVUM (ZYGOTE) to the ENDOMETRIUM (lining of the UTERUS), occurring seven to nine days after FERTILIZATION.
> During its journey through the FALLOPIAN TUBE into the uterus, the cells of the zygote have begun to divide, developing into a two-layered ball of cells. The outer layer is called the *trophoblast;* the inner layer, the *blastocyst.* The trophoblast attaches to the endometrial surface, eventually developing into one of the embryonic membranes, the chorion. The blastocyst burrows into the endometrium until it is completely covered. In time, it becomes the EMBRYO and the other embryonic membrane, the AMNION. The uterine lining thickens beneath the implanted blastocyst, and the cells of the trophoblast grow down into the thickened lining, forming *villi.* Eventually these villi will become the PLACENTA, the source of nourishment and oxygen for the developing embryo.

Successful implantation requires PROGESTERONE, secreted by the corpus luteum, to enrich the endometrium with nutrients for the zygote. When this mechanism fails, a disorder called luteal phase defect, the zygote may not implant or it may not survive. Luteal phase defect occurs in 3 to 5% of infertile women and accounts for approximately one-third of habitual early MISCARRIAGES. Progesterone therapy administered at the critical point in the cycle may help achieve implantation.

impregnation
See FERTILIZATION; also ARTIFICIAL INSEMINATION.

inborn error of metabolism An inherited deficiency of a specific enzyme needed for normal metabolism of specific chemicals. The most common of these is PHENYLKETONURIA (PKU), occurring at a rate of 1 in 12,000 live births worldwide. It occurs most often in white population groups from northern Europe and the United States, and is seldom seen in African, Jewish, or Japanese people. All newborns in the United States are screened routinely for PKU. When detected, the disorder can be corrected by dietary means. Untreated, it leads to progressive mental retardation.

incompetent cervix Also *incompetent cervical os, dysfunctional cervix*. Premature dilatation of the CERVIX, usually during the fourth or fifth month of PREGNANCY, followed by spontaneous ABORTION (MIS-CARRIAGE). This condition is often associated with habitual second TRIMESTER miscarriage, occurring in 1% or less of pregnancies. Causes include anatomical defects of the cervix or UTERUS, some of which result from maternal exposure to DIETHYLSTILBESTROL (DES), trauma to the cervix during previous deliveries, or surgical procedures such as DILATATION AND CURETTAGE (D&C).

The most widely used treatment is a surgical procedure called *cerclage,* a reinforcement of the cervix with a "purse-string" SUTURE, performed between 14 and 18 weeks' GESTATION. If CESAREAN DELIVERY is planned, the suture is left in place for possible future pregnancies. Otherwise the suture is removed about the 38th or 39th week, or when LABOR begins, so that vaginal birth can occur. Cerclage is 80 to 90% successful in enabling a woman to carry the pregnancy to term. If it fails, however, the suture must be removed quickly to prevent injury to the cervix.

incomplete miscarriage
  See ABORTION.

increment   Increase or buildup, as in a uterine CONTRACTION; the opposite of DECREMENT.

induction of labor   Also *induced labor.* Medical or surgical stimulation of uterine CONTRACTIONS in order to hasten DELIVERY of the FETUS. Although sometimes necessary when delayed delivery jeopardizes either mother or baby, induction of LABOR entails serious risks to both and should not be performed for minor or controversial reasons. Risks to the mother include emotional crisis due to fear and anxiety, PRO-LONGED LABOR, traumatic labor with contractions powerful enough to cause premature separation of the PLACENTA, laceration of the CERVIX or uterine rupture, and POSTPARTAL HEMORRHAGE. Risks to the baby include possible prematurity, oxygen deprivation caused by PRO-LAPSED CORD leading to permanent brain damage, other birth injury, or death due to traumatic labor.

The two most widely used methods of inducing labor are rupturing the membranes (AMNIOTOMY) and intravenous administration of OXYTOCIN. These two methods are most effective when used together. Successful induction requires that the cervix be ripe, that is, softened, and that it be more than 50% effaced and dilated sufficiently to at least 2 centimeters (¾ inch) so that the examiner's index finger can be easily inserted. Unless the cervix is ripe, sufficiently effaced, and dilated, rupturing the membranes may not induce contractions. Even if contractions begin, labor may be prolonged. See EFFACEMENT; PRO-LONGED LABOR.

If the cervix is not ripe and labor must be induced because of a health problem such as DIABETES mellitus, PROSTAGLANDINS may be administered to promote ripening. Research shows that one of the prostaglandins, PGE2, administered vaginally or applied as a local extra-amniotic (outside the amniotic membrane) gel, is most effective in ripening the cervix. Mechanical devices such as LAMINARIA are less effective and may increase the risk of infection. Limited studies have been done using ESTROGEN for cervical ripening; results are inconclusive, however, when compared with prostaglandin administration.

Induction of labor with oxytocin is absolutely contraindicated when the baby is very large (more than 4,000 grams, or 8.8 pounds), in cases of TRANSVERSE LIE (abnormal horizontal position of the fetus in utero) or PLACENTA PREVIA, or in the presence of a uterine scar from previous CESAREAN DELIVERY or other abdominal surgery. Relative contraindications include BREECH presentation, POLYHYDRAMNIOS, MULTIPLE PREGNANCY, or previous birth of five or more INFANTS.

infant   A child less than one year old.

infant death (mortality) rate   The number of children who die before their first birthday per 1,000 live births in a given population per year.

infant of a diabetic mother (IDM)   Baby born to woman who has DIABETES mellitus. If her blood glucose levels have been strictly monitored and held within the normal range throughout PREGNANCY, the infant's risk of BIRTH DEFECTS or perinatal death is no greater than for infants of mothers without this condition. Untreated diabetes, however, carries a high risk of CONGENITAL ABNORMALITIES, HYPOGLYCEMIA, RESPIRATORY DISTRESS SYNDROME, and hyperbilirubinemia.
    See also DIABETES MELLITUS.

infertility   Also *subfertility.* Inability to conceive after one year of sexual intercourse without contraceptive measures, experienced by one in six couples in the United States. *Primary infertility* describes never having conceived, while *secondary infertility* refers to having conceived in the past but having difficulty in the present. STERILITY means complete inability to achieve conception.
    Authorities attribute the apparent increase in infertility to a number of causes, including delayed childbearing, use of INTRAUTERINE DEVICES (IUDS) for CONTRACEPTION, and a greater number of sexual partners leading to increased exposure to SEXUALLY TRANSMITTED DISEASES. Medications can also contribute to infertility; use of HORMONES, antibiotics, antihypertensive drugs, aspirin, ibuprofen, antidepressants, hallucinogens, and ALCOHOL may disrupt the reproductive process at different stages. Sometimes discontinuing use of the drugs reestablishes FERTILITY.
    The development and marketing of various assisted reproductive technologies has caused many couples to seek treatment rather than accept childlessness. Unfortunately, some unscrupulous clinicians and facilities exploit infertile couples, exacting a high price, both emotionally and financially. Thus couples seeking infertility evaluation and

treatment need to be aware that the "infertility industry" is unregulated, and that clinicians affiliated with major medical centers and/or teaching hospitals may offer greater expertise and higher ethical standards of practice than private infertility clinics. See Table I-1 (page 161). Resolve, Inc. is a national organization that assists infertile couples by providing medical referrals, fact sheets, newsletters, and an information hotline. Their address is 1310 Broadway, Somerville MA 02144; 617-623-0744.

A thorough evaluation is necessary to determine the cause of a couple's infertility. This is best done by a reproductive endocrinologist, an obstetrician-gynecologist with two or more years additional training in infertility. Because infertility is an emotional crisis, couples need a clinician whose medical and technical expertise is balanced by a sense of human compassion and understanding.

The probable cause of infertility can be established in 85 to 90% of couples and appropriate therapy will result in pregnancy for 50 to 60%, without such high-tech procedures as IN VITRO FERTILIZATION (IVF). In 15 to 20% of couples diagnosed as infertile, PREGNANCY will occur without treatment. Those remaining can assess their options as evaluation and treatment progress.

Both partners have a potential role in fertility, and both may be subfertile. In about 30% of cases, a male factor is the primary cause of infertility; in another 20 to 30%, a male factor is a contributing cause. In the remaining 40 to 50%, a female factor is responsible.

The evaluation (workup) begins with a careful medical history and physical examination of both partners, including BLOOD and URINE TESTS. Routine tests for the male include semen analysis (see under SPERM); for the female, a SIMS-HUHNER TEST of cervical mucus, HYSTEROSALPINGOGRAPHY to detect any blockage in the FALLOPIAN TUBES, and BASAL BODY TEMPERATURE charts or endometrial biopsy to determine whether OVULATION is occurring.

If the partner's semen analysis does not identify a problem, but the cervical mucus test reveals limited sperm or absence of sperm, changing the timing, techniques, and positions for intercourse may prove effective. If these measures do not achieve pregnancy, ARTIFICIAL INSEMINATION, with either partner or donor sperm, may be an option.

If the woman's cervical mucus is proving to be a barrier to sperm, the clinician may recommend estrogen therapy or insertion of the partner's sperm directly into the UTERUS. Ovulation disorders can be corrected by administration of clomiphene citrate or HUMAN MENO-

PAUSAL GONADOTROPIN (see FERTILITY PILL). Uterine FIBROIDS or blocked FALLOPIAN TUBES can be surgically corrected.

If pregnancy does not occur within six to nine cycles, female fertility factors should be reappraised. Women who agree to hormonal treatment for infertility need to realize that these are powerful drugs with potential for long-term consequences, such as increased risk for breast and/or ovarian cancer.

informed consent   A legal principle protecting an individual's rights to autonomy and self-determination by specifying that no action, including medical and surgical procedures, may be performed unless that individual fully understands the risks and benefits involved and has freely agreed or consented to that action. All too often, physicians explain clinical procedures or prescriptions in "medicalese" and patients consent without really understanding the full range of possibilities inherent in the procedures or drugs prescribed. It is every patient's right to ask questions until she or he clearly understands the explanation, and to receive a written copy of the explanation. It is also a patient's right to refuse during a procedure as well as before.

insufflation, tubal
    See RUBIN TEST.

insulin
    See DIABETES MELLITUS.

intensity   The strength of a uterine CONTRACTION at its acme (peak).

internal os   The inner opening or mouth; the opening between the CERVIX and the UTERUS.

intrapartum   The period from the beginning of LABOR until the end of DELIVERY of the INFANT and the PLACENTA.

intrauterine device (IUD)   A small contraceptive device that fits inside the UTERUS, with a barium coating that makes it visible in X-rays. How the IUD prevents pregnancy is not completely understood; however, it has only a 3% failure rate. During the 1960s, the IUD was used by about 10% of women in the United States, but that number has declined to less than 1% today. At the same time, 85 million women in other countries have turned to the IUD as a method of CONTRACEPTION, most of them in developing countries. Unfortunately, poor health and limited access to medical care increase the risk of complications from IUDs. In addition, the IUD provides no protection against SEXUALLY TRANSMITTED DISEASE (STDs) including AIDS.

Use of IUDs in the United States began before adequate research on long-term safety and effectiveness had been done. As a result, such major complications developed with some types of IUDs that they were pulled off the market. The Dalkon Shield serves as the most glaring example. Manufactured and marketed from 1971 to 1975 by the A. H. Robins Company, the Dalkon Shield soon became implicated in a large number of spontaneous septic ABORTIONS and PELVIC INFLAM-MATORY DISEASE (PID). Twenty U.S. women died as a result of septic abortions related to the Dalkon Shield. It was removed from the U.S. market in 1974 but continued to be sold abroad; however, none of the devices already sold were recalled by the company.

A class action lawsuit was filed against A. H. Robins by the National Women's Health Network in 1981 and again in 1983. The suit demanded a worldwide recall of the Shield, which by then was being used by 50,000 women in the United States and 500,000 women in other countries. Although the suit was unsuccessful, women learned that corporations should be held accountable for their defective products.

Today, only two IUDs are available in the United States: the TCU-380A (ParaGard) and the Progesterone T device (Progestasert). The TCU-380A is a plastic IUD with a thin copper wire wrapped around the vertical stem and a sleeve of copper on each "arm"; a clear or whitish string is attached to it. The use of copper tends to increase menstrual bleeding. This device should be replaced every four years.

Women who are using an IUD should have a PREGNANCY TEST after the first missed period. If the test is positive, the IUD should be removed at once since the chances of its causing a spontaneous ABOR-TION (MISCARRIAGE) are about 50%, and even higher during the second TRIMESTER. Carrying a pregnancy to term with an IUD in place increases the risk of premature delivery, a low-BIRTH-WEIGHT baby, or STILLBIRTH.

The Progesterone T device (Progestasert) is a plastic IUD containing a year's supply of synthetic PROGESTERONE; it has a blue-black double string attached. This IUD tends to decrease menstrual bleeding but is associated with a higher incidence of ECTOPIC PREGNANCIES than other IUDs. At the end of a year, this device must be replaced.

Clinicians recommend that IUDs be used with spermicidal cream, jelly, or foam for maximum effectiveness, and particularly for the first three months after IUD insertion.

Disadvantages of the IUD include the high rate of expulsion (from 2 to 20% of women expel the device during the first year of use). Other potential side effects include uterine perforation, ectopic pregnancy, pelvic inflammatory disease, impaired FERTILITY, or STERILITY.

intrauterine growth retardation (IUGR)   Delayed growth of the FETUS due to any cause, such as intrauterine infection, nutritional deficiency, or pregnancy-induced HYPERTENSION.

in vitro fertilization (IVF)   *Fertilization* of the female OVUM by SPERM in a laboratory container. *In vitro* is Latin for "in glass," hence the expression "test-tube baby" has been applied to infants resulting from this assisted reproductive technology. The first such baby, Louise Brown, was born in England in 1978; the first U.S. test-tube baby was born in 1981.

In vitro fertilization is an invasive, expensive, complicated procedure, still considered experimental by many authorities. Each attempt to achieve PREGNANCY by this method costs from $5,000 to $10,000 and is generally not covered by health insurance. The success rate, based on "take-home babies," ranges from 10 to 20%; thus many couples experience enormous financial loss and emotional disappointment if pregnancy and birth do not yield a healthy INFANT.

The growing number of couples with INFERTILITY problems is seen as an expanding market by many entrepreneurial clinicians, and has created a booming fertility "industry"—more than 20,000 couples undergo IVF every year in the United States. While some of the more than 200 IVF clinics are reputable and effective in treating infertility, others have been found guilty of unethical practices, such as misrepresenting their success rate and failing to fully inform women about the potential side effects of the drugs used. The American Fertility Society sets standards for such clinics, but because there are no state or federal regulations for these clinics, there is no way to enforce the standards. It is essential, therefore, that couples considering IVF should thoroughly and carefully investigate these clinics before deciding to undergo treatment. Resolve, Inc., can provide information on specific clinics (see INFERTILITY). Questions to ask about

(text continued on page 163)

Table I-1   Questions to Ask About
Assisted Reproductive Technology (ART) Programs

Deciding on which clinic to use for an IVF, GIFT, or ZIFT cycle is a major decision. The only resource for clinic-specific data and success rates is the SART Report (Society for Assisted Reproductive Technology). This report is available for $20 per region from the American Fertility Society, 1209 Montgomery Hwy., Birmingham AL 35216-2809, 207-978-5000. In this report you can see statistics for over 200 clinics. The data are divided into several statistical categories: women 39 years of age and younger; women 40 years of age and older; with and without male factor infertility. Statistics are also provided for GIFT and ZIFT, combination cycles using IVF and GIFT or ZIFT, unstimulated cycles, donor egg cycles, host uterus cycles, and frozen embryo cycles.

The following questions may also help you choose a clinic:

Credentials	Is the IVF staff affiliated with any major academic medical center? What are their credentials or training?
	Is the program an active or associate member of SART?
Success rates	Does the clinic report its results to the IVF registry and to SART?
	When did they start offering ART? How many patients undergo transfer per month? Clinics that have been involved with the procedure longest may have the best record of success.
In the last twelve months	How many successful ovulation inductions with egg retrievals have they had?
	How many clinical pregnancies (confirmed by ultrasound and fetal heartsounds) have they had relative to the number of embryo transfers?
	How many live births have they had relative to the number of transfers?
	How many of these are multiple pregnancies?
	What is the miscarriage rate for the program?
	If you are over 40 or have a male factor infertility problem
	If you have a particular diagnosis

Table I-1   Questions to Ask About
Assisted Reproductive Technology (ART) Programs (continued)

Services and costs	When does their ovulation induction program start? Are all patients synchronized or can you start at your own convenience?
	Do they use drugs to suppress your hormones (Lupron, for example) before stimulating ovulation?
	Do they freeze extra embryos? If not, can you choose to donate your eggs to a donor egg pool to be used by another couple?
	What are the clinic hours and lab hours? This is important if you work and need ultrasounds or other tests done before going to work. Are they open weekends and holidays?
	Does the clinic provide general infertility services as well? This is particularly important if you are not sure if you are an appropriate ART candidate.
	Is there an intake interview? Will you meet with a doctor, nurse, and/or financial manager? What is the fee for this appointment?
	What does each cycle cost, including drugs and any other expenses? How much is covered by insurance? Do you have to pay up front or can you pay in divided payments? If a cycle is canceled because of poor ovulation response, what is your financial responsibility?
Support services	Are there counseling and support services available?
	Do they have a "contact system" of patients who have completed their program, successfully or not, with whom you can speak?

Suggested reading:

"A Patient's Guide to the Assisted Reproductive Technologies." This booklet is available from the American Fertility Society for $1.00 (1209 Montgomery Hwy., Birmingham AL 35216-2809).

American Fertility Society, "InVitro Fertilization/Embryo Transfer in the United States: 1990 Results Taken from the National IVF/ET Registry," *Fertility & Sterility.* 59:1, January, 1992, pp. 15–25.

Sher, Geoffrey, M.D., V. Marriago, J. Stoess. *From Infertility to InVitro Fertilization.*

Table I-1   Questions to Ask About
Assisted Reproductive Technology (ART) Programs (continued)

New York: McGraw Hill Publishing Company, 1988.

Silber, Sherman, M.D. *How to Get Pregnant with the New Technology.* New York: Warner Books, 1991.

"Overview of the Assisted Reproductive Technologies," Resolve fact sheet available through National Resolve.

Source: Resolve, Inc., © 1993. All rights reserved. Reproduced with permission.

---

assisted reproductive technology (ART) programs are summarized in Table I-1.

See FERTILITY PILL; GAMETE INTRAFALLOPIAN TRANSFER.

In vitro fertilization is most successful for women between the ages of 20 and 35 with normal ovarian and uterine function, but with blocked or malfunctioning FALLOPIAN TUBES. Screening candidates for this procedure often includes psychological tests and counseling for the couple to assess their ability to deal with the emotional pressures involved. Once accepted for treatment, the woman is given fertility drugs so that more than one ovarian FOLLICLE will mature (see FERTILITY PILL). ULTRASOUND and frequent BLOOD TESTS are used to monitor HORMONE levels, often ruling out 20% or more of IVF candidates. At the time judged to be optimal for fertilization, the eggs are removed from the OVARY by means of needle aspiration, either through the upper vaginal wall or through LAPAROSCOPY (a small abdominal incision). The eggs are then mixed with sperm in a laboratory container and put into a protected environment for 36 hours. If fertilization has occurred during that period, the EMBRYOS (from two to eight) are inserted into the woman's UTERUS. Additional embryos may be frozen for possible later use if the couple has agreed to this. If the IVF cycle fails, the frozen embryos can be thawed and used. Only about half of frozen embryos survive the thawing process, of which only 10% result in pregnancy.

Twelve to fourteen days after the eggs have been inserted into the uterus, a PREGNANCY TEST is performed. If the test is positive, PROGESTERONE shots may be continued as long as 12 weeks to help ensure continuation of the pregnancy.

About 20 to 25% of women become pregnant after the first IVF procedure; nearly one-fourth of them miscarry, however. Pregnancy is achieved in about 50% of women undergoing three IVF procedures, but the success rate does not improve much even after additional attempts. Many clinicians recommend that couples agree on a time limit for attempting IVF in order to be realistic about their chances for parenthood.

The risks involved in IVF include MISCARRIAGE, ECTOPIC PREG-NANCY, and a high rate of MULTIPLE PREGNANCY, which carries far greater potential for complications than single pregnancy. One out of three IVF pregnancies results in twins, one out of ten results in triplets. Some hormones cause both short-term and long-term side effects, including increased risk for breast and ovarian cancer.

involution, uterine   Shrinking of the UTERUS to its pre-pregnant size following DELIVERY. Involution begins as soon as the baby emerges, even before the PLACENTA is expelled, largely the result of uterine CONTRACTIONS which continue for 48 hours after birth. BREASTFEEDING accelerates the process since it triggers additional contractions as the baby nurses. Within 10 days after birth, the uterus has normally de-scended within the PELVIS so that it cannot be felt by palpating the abdomen. At the end of six weeks, it will have returned to its original pear-like shape, weighing about two ounces.

ischial spines
    See PELVIMETRY.

itching   Also *pruritus*. Irritation of the skin, sometimes relieved by scratching. Itching can have many causes for both men and women, including allergies, DIABETES, exposure to poison ivy or poison oak. Two types of itching disorders only affect women. The first type, called *cholestasis of pregnancy*, occurs during the third TRIMESTER and involves intense itching, sometimes accompanied by JAUNDICE. Trig-gered by hormonal effects on liver function, the condition disappears spontaneously after DELIVERY. It is likely to recur in subsequent preg-nancies or if an ORAL CONTRACEPTIVE containing high levels of ESTRO-GEN is used. The second type of itching disorder affects the VULVA and VAGINA, referred to as VULVITIS and VAGINITIS, respectively. This type of itching may be caused by inflammation and/or infection (such as a YEAST INFECTION), or by dry skin and MUCOUS MEMBRANES. When the infection is appropriately treated, the itching usually stops. If it per-sists, however, cortisone ointment may prove helpful.

J

jaundice
>See NEONATAL JAUNDICE.

jelly, contraceptive
>See under SPERMICIDE; also LUBRICANT.

K

karyotyping   A genetic diagnostic test to determine the cause of BIRTH DEFECTS, STILLBIRTH, or HABITUAL MISCARRIAGE. The test involves photographing CHROMOSOMES from a woman's blood or body tissue, or from fetal or placental tissue, then enlarging the photographs so that chromosomes can be cut out and arranged in pairs according to size and structure on a chart called a karyotype. This process enables the geneticist to detect missing, broken, or otherwise abnormal chromosomes that are responsible for such genetic disorders as DOWN SYNDROME.

See also CHROMOSOME.

Kegel exercises   Exercises that strengthen the pubococcygeus muscle, the major pelvic floor muscle that supports all the pelvic organs. Good tone in this muscle increases its elasticity and helps prevent urinary incontinence, the involuntary release of urine (see STRESS INCONTINENCE). Named for Arnold Kegel, the physician who developed the exercises, they involve contracting and relaxing the pubococcygeous muscle. This muscle can be identified easily by stopping and starting the flow of urine. Kegel exercises should not be done during urination, however, since this practice has been associated with urinary tract infection. These exercises are important throughout PREGNANCY as well as in the POSTPARTUM period.

kernicterus   Severe NEONATAL JAUNDICE caused by high levels of bilirubin that lodge in the brain, leading to severe neurologic damage or death. This condition can usually be prevented by early administration of PHOTOTHERAPY and, in cases of Rh incompatibility, exchange blood transfusions.

Kerr incision
   See under CESAREAN DELIVERY.

Klinefelter's syndrome   A chromosomal disorder causing ambiguous genitalia in males (imperfectly formed GENITALS having both male and female characteristics), occurring in 1 out of 1,000 live male births. It can be detected by AMNIOCENTESIS and has been associated with advanced maternal age (35 or older). Instead of having two CHROMOSOMES, one X and one Y, males with Klinefelter's syndrome have three chromosomes, X, X, and Y. These males generally have a small PENIS and TESTES, poorly developed SECONDARY SEX CHARACTERISTICS (beard, pubic hair, chest hair, deep voice), and in many cases are mentally retarded. In some cases, female-like BREAST development occurs at PUBERTY; men with this disorder also face a high risk of BREAST CANCER, 66 times greater than men without the disorder. Surgery to remove breast tissue helps reduce this risk. Klinefelter's syndrome does not respond to hormonal therapy.

Kronig-Selheim incision
   See under CESAREAN DELIVERY.

K-Y jelly
   See under LUBRICANT.

L

labia   Two sets of tissue flaps that surround the vaginal opening, from the Latin word meaning "lips." The outer set is called the *labia majora;* the inner set is called the *labia minora.* Both sets have sebaceous (oil) glands, and are very sensitive.

The *labia majora* consist primarily of fatty tissue and correspond to the male SCROTUM. They extend back from the MONS PUBIS to the PERINEUM (the area between the inner lips and the anus [opening to the rectum]). In girls and women who have not borne children, they are usually close together, concealing the underlying structures. In women who have had children, the labia majora often are spread apart.

The *labia minora* (inner lips) are flat, reddish flaps of tissue that extend down from the CLITORIS, resembling MUCOUS MEMBRANE. At the upper end of these labia, each divides into separate flaps, forming the PREPUCE (foreskin) surrounding the clitoris. They vary greatly in size and shape, depending on whether the woman has borne children. Prior to childbirth, the labia minora are generally concealed by the outer lips; afterward, they may extend beyond the outer lips.

labor   Also *childbirth, confinement, parturition.* The process by which the baby leaves the UTERUS and emerges into the world. The actual birth is called DELIVERY. What causes labor to begin is not known. See INDUCTION OF LABOR.

Labor is well named; it is strenuous physical work. It is influenced by four critical factors: *the passage* (the bony and soft tissues of the mother's PELVIS), *the powers* (the CONTRACTIONS or forces of the uterine muscles), *the passenger* (the baby), and the *psyche.* Problems with one or more of these factors can cause complications in the process and the outcome of labor.

The passage, the bony pelvis and the soft tissues of the BIRTH CANAL, must be carefully assessed by the clinician prior to the onset of labor. This assessment includes PELVIMETRY and vaginal examination, and comparison of the measurements with estimated measurements of the fetal head. In cases where the fetal head appears just small enough to pass through the pelvic inlet, the clinician may order a trial of labor; if labor does not progress well, CESAREAN DELIVERY may be performed.

The powers are the contractions of the uterine muscles, which increase in frequency, duration, and intensity as labor progresses.

The passenger is the baby, whose malleable head must pass through the pelvic inlet for delivery to be accomplished. If the head is too large to pass safely through the mother's pelvis, cesarean delivery is the only option.

The psyche of the mother and her labor partner or coach can have a major impact on the course of labor. Studies have shown that anxiety and fear can trigger a cycle of pain and dysfunctional labor, eventually complicating the process to such an extent that cesarean delivery is required. Prenatal classes help the pregnant couple know what to expect, thus alleviating fear and building confidence in their ability to give birth without extensive medical and technological intervention. Research continues to validate that psychosocial support during labor helps reduce the need for FORCEPS or cesarean delivery.

Depending on the choice of a BIRTH ATTENDANT, labor may be viewed either as a continuous process, the length and rhythm of which is unique to each individual, or as a three-stage process with standard parameters for each stage, determined by the clinician and the institution in which he or she practices. MIDWIVES tend to approach labor as a continuous process, while physicians divide it into three stages. The first stage is the time it takes for the CERVIX to become dilated to 10 centimeters; the second is the delivery of the baby; and the third stage is the delivery of the PLACENTA. Since the majority of births are attended by physicians in hospitals or BIRTH CENTERS, this discussion takes the three-stage approach (Table L-1).

The *first stage* begins with the first uterine contraction and ends when the cervix has dilated to 10 centimeters (4 inches) in diameter. *True labor* can be distinguished from *false labor* by the strength and duration of the contractions (Table L-2). In true labor, contractions are regular, becoming stronger, longer, and more frequent as time passes, and are accompanied by DILATATION and EFFACEMENT of the cervix. In false labor, contractions are brief, irregular, and inconsistent in length, duration, and strength, and cause no change in the cervix.

Table L-1   Summary of Stages of Labor

True labor	False labor
Contractions are at regular intervals	Contractions are irregular
Intervals between contractions gradually shorten	Usually no change
Contractions increase in duration and intensity	Usually no change
Discomfort begins in back and radiates around to abdomen	Discomfort is usually in abdomen
Intensity usually increases with walking	Walking has no effect or lessens contractions
Cervical dilatation and effacement are progressive	No change

Source: From *Maternal Newborn Nursing,* Fourth Edition, by S. Olds, M. London, and P. Ladewig. © 1992 by Addison-Wesley Nursing. Reprinted by permission.

The average length of time for the first stage of labor is 8 to 12 hours for women having their first baby, and 6 to 8 hours for second and subsequent babies. Women who are encouraged to stand, walk, or sit upright, changing positions frequently, have stronger, more effective contractions, less discomfort, and overall, a shorter course of labor with reduced need for EPISIOTOMY and forceps or cesarean delivery. Unfortunately, some hospitals and clinicians do not encourage activity during the first stage, but instead, confine the laboring woman to bed in a supine (on her back) position. Such positioning works against the forces of gravity and compresses major blood vessels, thereby compromising the flow of oxygen to the FETUS. See BIRTHING BED; BIRTHING CHAIR.

The amniotic membranes generally rupture during the first stage of labor, although about 10% of women experience early RUPTURE OF MEMBRANES before labor begins. Once the membranes rupture, 9 out of 10 women begin labor within 24 hours. Since the membranes are the principal protection against infection, many clinicians will hospitalize women once the membranes rupture. It is important for women whose membranes have ruptured to avoid putting anything into the VAGINA:

Table L-2   True vs. False Labor

Stage/phase of labor	Cervical changes	Length of contractions	Interval between contractions	Duration of stage/phase
First stage				2 to 36 hours
Early labor latent phase	Cervix effaces and dilates to 3 to 5 cm	Increasing: 30 to 45 seconds	Decreasing: 20 to 5 minutes	6 to 8 hours
Active phase	Cervix dilates from 3 to 5 to 7 to 8 cm	Increasing: 45 to 75 seconds	Decreasing: 7 to 2 minutes (average 5 to 3 minutes)	2 to 3 hours
Transition phase	Cervix dilates from 7 to 8 to 10 cm	Increasing: 60 to 120 seconds	Variable: 3 to 2 minutes	½ hour to 2 hours
Second stage	Birth of baby	60 seconds	Variable: 5 to 2 minutes	A few minutes to 2 or more hours
Third stage	Delivery of placenta	Variable	Variable	10 to 20 minutes

Source: Alternative Birth: The Complete Guide by Carl Jones. Tarcher, 1991; adapted from *The Birth Partner's Handbook* by Carl Jones, Meadowbrook, 1989, page 21.

no sexual intercourse, baths, or pelvic exams. They should also drink plenty of fluid and take their temperature regularly.

The end of the first stage of labor is sometimes called *transition*. Some women experience slowed contractions at this point, giving their bodies time to rest. Others have such frequent contractions that they seem to run together. During this period, women may experience NAUSEA, vomiting, irritability, and tremors, symptoms usually lasting no more than 30 minutes.

The *second stage* of labor, delivery, can last from a few minutes up to one or two hours. Recent studies indicate that this time limit is artificial and that deliveries taking longer than two hours may not indicate complications. As long as there is no evidence of FETAL DISTRESS, the second stage may take as long as five hours.

The second stage begins when the cervix is fully dilated, and ends when the baby emerges (delivery). During this stage, the baby gradually moves down through the vagina, normally head first (VERTEX presentation). Women may feel the urge to push or bear down, as taught in some childbirth preparation classes. Recent research has shown that overly strenuous pushing does not shorten the second stage and in fact may be harmful to both the baby and the mother. Short pushing efforts interspersed with periods of panting may prove more effective. The more gradual the baby's descent, the more the perineal tissues relax. This allows them to stretch more easily without tearing and without the need for an episiotomy, reducing the pressure on the baby's head. Episiotomy is unnecessary except in cases of fetal or maternal distress, or when the PERINEUM fails to permit adequate progress in labor.

Women who are able to choose an upright position for delivery (sitting, squatting, or kneeling) are more likely to have a spontaneous birth and less likely to need episiotomy, forceps, or other obstetric intervention. Spontaneous delivery also reduces the incidence of shoulder dystocia (difficulty with delivery of the shoulders).

When the PRESENTING PART (the head) appears at the opening of the vagina (CROWNING), delivery is imminent. After the head emerges, the shoulders are delivered, followed by the rest of the body. If the baby is a BREECH, either the feet or buttocks present first, followed by the trunk, shoulders, and head, the largest part of the body. Breech babies are at much higher risk, and thus are often delivered by cesarean section, unless the clinician is able to rotate the baby by external means. See BREECH PRESENTATION, PROLAPSED CORD.

The *third stage* of labor consists of the expulsion of the placenta after it separates from the wall of the UTERUS. After the baby emerges, the uterus continues to contract, forcing the placenta down and out. As it descends, the placenta strips the remaining amniotic membranes from the uterine wall. While the third stage is something of an anticlimax, especially for the mother who is now preoccupied with her newborn infant, it holds high risk for POSTPARTAL HEMORRHAGE, still an important cause of maternal mortality. Thus many clinicians practice active management of this stage by early clamping of the UMBILICAL CORD and use of oxytocic drugs to strengthen contractions and reduce the risk of hemorrhage.

lactation   Production of milk by the BREASTS. Lactation is regulated by the HORMONES, PROLACTIN and OXYTOCIN, produced by the anterior and posterior PITUITARY respectively, but also depends on the POSTPARTUM drop in ESTROGEN and PROGESTERONE levels. As the baby nurses, additional prolactin is released, producing more milk; at the same time, oxytocin is released, causing the LETDOWN REFLEX or release of milk from the NIPPLE, plus uterine CONTRACTIONS that help return the uterus to its pre-pregnant size. Generally, the more the baby suckles, the more the milk supply increases. Thus it is important to empty both breasts at each feeding so the milk supply will continue. If the baby is not hungry enough to use all this milk, a breast pump may be used. If a woman chooses not to BREASTFEED, however, the milk supply will dry up within a few days after birth as long as the breasts are not stimulated by suckling.

The breasts are prepared for lactation during PREGNANCY when high levels of estrogen and progesterone promote the development of breast ducts, lobules, and alveoli. This development enlarges the breasts from 200 to 400 grams (7 to 14 ounces) during pregnancy. During the second TRIMESTER, the breasts start to secrete *colostrum*, a yellowish fluid that is rich in proteins, minerals, vitamin A, and natural ANTIBODIES to protect the infant from disease. After birth, this secretion continues for two to three days until lactation begins.

When milk replaces the colostrum, the breasts increase in size and become hard, a process called *engorgement*. The breasts may be tender and painful until breastfeeding begins. Ice packs or hot showers help relieve the discomfort of engorgement. A well-fitted nursing bra is essential to support enlarged breasts. Whenever possible, the flaps on the bra should be left open, exposing the nipples to the air in order to prevent irritation. If nipples do become sore or cracked, a small amount of vitamin E applied directly from a vitamin E capsule will promote healing. Nipples should be washed *only* with water, never with soap or other commercial product. Measures to relieve breastfeeding problems are listed in Table L-3.

Once lactation is established, prolactin secretion decreases and the milk supply is stimulated by oxytocin and suckling. Lactating
(text continued on page 176)

Table L-3   Measures to Prevent or Relieve Breastfeeding Problems

Abnormal nipples	Use Hoffman's exercises antepartally to increase protractility.
	Use special breast shields such as Woolrich or Eschmann.
	Use hand to shape nipple when beginning to nurse.
	Apply ice for a few minutes prior to feeding to improve nipple erection.
	Use electric or hand pump to cause nipple prominence and express a few drops of breast milk, then switch to regular nursing.
Inadequate letdown	Massage breasts prior to nursing.
	Feed in a quiet, private place, away from distraction.
	Take a warm shower before nursing to relax and stimulate letdown.
	Apply warm pack for 20 minutes before nursing.
	Use relaxation techniques and focus on letdown.
	Drink water, juice, or noncaffeinated beverages before and during feeding.
	Avoid overfatigue by resting when the baby sleeps, feeding while lying down, and having a quiet time alone.
	Develop a conditioned response by establishing a routine for starting feedings.
	Allow the baby sufficient time (at least 10 to 15 minutes per side) to trigger the letdown reflex.
	Use breast alternating method.
	If all else fails, obtain a prescription for oxytocin nasal spray from the health care provider.
Nipple soreness	Ensure that infant is correctly positioned at the breast, with ear, shoulder, and hip in straight alignment.
	Rotate breastfeeding positions.

Table L-3   Measures to Prevent or Relieve Breastfeeding Problems (continued)

Use finger to break suction before removing infant from the breast.

Hold baby close when feeding to avoid undue pulling on nipple.

Do not allow baby to sleep with nipple in mouth.

Nurse more frequently.

Begin nursing on less sore breast.

Apply ice to nipples and areola for a few minutes prior to feeding.

Protect nipples to prevent skin breakdown:
  — Clean nipples gently with warm water.
  — Allow nipples to air dry, or dry nipples with hair dryer set to low heat, or expose nipples to sunlight.

If clothing rubs nipples, use ventilated shields to keep clothing away from skin.

To promote healing, apply a small amount of breast milk to nipple and areola after nursing and allow to dry.

The routine application of ointment to nipple, areola, or breast (e.g., lanolin, Massé cream, or A & D ointment) should be discouraged.

Apply tea bags soaked in warm water.

Change breast pads frequently.

Nurse long enough to empty breasts completely.

Alternate breasts several times during feeding.

Cracked nipples   Use interventions discussed under sore nipples.

Inspect nipples carefully for cracks or fissures.

Temporarily stop nursing on the affected breast and hand express milk for a day or two until cracks heal.

Table L-3   Measures to Prevent or Relieve Breastfeeding Problems *(continued)*

	Maintain healthy diet.
	Use a mild analgesic such as acetaminophen for discomfort.
	Consult health care providers if signs of infection develop.
	A nipple shield should be tried before the nursing on a breast is stopped, but it should be used only as a last resort. A consultation with a lactation specialist prior to use is advised.
Breast engorgement	Nurse frequently (every 1½ to 3 hours) around the clock.
	Wear a well-fitting supportive bra at all times.
	Take a warm shower or apply warm compresses to trigger letdown.
	Massage breasts and then hand express some milk to soften the breast so the infant can "latch on."
	Breastfeed long enough to empty breast.
	Alternate starting breast.
	Take a mild analgesic 20 minutes before feeding if discomfort is pronounced.
Plugged ducts (caked breasts)	Nurse frequently and for long enough to empty the breasts completely.
	Rotate feeding position.
	Massage breasts prior to feeding, in a warm shower when possible.
	Maintain good nutrition and adequate fluid intake.

Source: From *Maternal Newborn Nursing,* Fourth Edition, by S. Olds, M. London, and P. Ladewig. © 1992 by Addison-Wesley Nursing. Reprinted by permission.

mothers should drink plenty of fluids and continue to eat a balanced DIET, increasing their daily caloric intake about 500 calories above their pre-pregnancy requirements.

lacto-ovovegetarians   Vegetarians whose DIETS include milk and other dairy products, eggs, and occasionally fish, poultry, and liver. Vegetarians tend to have lower incidence of HYPERTENSION (high blood pressure), coronary artery disease, osteoporosis, gallstones, kidney stones, and diverticulitis than nonvegetarians; their weight tends to be closer to recommended levels.

Pregnant women who are vegetarians need to eat a proper combination of foods to obtain adequate nutrition for themselves and their developing baby. Ample and complete proteins can be obtained from dairy products and eggs. If plants containing protein (beans and greens) are eaten with dairy products and eggs, they yield additional protein. A diet containing less than four servings of milk or milk products may require calcium supplements.

lactose intolerance   Difficulty in digesting milk and milk products.

lacto-vegetarians   Vegetarians whose DIETS include milk and other dairy products but no eggs, poultry, fish, or liver. This diet can provide adequate nutrients for the pregnant woman; however, it requires careful planning of combinations of foods.

See also LACTO-OVOVEGETARIANS.

La Leche League   International organization that provides information on and assistance with BREASTFEEDING. Local chapters can be found in most cities. For information, call or write La Leche League International, 9616 Minneapolis Avenue, Franklin Park IL 60131; 708-455-7730.

Lamaze method
See PSYCHOPROPHYLACTIC METHOD.

laminaria   A kind of seaweed that expands to three to five times its normal size when wet, which is often used for gradual, painless dilation of the CERVIX.

lanugo   Fine, downy hair that covers the body of the FETUS (except for the palms of the hands and soles of the feet) after 20 weeks' gestation. It begins to disappear at 36 weeks and is usually absent from full-term newborns.

laparoscopy Also *Band-Aid surgery, belly-button operation*. Insertion of a laparoscope, a long, slim optical instrument, through a small incision in the abdominal wall just below the navel, to examine the pelvic organs. This procedure is used to detect causes of PELVIC PAIN, such as ovarian CYSTS, obstructed FALLOPIAN TUBES, ECTOPIC PREGNANCY, and ENDOMETRIOSIS. It is also used for TUBAL LIGATION, a STERILIZATION procedure.

To improve visibility and access, carbon dioxide is injected into the ABDOMEN to lift the abdominal wall up and away from the underlying structures. Other surgical instruments can then be passed through the laparoscope to collect tissue samples for biopsy, remove POLYPS or tumors, retrieve an INTRAUTERINE DEVICE (IUD) that has migrated from the UTERUS, or perform a tubal ligation. Once the procedure is completed, the instruments and carbon dioxide are removed and the incision closed with a single SUTURE. The site is covered with a Band-Aid; thus the name, "Band-Aid Surgery."

Laparoscopy has great advantages over surgery through a large abdominal incision (see LAPAROTOMY). It can be performed under regional ANESTHESIA, shortening the recovery period for the patient to a matter of hours. It requires a skilled surgeon, experienced in the procedure, to reduce the risk of infection and possible perforation of the stomach or intestine. Some women experience heavy menstrual bleeding following laparoscopy, a few of whom require repeated DILATATION AND CURETTAGE (D & C) or even HYSTERECTOMY.

Laparoscopy is CONTRAINDICATED in women with intestinal obstruction, extensive abdominal cancer, or a serious heart disorder. Women near the age of MENOPAUSE are advised to choose safer contraceptive measures.

laparotomy Abdominal surgery performed to diagnose or treat certain disorders. It is major surgery involving general ANESTHESIA and a crescent-shaped incision in the lower ABDOMEN, just above the pubic hair. Laparotomy is performed when serious problems such as ECTOPIC PREGNANCY, ovarian or uterine cancer, or pelvic infection are suspected. It is also used for removal of FIBROID tumors, or for other procedures too extensive to be done through LAPAROSCOPY. Recovery from laparotomy generally requires several days in the hospital plus two or more weeks of rest at home.

See also TUBAL LIGATION.

large for gestational age (LGA)   Accelerated fetal growth, exceeding normal standards for the gestational time period; babies whose birth weight exceeds 4,000 grams (8 pounds 12 ounces). This condition is most commonly associated with maternal DIABETES mellitus; however, only a small percentage of LGA babies are in this category. Other causes include genetic influence (large parents have large babies), ERYTHROBLASTOSIS FETALIS, Beckwith-Wiedemann syndrome (genetic disorder associated with neonatal HYPOGLYCEMIA and hyperinsulinism), and transposition of the great vessels (a serious congenital heart disorder requiring surgical correction).

last menstrual period (LMP)   The final normal menstrual period prior to PREGNANCY. This date is sometimes used to calculate gestational age.

late decelerations
   See DECELERATION.

LDRP (labor, delivery, recovery, postpartum room)   A hospital room equipped and staffed to meet the needs of the laboring woman throughout the birth experience.
   See also BIRTHING ROOM.

Leboyer method   Also *birth without violence, gentle birth.* A method of childbirth pioneered during the 1970s by Frederick Leboyer, a French OBSTETRICIAN, designed to ease the newborn's transition from intrauterine to extrauterine life. This approach replaced the bright lights of the typical delivery room with subdued lighting; eliminated sudden, loud noises from the birth environment; and immersed the infant in a warm bath immediately after delivery. Some hospitals and BIRTHING CENTERS have adopted the general principles of this approach.

leiomyoma
   See FIBROID.

Leopold's maneuvers   A series of maneuvers to determine the position and presentation of the FETUS by carefully palpating the mother's ABDOMEN in four different areas, beginning with the upper area.

lesbian   A female HOMOSEXUAL, that is, a woman who prefers a woman as a sexual partner. The name comes from Lesbos, a Greek island where the poet Sappho lived and wrote of her love for women. For many years lesbians were thought to be mentally ill, as were male homosexuals; in 1974, however, the American Psychiatric Association reclassified homosexuality as a type of sexual behavior rather than a mental illness. Nevertheless, considerable prejudice toward all homosexuals still exists within the HETEROSEXUAL ("straight") population.

No significant physical differences have been found between lesbians and heterosexual women. Both experience the same developmental cycle of PUBERTY, menstruation, and MENOPAUSE. The only difference is in their sexual preference, a preference sometimes discovered at varying times in life. Some lesbians recognize and acknowledge their preference for other women as adolescents. Others make this discovery much later, sometimes after years of heterosexual marriage and childbearing.

Today, increasing numbers of lesbians are choosing to establish a family unit by having babies together, either through ARTIFICIAL INSEMINATION or heterosexual intercourse. Depending on the community in which they live, lesbians who want to become pregnant may encounter either prejudice and resistance or nonjudgmental understanding and support. Thus, a lesbian couple may need to change clinicians in order to find acceptance and supportive care.

Lesbian couples need to understand the medical, legal, and psychological implications of artificial insemination. The health of the donor, custody and visitation rights, and financial responsibility are critical issues to be discussed ahead of time.

See also ARTIFICIAL INSEMINATION.

lesion   Body tissue that is changed from its normal state and from that of the surrounding area by disease or injury. Examples include a cut, burn, bruise, pimple, wart, or ABSCESS.

letdown reflex   Also *milk ejection reflex*. A process of stimulation, HORMONE release, and muscle contraction that forces milk through the ducts of the BREAST and into the NIPPLES. A woman who is lactating may experience a momentary feeling of tingling or tightening when the letdown reflex occurs. It is triggered by release of the hormone OXYTOCIN, which can result from suckling or the thought of suckling, or the baby's cry. This reflex is most noticeable during the first weeks of BREASTFEEDING, and generally simultaneous in both breasts. If a mother is not near her infant when letdown occurs, pressing lightly with the palm of her hand on the nipple area may prevent leaking; however, absorbent breast pads offer extra protection against leaking.

See also BREASTFEEDING; LACTATION.

leukorrhea
See VAGINAL DISCHARGE.

libido   Also *sex drive*. The desire for sexual intercourse or other sexual activity. It is highly individual from person to person and within the same individual from time to time, depending on circumstances. Defining what level of desire constitutes "normal" libido is impossible. Hormonal changes can dramatically affect libido. Adolescence is one example; PREGNANCY is another. Some pregnant women become much more interested in sexual activity; others tend to withdraw from it, perhaps fearing injury to the baby or sometimes being preoccupied with the pregnancy to the exclusion of the partner. Unless the clinician advises otherwise, however, pregnancy need not interfere with sexual activity.

Loss of libido can be triggered by psychological factors such as work-related stress, marital conflict, or GRIEF, as can such physical problems as fatigue, illness, or medications, particularly tranquilizers or antihypertensive drugs. ORAL CONTRACEPTIVES may either increase or decrease desire, depending on the individual.

lie, fetal   The relationship of the baby's head-to-toe dimension or axis to the mother's head-to-toe dimension. The lie may be *longitudinal* (the normal lie, in which the baby's spine is parallel to the mother's spine), *transverse* (the baby's spine is at right angles to the mother's spine), or *oblique* (the baby's spine is at less than a 45-degree angle to the mother's spine).

lightening   Also *dropping, engagement*. Downward movement of the FETUS and UTERUS into the pelvic cavity a few weeks before LABOR begins. When lightening occurs, the abdomen appears less protuberant and the lower portion more droopy. The baby's head becomes fixed (engaged) in the pelvic inlet in preparation for birth. Lightening often relieves difficult breathing caused by pressure of the uterus on the rib

cage; however, the pressure on lower organs increases, causing URI-
NARY FREQUENCY and, in many women, leg cramps.

linea nigra   A line of darker pigmentation extending from the navel
to the pubic hair during the later months of PREGNANCY.

lithotomy
> See DORSAL LITHOTOMY.

LMP
> See LAST MENSTRUAL PERIOD.

local anesthesia
> See under ANESTHESIA.

local infiltration   Injection of a local (regional) anesthetic into the
subcutaneous tissue in a fanlike pattern.

lochia   Vaginal discharge during the POSTPARTUM period. For three or
four days after DELIVERY, lochia is bloodstained, resembling menstrual
flow and is termed *lochia rubra*. It then becomes pinkish *(lochia
serosa)* and, from the 10th to about the 21st day, white or yellowish
white *(lochia alba)*. Normal lochia smells much like menstrual flow
(musty, stale, but not offensive), and does not contain large clots. Any
foul smell or the presence of clots larger than a nickel should be
reported to the clinician immediately so the cause can be determined.

loss
> See GRIEF.

L/S ratio   The ratio of two phospholipids, lecithin and sphin-
gomyelin, produced by the fetal lungs, used to assess the maturity of
fetal lungs and the baby's ability to survive outside the UTERUS.

lubricant   Any substance that reduces friction. Sexual arousal
causes the lining of the VAGINA to secrete mucus, a lubricant that aids
sexual intercourse. Unless the vagina is well-lubricated, intercourse
can be painful. This is a constant problem for some women, particularly during LACTATION or after MENOPAUSE. Sometimes the problem
can be eliminated by a longer period of foreplay or by use of saliva. If

neither is effective, water-soluble products such as K-Y jelly, Lubri-fax, Replens, or Astroglide will generally solve the problem. HORMONE creams or pills also may be effective, but the risks may outweigh the benefits. Vaseline (petroleum jelly) should not be used since it is not water-soluble.

luteinized unruptured follicle   Also *trapped egg syndrome*. A disruption in the ovulatory process caused when the surface of an ovarian FOLLICLE does not rupture and release the egg. This is associated with taking FERTILITY drugs and also with PELVIC INFLAMMATORY DISEASE.

luteinizing hormone (LH)   A pituitary HORMONE that stimulates ovulation and development of the corpus luteum.
     See also OVULATION.

lymphogranuloma venereum
     See GRANULOMA INGUINALE.

macrosomia Neonatal condition involving large body size and large birth weight, such as found in INFANTS born to mothers with DIABETES.

magnetic resonance imaging (MRI) A noninvasive diagnostic test that produces cross-sectional images of interior body structures, using a combination of radio waves and magnetic fields. Because it does not involve ionizing radiation, MRI can be used during PREGNANCY for PELVIMETRY, for determining the location of the PLACENTA, and for confirming fetal abnormalities suggested by ULTRASOUND examination. The disadvantages of MRI include its expense (each machine costs more than $1 million and each scan costs more than $1,000), performance time (45 to 60 minutes for scanning), and occasional claustrophobia on the part of the patient being scanned. If the FETUS is very active, MRI is largely ineffective since it only produces static (still) images.

An MRI scan requires that the woman lie on her back on a sliding table which then moves into a large cylindrical unit. The outer layers of the unit contain coils of wire which create a magnetic field when electricity is passed through them. The inner layers also contain coils of wire that act as radio antennae, transmitting and receiving radio waves to and from the woman by creating a magnetic field and thereby producing images of the area of the body being scanned.

No harmful effects of MRI have been reported in the medical literature; however, the patient must sign an informed consent form before the procedure is performed.

male contraceptive Any drug or device used by the male to prevent CONCEPTION. These drugs and devices work by impairing the normal production, storage, chemical makeup, or transport of SPERM. The primary device is the CONDOM, a rubber sheath that collects the ejaculated

SEMEN containing the sperm. The only other method available in the United States is VASECTOMY, surgical STERILIZATION that is usually not reversible. One recent controversial study indicates an association between vasectomy and prostate cancer; additional studies are underway, however, as are studies of HORMONE compounds for contraception.

malposition   An abnormal position of the FETUS in the BIRTH CANAL. If the clinician is unable to rotate the fetus to a normal position, CESAREAN DELIVERY is usually performed to minimize risk to mother and baby.

malpresentation   An ABNORMAL PRESENTATION of the FETUS in the BIRTH CANAL in relation to the mother's PERINEUM. Normally, the top or crown of the baby's head presents first (VERTEX presentation), followed by the shoulders and the remainder of the body. In malpresentation, the baby's brow, face, shoulder, or rump (BREECH) present first, making DELIVERY difficult. CESAREAN DELIVERY is commonly performed for most malpresentations.

mammogram   An X-RAY of the BREAST to detect tumors before they can be felt. Currently, mammography is the only available technology for screening women for BREAST CANCER, although researchers are seeking a BLOOD TEST that will detect cancer cells before they form a lump. BREAST SELF-EXAMINATION and annual clinical examination by a physician or nurse practitioner are recommended for all women over the age of 16. In premenopausal women, mammography has limited effectiveness because of the density of breast tissue. Both breast tissue and tumors appear white on a mammogram; thus, they can be difficult or impossible to find in younger women with dense breast tissue. Mammograms should not be performed during PREGNANCY because of the potential for radiation damage to the FETUS. If a breast lump appears during pregnancy (a rare occurrence), the woman should consult a breast health specialist as well as her OBSTETRICIAN to determine how best to manage the situation.

To obtain a mammogram, the woman's breast is placed on a metal plate and another plate is pressed down on the breast, holding it firmly so that the mammogram will be clear. Then the technician takes two pictures of the breast, one from the top and the other from the side. The procedure is then repeated on the other breast. Most women find having a mammogram only slightly uncomfortable; a few find it pain-

Table M-1   American Cancer Society Guidelines for Screening Mammography *

Age 40	Baseline mammogram
Age 40–50	Mammogram every 1 or 2 years
Age 51 and up	Mammogram annually

*The American College of Surgeons has declined to endorse these guidelines; The American College of Physicians and the U.S. Preventive Services Task Force, an advisory panel to the Department of Health & Human Services, openly oppose these guidelines, and recommend that mammograms begin at age 50. Women who are at higher risk for breast cancer should consult a breast health specialist.

ful. It takes only a few minutes, however, and it can be a lifesaving procedure, since early detection of breast cancer is the most important factor in successful treatment.

The age at which women should begin having mammograms remains controversial. Studies in Canada and Europe have shown that screening mammograms do not alter survival rates in women under age 50; however, if every woman over age 50 had an annual mammogram, the death rate from breast cancer could be reduced by one-third. The American Cancer Society's guidelines for screening mammograms are shown in Table M-1.

Not all mammography facilities are alike; some use obsolete equipment and employ technicians and radiologists without adequate training. Women seeking a mammogram should be sure that the facility is accredited by the American College of Radiology; this will help ensure that the mammogram will be properly performed and interpreted, with minimal radiation exposure. To find out if a facility is accredited, call 1-800-4-CANCER. If possible, all women at high risk for breast cancer should seek care at a special breast health center, available in most major cities.

mask of pregnancy
See CHLOASMA.

mastalgia   Also *mastodynia, mammalgia.* BREAST pain. Mastalgia can have several causes including premenstrual EDEMA (fluid retention), injury, infection, engorgement (see LACTATION), CYSTS, or BREAST CANCER. Brassieres that are not well-fitted can also cause breast pain. While women with small breasts may be more comfortable without a bra, women with heavy breasts may find lack of proper support uncomfortable. Cysts in the breasts can be painful, but usually do not indicate breast cancer (see BREAST). However, some breast cancers do cause pain; therefore, any persistent breast pain or lump should be thoroughly investigated. Following MASTECTOMY, women generally experience considerable postoperative pain.

mastectomy   Surgical removal of the BREAST.
     See also BREAST CANCER.

mastitis   Inflammation of the BREAST due to infection, usually occurring during BREASTFEEDING. The infectious organism is most frequently *Staphylococcus aureus*. Symptoms include pain, tenderness, and swelling, usually accompanied by fever and sometimes chills. Oral antibiotics are prescribed to eliminate the infection, and warm compresses are recommended to relieve the pain and swelling, usually within 48 hours. If these measures are not effective, the infection becomes localized and can develop into an ABSCESS that requires surgical drainage. Clinicians no longer recommend that women who develop mastitis during breastfeeding stop nursing, since the bacteria probably came from the baby's mouth. Nursing also relieves some of the pain by emptying the breast.

masturbation   Sexual stimulation of one's own GENITALS or those of another by manual means. Once considered perverted and unhealthy, especially for women, masturbation is now considered by most authorities a normal outlet for sexual desires. Research indicates that women who masturbate to ORGASM often experience more intense contractions than during intercourse with a partner. Some couples find mutual masturbation a satisfying sexual practice as well as an alternative to vaginal intercourse during illness or a fertile period.

maternal mortality   Number of maternal deaths (at any time during PREGNANCY, DELIVERY, or POSTPARTUM) per 100,000 live births.

maternity center
     See BIRTH CENTER, BIRTHING ROOM.

McDonald's sign   One of the PROBABLE SIGNS OF PREGNANCY, characterized by an ease in flexing the body of the UTERUS against the CERVIX.

measles   Also *rubeola*. A highly contagious viral infection primarily affecting children. Symptoms include fever, cough, eye inflammation (conjunctivitis), and a rash that spreads over the entire body. Not a serious disease in itself, measles can result in such life-threatening complications as pneumonia and encephalitis. It can be prevented by vaccination. Measles is rare in adults; however, it is critical to differentiate measles from German measles or RUBELLA, a related disease that can cause severe BIRTH DEFECTS in a baby whose mother is infected during PREGNANCY.

meconium   Dark green or black fecal material in the large intestine of the FETUS; the first stools passed by a newborn infant. Meconium consists of undigested material from the amniotic fluid swallowed by the fetus and other substances shed by the developing baby's gastrointestinal tract. If the baby's oxygen supply is seriously impaired, the baby will release meconium into the amniotic fluid. Thus any sign of meconium in the amniotic fluid signals a problem, and the FETAL HEART RATE should be carefully monitored. In addition, meconium in the amniotic fluid may be aspirated into the baby's lungs, causing a severe irritation, meconium aspiration pneumonitis. This condition is the second leading cause of newborn respiratory distress. (HYALINE MEMBRANE DISEASE is the leading cause.)

  After delivery, the baby's first few bowel movements consist of meconium. It is soft, dark greenish, and usually odorless. Once formula or BREASTFEEDING has begun, the feces change to a light yellow color.

membrane rupture
  See AMNIOTOMY; RUPTURE OF MEMBRANES.

menarche   The beginning of menstruation and female reproductive function, usually occurring between ages 9 and 16. Menstruation beginning prior to age 9 may be either *precocious puberty* (abnormally early development of secondary sex characteristics) or a sign of endocrine dysfunction. The average age for menarche in the United States is 12.6 years.

  Menarche generally follows the onset of PUBERTY by three to four years; thus most girls have attained 90% of their adult height and weight by the time menstruation begins. The first few years of menstruation are often characterized by irregular periods with varying amounts of menstrual flow.

See also AMENORRHEA.

menopause   Also *change of life, climacteric, the change.* The end of menstruation, usually sometime between age 40 and 55. In the United States, the average age ranges between 45 and 53 years. Natural menopause generally occurs over a period of several years. Symptoms include changes in the MENSTRUAL CYCLE: periods may become irregular and/or with much lighter or heavier menstrual flow. Hot flashes are also a common symptom, thought to be caused by decreased ESTROGEN levels. Other symptoms vary widely among individual women but include vaginal dryness, insomnia, osteoporosis (decreased bone density), EDEMA, HEADACHES, and MOOD SWINGS. Estrogen replacement therapy (ERT) can relieve menopausal symptoms, but remains controversial since some studies show it increases the risk of BREAST CANCER.

menorraghia   Excessive menstrual flow. It can result from several causes, including ECTOPIC PREGNANCY, cervical or endometrial POLYPS, PELVIC INFLAMMATORY DISEASE, an ovarian CYST or other tumor, a uterine FIBROID, or an INTRAUTERINE DEVICE (IUD). Since persistent heavy bleeding can be potentially dangerous, it should be investigated and treated. Treatment may be either medical (administration of PROGESTERONE alone, or a combination of progesterone and ESTROGEN) or surgical DILATATION AND CURETTAGE (D&C).

menstrual cycle   The regular, periodic buildup of the uterine lining, followed by OVULATION and shedding of the lining every 29 days in females who are not pregnant. The length of the cycle and amount of the menstrual flow is different for each woman each month. Some women's periods are as regular as clockwork; others' are highly irregular and erratic.

See also AMENORRHEA; FOLLICLE; GRAAFIAN FOLLICLE; OVULATION.

mentum   The fetal chin.

mesoderm   The middle section of the primary germ cell layers, which eventually develops into the skin, bone, cartilage, muscles, cardiovascular system, lungs, kidneys, and GENITALS of the FETUS.

metabolic toxemia of pregnancy
    See ECLAMPSIA.

metabolism   The body's physical and chemical processes for converting food into living tissue and energy. It includes the chemical processes that transform complex substances into simpler ones that can be used by the body. *Basal metabolism* is the minimum energy required to maintain breathing, circulation of blood, muscle tone, body temperature, endocrine function, and other basic functions that continue even when the body is at rest. The *basal metabolic rate (BMR)* is measured by a calorimeter and is expressed in calories per hour per square meter of body surface. Metabolic disorders—the inability to metabolize (use) certain nutrients and energy—can be either genetic, CONGENITAL, or acquired. One such disorder is DIABETES, although the means of inheritance is not clearly understood.

midwife   A person other than a physician who is trained to assist women in childbirth. The training may be either formal or informal. Two kinds of midwives practice in the United States, *certified nurse-midwives* and *lay midwives* (also called *independent midwives)*. Laws regulating their practice differ from state to state. In some states, it is illegal for lay midwives to practice; in others, they must be licensed and must pass an examination to qualify for a license. Certified Nurse-Midwives (CNMs) are gaining recognition and acceptance among consumers and professionals alike. CNMs have prescription-writing privileges in about one-half of the states in the United States and, in many areas, have been granted hospital privileges. The education and training of lay midwives and of CNMs is different; however, both groups share a similar philosophy of PREGNANCY and birth as normal, healthy life processes rather than illnesses requiring high-tech medical interventions.
    Throughout history, midwives have assisted women in childbirth; in many countries, midwives continue to deliver the majority of babies. In the United States and England, however, when men began to enter obstetrics as physicians, the practice of midwifery was discouraged, probably because of the competition for patients. As childbirth moved out of the home and into the hospital, midwifery disappeared except for in rural areas where doctors were scarce. The *granny midwife* was a familiar figure in the southern United States; up until the 1950s, most Black babies in the South were delivered

by granny midwives. Today midwives care for less than 1% of child-bearing women, having been legally eradicated or forced under-ground. The white granny midwives of Appalachia and the Hispanic grannies of the southeastern United States have met with a similar fate.

lay midwife   Also *independent midwife, direct-entry midwife.* A mid-wife who chooses this occupation because she wants to help families participate in HOME BIRTHS. Most lay midwives learn by assisting phy-sicians or experienced midwives until they feel confident enough to work alone. During the 1970s, lay midwives became very popular in the western United States, especially California, among the newly formed communes and other counter-culture groups. Couples choos-ing home births often select a lay midwife as BIRTH ATTENDANT. Lay midwives can serve as birth partners or labor coaches during hospital births but only unofficially by private agreement with the expectant mother or parents. The lay midwife's approach is generally one of support rather than intervention; many of them describe their practice as "catching" a baby rather than "delivering" it. Their concern also extends beyond the pregnancy and birth to the total health of the woman and her family. Ordinarily, any suspected complication either in the pregnancy or the birth signals the need for the mother to seek the care of a physician.

The practice of lay midwives is unregulated in many states and their experience, training, and competence vary from person to per-son; thus it is difficult to know ahead of time whether a particular midwife is sufficiently capable and knowledgeable to provide a safe standard of care. The official network of lay midwives is Midwives Alliance of North America (MANA); their address is P.O. Box 1121, Bristol VA 24203; 615-764-5561.

Certified Nurse-Midwife (CNM)   A registered nurse with special postgraduate preparation in gynecology and obstetrics, qualified to manage independently the care of essentially normal women and new-borns, before, during, and after birth, and/or gynecologically. A CNM practices within the framework of a medically directed health service, in accordance with the *Standards for the Practice of Nurse-Midwifery* as defined by the American College of Nurse-Midwives in 1987. She may practice in a hospital or clinic that can provide medical consulta-tion, collaborative management, and referral, but may also attend home birth.

In 1988, the Institute of Medicine recommended that physicians and state legislatures encourage hospital privileges for nurse-midwives. That same year, the National Commission to Prevent Infant Mortality urged state universities to expand their nurse-midwifery programs. In 1991, there were about 4,200 CNMs practicing in the United States, with fewer than 200 new graduates entering the field each year.

In the state of Kentucky, nurse-midwives have been demonstrating the quality of their care to women, families, and communities since 1925 when the Frontier Nursing Service (FNS) was founded by Mary Breckinridge. Staffed entirely by nurse-midwives, the first ones having been trained in England, the Frontier Nursing Service has dramatically reduced maternal and infant mortality and morbidity while improving the overall health of the communities in rural Kentucky. In 1935, the FNS opened its own college of nurse-midwifery, admitting a class of 12 to 15 students annually. During the 1980s, as OBSTETRICIANS began to close their practices in fear of malpractice litigation, the demand for nurse-midwives far exceeded the supply. In response to this demand, in 1990 the FNS replaced its small residential program with a new nurse-midwifery education program, the Community-Based Nurse-Midwifery Education Program (C-NEP). Using advanced technology and regional faculty, this "school without walls" can now admit more than 90 students annually, thus boosting the still-limited national supply of CNMs.

Many women who can afford a choice of caregivers are choosing nurse-midwives for pregnancy and childbirth, not only for the quality of care provided, but for the recognition of birth as a normal, family-centered event. Depending on where the CNM practices, however, she may not be allowed to assist at a home birth, since she works under a doctor's supervision. Furthermore, some medical insurance plans do not reimburse deliveries by a nurse-midwife, even though her fee may be much lower than that of an obstetrician.

milia   Tiny, white bumps on the skin of a newborn, resulting from unopened sebaceous glands. They disappear without treatment during the first few weeks after birth.

milk leg
    See PHLEGMASIA.

miscarriage   Also *spontaneous abortion*. Loss of a pregnancy during the first 20 weeks' gestation.
> See also ABORTION; HABITUAL MISCARRIAGE.

mitleiden   Development of pregnancy-like symptoms on the part of the expectant father, including weight gain, NAUSEA, and miscellaneous aches and pains.

molding   Shaping of the fetal head by movement of the overlapping cranial bones, making possible its passage through the BIRTH CANAL during LABOR.

Mongolian spot   Dark birthmark on the lower back and buttocks of some infants. Generally, this disappears by age five or six years.

mongolism, mongoloid   Outdated terms relating to DOWN SYNDROME.

moniliasis
> See YEAST INFECTION.

mons pubis   Also *mons veneris, pubis, pubic mound*. A pad of subcutaneous fatty tissue that covers the symphysis pubis, or pubic bone. After puberty, it is covered with pubic hair.

mood swings   Dramatic shifts in mood from sadness to happiness and back again. Mood swings are a normal part of PREGNANCY, especially in the first TRIMESTER, in part because of the major hormonal shifts that take place during the course of pregnancy and birth. Women who experience PREMENSTRUAL SYNDROME (PMS) are more likely to have similar mood swings during pregnancy. Although mood swings cannot be eliminated, they can be helped by avoiding sugar, chocolate, and caffeine; eating a healthful DIET; getting plenty of rest and exercise; and receiving support from your partner and/or family.

A few women experience mild to moderate depression during pregnancy, particularly if they feel unsupported by their partner or have mixed feelings about being pregnant. Financial difficulties, physical complications, or anxiety about the baby's health can also contribute to feelings of depression. If depression persists, it helps to seek counseling. Antidepressant drugs may not be safe for the FETUS.

morning-after pill A pill given to prevent conception after unprotected intercourse. The most commonly prescribed morning-after pill is Ovral, a combination of high-dose estrogens and progesterone, which must be started within three days of unprotected intercourse. Clinicians generally recommend a dosage of 200 milligrams (100 milligrams within 72 hours of unprotected intercourse, and another 100 milligrams 12 hours after the first dose). Side effects include nausea, vomiting, headache, and breast tenderness.

Some doctors still prescribe DIETHYLSTILBESTROL (DES) as a morning-after pill, even though the long-term side effects of even a single dose have not been adequately studied. The Food and Drug Administration has never approved of the use of any oral contraceptive as a "morning-after" pill. Any woman who becomes pregnant after taking morning-after pills may want to consider terminating the pregnancy because of the high risk of serious damage to the fetus.

morning sickness The NAUSEA of early PREGNANCY, experienced by more than half of all pregnant women between the second and twelfth weeks of pregnancy. Officially called nausea gravidarum, this problem is thought to be caused by the rapid increase of HCG (HUMAN CHORIONIC GONADOTROPIN), and generally disappears after the first three-and-a-half months of pregnancy. A few women have problems with nausea throughout their pregnancy, either continuously or occasionally.

Although termed "morning sickness," nausea gravidarum can occur at any time of the day, and is sometimes accompanied by vomiting. The most effective remedies are light, dry foods (crackers or toast); small, frequent meals; plenty of fluids between meals; and avoidance of fatty foods. Some women have also experienced relief from nausea by wearing acupressure wrist bands. Several of the medications formerly prescribed for morning sickness have come under scrutiny as possible causes of BIRTH DEFECTS. Thus, unless the problem is severe enough to cause malnutrition, dehydration, or fluid-electrolyte imbalance, no medication of any kind should be used. Very severe nausea and vomiting is called *hyperemesis gravidarum* and may require hospitalization.

Moro reflex Also *startle reflex*. A reflex in the newborn, elicited by a sudden noise or movement, involving flexion of the knees and thighs, and accompanied by fingers that spread, then clench, as the arms are spread and then brought together as though hugging something.

motility, sperm   The ability of SPERM to move or swim, essential for CONCEPTION to occur, since sperm must journey from the VAGINA through the cervical canal to the UTERUS and FALLOPIAN TUBES to fertilize an OVUM. At least 60% of the sperm in a SEMEN sample must be moving four hours after EJACULATION for a man to be considered fertile. Motility can also be impaired by heat in the region of the TESTES (for example, hot tubs, saunas), by hormonal factors, infections, and prostate disorders.
        See also SPERM.

mottling   Irregular discoloration of the skin, as occurs with chilling, poor circulation, or hypoxia (oxygen deprivation).

mucous membrane   Also *mucosa.* Glandular tissues that secrete mucus, a thick, sticky lubricant. Mucous membranes line the mouth, nose, rectum, and VAGINA, as well as the surfaces of many internal organs.

mucus method
        See CERVICAL MUCUS METHOD.

mucus plug   Also *operculum.* A collection of thick mucus that blocks the opening of the CERVIX during PREGNANCY. Its passage through the VAGINA, usually with a small amount of blood, is called *bloody show* and frequently signals the onset of LABOR.

multigravida   A woman in her second or subsequent PREGNANCY.

multipara   A woman who has had more than one PREGNANCY producing a viable FETUS.

multiple pregnancy   A PREGNANCY involving more than one FETUS, that is, twins, triplets, quadruplets, and so on. There are two types of multiple pregnancy: *monozygotic,* or *identical,* in which a single fertilized egg divides into two or more individuals; and *dizygotic,* or *fraternal,* in which two or more eggs are fertilized during the same menstrual cycle. Monozygotic pregnancy involves one SPERM and one egg; dizygotic involves two or more eggs and sperm. In both situations, two or more babies can result. Triplets can develop from one, two, or three eggs; however, single-egg triplets are rare. Usually triplets develop from two eggs, one of which develops into a single fetus, the other into twins.

The most common multiple pregnancy is twins, about one-third of which are identical (monozygotic). The remaining two-thirds are fraternal, and may be no more like each other than other single children of the same parents. They may be of the same or opposite sexes, while identical twins are always the same sex. On rare occasions, the EMBRYO does not completely divide, resulting in twins that are born joined, sharing some of the same organs. This phenomenon is known as *Siamese twins,* occurring once in every 50,000 births and once in every 400 pairs of monozygotic twins. These twins can sometimes be successfully separated by surgery. Forty percent of Siamese twins are STILLBORN.

Identical twins occur once in every 200 pregnancies, and are thought to be a random event. Fraternal twins, however, are related to the secretion of FSH (FOLLICLE-STIMULATING HORMONE), and their incidence has risen significantly since various types of FERTILITY PILLS (a stimulant of FSH production) have been prescribed more frequently. These drugs can result in as many as nine fetuses. The same is true of IN VITRO FERTILIZATION, in which several EMBRYOS are transferred into a woman's UTERUS to increase the possibility that at least one will develop into a viable fetus. Fraternal twins occur more often in Blacks than in whites, and less often in Asians. A family history of fraternal twins increases the probability of more twins, perhaps because the trait of releasing more than one egg at OVULATION (polyovulation) is hereditary.

The likelihood of conceiving fraternal twins rises with the mother's age and the number of previous pregnancies. At age 20, the odds are 4 in 1,000; at age 40, they are 16 in 1,000, after which they drop markedly. The incidence of fraternal twins also rises with weight; fat women are more likely to have twins than are thin women, perhaps because of higher levels of ESTROGEN and other HORMONES.

Any multiple pregnancy is considered high risk for both mother and babies. The perinatal morbidity and mortality rates for twins are almost double those of singleton pregnancies, and the mortality rate for monozygotic twins is three times that of fraternal twins. Preterm birth is 12 times that of singleton births and only 5% of twins reach the full 40 weeks' GESTATION.

maternal risks Women with twin pregnancies have an 83% chance of prenatal complications as compared to an incidence of 32% in singleton pregnancies. These complications include: spontaneous ABORTION; maternal ANEMIA; pregnancy-induced HYPERTENSION (PIH); third-TRIMESTER bleeding from PLACENTA PREVIA and ABUPTIO PLACENTAE; and HYDRAMNIOS. The mother may also experience such physical discomforts as shortness of breath, feeling faint and "lightheaded," backaches, and swollen feet. Complications that can occur during LABOR include: PRETERM LABOR; uterine dysfunction due to an over-extended myometrium, and abnormal fetal presentations. If multiple pregnancies are not diagnosed until birth, the family may be physically, psychologically, and financially unprepared for two babies, particularly if they need intensive care.

fetal-neonatal risks Multiple pregnancy carries a high risk of CONGENITAL ABNORMALITIES, more than twice that of singleton pregnancy. More than 10 times as many twins are premature as compared with singletons, and half of all twins weigh less than 2,500 grams at birth.

Identical twins whose placentas developed from the same chorionic layer (monochorionic) are at high risk for transfusion syndrome in which one twin causes the other to bleed to death in utero. Those identical twins who share the same AMNIOTIC SAC are at increased risk of becoming entangled in each other's UMBILICAL CORDS, resulting in a stillborn rate of 50%. They are also at higher risk for physical and mental developmental problems after birth.

Multiple pregnancy demands comprehensive PRENATAL CARE to prevent or treat problems that threaten maternal or fetal well-being. Thus, it is important to detect the presence of twins or other multiple pregnancy very early; the first sign is a larger than normal uterus based on the LAST MENSTRUAL PERIOD. High levels of ALPHA-FETOPROTEIN can reveal twins at 16 weeks; ULTRASOUND can detect twins at 20 weeks. It may be difficult to detect two heartbeats as early because the fetuses are smaller than in a singleton pregnancy of the same GESTATION.

If infertility treatment results in a multiple pregnancy, the couple may choose to have the clinician perform an ethically controversial technique called *selective fetal reduction* or *selective reduction of pregnancy*. This procedure involves injecting a lethal substance into one or more of the fetuses in utero to give the remaining ones (usually twins) a better chance for survival. It must be performed before 12 weeks' gestation, and may cause MISCARRIAGE of all the fetuses.

Some clinicians recommend restricted activity for women pregnant with twins beginning at 20 weeks, and modified bed rest beginning at 24 weeks. During the last two months, women carrying twins must be monitored carefully for signs of preeclampsia and PRETERM LABOR. Extra rest, careful adherence to dietary restrictions, and more frequent physician visits are advisable.

Labor may progress very slowly or very quickly, and the decision about vaginal birth versus cesarean may not be made until LABOR occurs. Maternal complications such as placenta previa, abruptio placentae, or severe PIH usually require CESAREAN DELIVERY. Fetal problems such as severe INTRAUTERINE GROWTH RETARDATION, preterm birth, FETAL DISTRESS, congenital abnormalities, or unfavorable fetal position or presentation also mandate cesarean delivery.

The first baby may emerge in normal VERTEX presentation; the second, however, may be a BREECH or in a TRANSVERSE LIE, in which case the clinician will attempt external VERSION (turning the baby into vertex presentation). If successful, the second baby can be delivered vaginally; if not, a cesarean section may be necessary.

Sometimes the overstretched uterine muscle fibers stop contracting after the birth of the first baby, and clinicians disagree about how long to wait for delivery of the second baby. Most seem to believe that waiting more than 15 minutes jeopardizes the second baby, and favor proceeding with delivery. FORCEPS or other instruments may be necessary to accomplish this.

muscular dystrophy   An inherited chronic disease, affecting both children and adults, characterized by a gradual and progressive weakening of the voluntary muscles. The most common form is *Duchenne muscular dystrophy,* a sex-linked recessive-gene disorder (see BIRTH DEFECTS) that primarily affects boys (1 in every 3,000 to 4,000 live births). Initial symptoms are muscle weakness in the hips, shoulder, and spine, usually appearing before age four. Eventually the disease affects all muscles, including those of the respiratory and cardiovascular system. Death from respiratory infection or heart failure usually occurs before age 20.

Muscular dystrophy can be detected by a BLOOD TEST that measures creatinine phosphokinase (CPK), an enzyme normally found in muscle tissue. As muscles weaken and atrophy, they release CPK into the blood. By using the CPK test and a genetic test to detect the recently identified gene responsible for muscular dystrophy, clinicians can predict with nearly 100% accuracy whether or not a woman is a carrier of the muscular dystrophy gene. Identification of this gene holds promise for an eventual ability to cure or even prevent muscular dystrophy.

myometrium   The muscular structure of the UTERUS.

N

Nabothian cyst
See CYST.

Nagele's Rule   A method for predicting the estimated day of delivery (EDD). It involves subtracting three months from the first day of the LAST MENSTRUAL PERIOD (LMP) and adding seven days. For example, with an LMP of July 14, the EDD is April 21. This rule is based on a normal 28-day cycle. Women with longer cycles need to add the usual seven days, plus the number of days their cycle extends beyond 28 days.

natural childbirth   Also *prepared childbirth.* This approach includes physical and emotional preparation of the childbearing woman and her partner ("coach") to give birth with minimal use of technology, medical or surgical procedures, and drugs during normal LABOR. Natural childbirth is based on the concept that education and preparation can reduce or eliminate the maternal fear that results in tension, which in turn causes pain that can interfere with the progress, as well as intensify the discomforts, of normal LABOR and DELIVERY.

Natural childbirth does not necessarily mean painless or drug-free labor and delivery, but lower doses of medication are generally used and the labor is made easier when a woman is informed, relaxed, and confident. The two most popular methods of natural childbirth are Lamaze and Leboyer.

See also LEBOYER METHOD; PSYCHOPROPHYLACTIC METHOD.

natural family planning   Also *biological birth control, calendar method, fertility awareness, periodic abstinence, rhythm method.* FAMILY PLANNING or birth control without the use of contraceptive drugs or devices (for example, birth control pill, CONDOMS, INTRAUTERINE DE-

VICE (IUD)), designed either to achieve or avoid PREGNANCY by determining a woman's time of OVULATION and scheduling intercourse accordingly. Natural family planning methods include (1) the Calendar Method; (2) BASAL BODY TEMPERATURE (BBT) method; (3) CERVICAL MUCUS METHOD; and, (4) determining the LUTEINIZING HORMONE (LH) peak in blood specimens. These methods are the only methods of birth control approved by the Roman Catholic church. However, many factors contribute to their high failure rate, including irregular cycles and the variables that influence fluctuations in body temperature and hormonal levels, such as infections and emotional stress.

The Calendar Method predicts the day of ovulation using a formula based on the woman's menstrual pattern recorded over a period of several months. Ovulation usually occurs 14 days before the first day of the next menstrual period. A woman should be assumed to be fertile from at least two days before the first day of the next menstrual period. A woman should be assumed to be fertile from at least two days before to no less than two days after ovulation. *Periodic abstinence,* that is, abstinence from intercourse during the fertility interval, plus one to two days either way, increases the likelihood of avoiding pregnancy. Referring to the remaining time as the safe period (for intercourse without conception) is not accurate, however, since the Calendar Method is the least reliable method of family planning.

Determining the luteinizing hormone peak in serum specimens is the most accurate method of determining ovulation time. LH is produced in the PITUITARY GLAND and is responsible, along with FOLLICLE-STIMU-LATING HORMONE (FSH), for triggering the ovulation process. However, because of the cost and amount of time required for the series of measurements of LH that are essential to indicate its peak, this method is impractical as a method of birth control. It is more frequently used in the evaluation and treatment of INFERTILITY, when knowing the best time for coitus or ARTIFICIAL INSEMINATION is of great importance.

nausea Also *morning sickness.* A sensation of discomfort in the stomach region, with aversion to food and a tendency to vomit. Nausea is common during the first TRIMESTER of PREGNANCY, though it can extend into the second and third trimesters.

See also MORNING SICKNESS.

neonatal jaundice Also *hyperbilirubinemia, icterus neonatorum.* Jaundice in the newborn, characterized by yellowish skin tones, caused by excessive bilirubin, the principal pigment of bile, in the blood. This is the most common physical abnormality in newborns, occurring in about half of all full-term babies and in 8 out of 10 premature babies. It is caused by failure of the liver to metabolize bilirubin, an orange or yellowish pigment that results from the breakdown of surplus red blood cells. If the newborn's liver is not fully developed, the levels of bilirubin can rise to dangerous levels (hyperbilirubinemia), causing permanent brain damage. When hyperbilirubinemia is suspected, a simple BLOOD TEST will confirm the diagnosis. Treatment consists of blindfolding the baby and exposing him or her to bright lights (PHOTOTHERAPY). If phototherapy does not resolve the problem, a blood transfusion may be necessary. Follow-up and monitoring until the levels of bilirubin decrease is important, as hyperbilirubinemia can indicate serious disease and can cause permanent brain damage. Parents who choose HOME BIRTH or other nonhospital settings for childbirth should be aware of the risks of hyperbilirubinemia and seek routine medical examination and evaluation for the newborn soon after DELIVERY to rule out potential life-threatening conditions.

neonatal mortality rate   The number of recorded deaths among IN-FANTS under one month of age per 1,000 recorded live births in a given population in a calendar year.

The neonatal mortality rate is directly related to the living standards of the community or socioeconomic group into which the infant is born. Rates of death are consistently lower in the most affluent, best educated, and best housed segments of the population. Rates also vary considerably from country to country, between different ethnic groups, and according to the duration of GESTATION and the size and weight of the infant.

Neonatal mortality rates are calculated for specific regions using local data, as well as for entire countries, using data compiled from all regions of the country. The neonatal mortality rate in the United States, based on data from 1990, is 10 in 1,000 live births. Though the United States government publicly expresses concern about the neonatal mortality rate, the United States has dropped to 19th among developed countries in infant mortality. These statistics can be attributed directly to the fact that as many as one-third of pregnant women in the United States do not receive PRENATAL CARE. Japan has the lowest infant mortality of any developed country.

neonate   An INFANT from birth to 28 days of age.

neonatology   The study and science of the newborn or NEONATE, focused on high-risk conditions.

neural tube defects   A category of common, severe BIRTH DEFECTS related to impaired development of the neural tube, the embryonic structure from which the brain and spinal cord are formed. The two most common types of neural tube defects that occur are *meningomylocele* and *meningocele.*

meningomyelocele   Also *myelomeningocele, spina bifida.* The most obvious manifestation of this defect is a sac-like bulging of neural elements (nerve fibers, spinal cord, vertebrae) through a defect in the vertebral column, usually protruding through an opening in the skin of the back.

Meningomyelocele is the more common of the two neural tube defects and also the most common severe birth defect in all newborns. It occurs approximately two to eight times per 10,000 live births in the United States, and is more common in females. Women who give birth to one child with meningomyelocele have an increased risk of producing another child with the same defect. The risk increases proportionately if the woman has two children with the defect, if the woman herself suffers from meningomyelocele, or if a maternal aunt has the condition.

There is strong evidence that a dietary deficiency of FOLIC ACID (found in leafy green vegetables, liver, and yeast) in the mother before PREGNANCY may play a major role in the development of this birth defect. Because the vitamin is cheap and safe, many doctors recommend that women at risk for this defect take folic acid supplements orally for several weeks before attempting to become pregnant.

Treatment of spina bifida ranges from comfort measures in cases so severe that death appears imminent, to a highly aggressive, multi-specialty approach, including immediate neurosurgical intervention to close the defect. All decisions about treatment must be made in the child's best interests, depending upon the severity of the condition, any concurrent complications, and an estimation of the long-term expected quality of life.

meningocele   An outpouching of skin and the lining of the spinal cord (dura) similar to spina bifida, but without other abnormality of the nervous system. These children are neurologically intact and prognosis for survival without disability is excellent.

Prenatal diagnosis of the neural tube defects that involve leakage of fetal spinal fluid (meningomyelocele and meningocele) can be made by AMNIOCENTESIS at 14 weeks' GESTATION. ULTRASOUND can usually detect almost all neural tube defects. The postnatal diagnosis of neural tube defects is, with rare exception, immediately obvious at birth.

nevus flammeus   Also *port wine stain; salmon patch.* A common birthmark involving tiny blood vessels, appearing as a sharply defined, flat, irregularly shaped patch, ranging in color from faint pink to orange (salmon patch) to dark red-purple (port wine stain), usually found on the face and neck. The paler types tend to fade during childhood, while the darker ones persist.

nevus vasculosus   Also *strawberry hemangioma* or *strawberry mark.* A birthmark caused by localized overgrowth of dilated, but otherwise normal, thin-walled blood vessels, creating areas of flat or raised redness of various sizes.

newborn screening tests   A group of tests that help rule out the possibility of BIRTH DEFECT or disease in the newborn. These screening tests usually include:

(1) An initial, brief physical evaluation immediately following DELIVERY to rule out any life-threatening conditions that may require immediate attention. The most important factors at this point are ensuring a clear airway for breathing and determining that breathing is normal for adequate ventilation. APGAR scoring is also performed at one and five minutes following birth.

(2) A more complete physical examination should be done after a transition period of one to six hours, during which the INFANT is observed for stability of temperature and vital signs. Weight, length, and head circumference are carefully recorded.

Another complete physical exam should be performed within 24 hours of delivery, but after the six-hour transition period, when the infant will have stabilized. Any abnormal findings during the transition period will indicate whether the infant requires more immediate evaluation.

(3) Laboratory testing to screen for potential medical problems is part of routine newborn care. Some tests are required by law, and should include the following:

a. Blood types for mother and infant, and a direct COOMBS' TEST for the infant (to detect blood group incompatibilities caused by ANTIBODY formation).

b. BLOOD TEST for SYPHILIS.

c. Whole blood screen for phenylalanine (an amino acid essential in human nutrition), commonly called PKU (PHENYLKE-TONURIA) screening. PKU is a hereditary metabolic disorder in which increased levels of phenylalanine are present in the blood. Left untreated, the disorder can result in mental retardation, eczema, fair hair, and occasionally, seizures. This test is a standard requirement in the United States. Some states also require testing for other amino acid abnormalities.

d. THYROID function tests.

e. SICKLE CELL and other abnormalities of hemoglobin (a blood component responsible for oxygenation of the blood).

f. Hematocrit screening.

g. Galactosemia in any infant with JAUNDICE. Galactosemia is a serious metabolic disorder of which jaundice is often an indicator.

The above laboratory testing involves a one-time drawing of blood, with the exception of the galactosemia screening which is a URINE TEST.

nidation   The implantation of a fertilized egg in the ENDOMETRIUM of the now-pregnant UTERUS.

nipple   The cylindrical projection in the center of the BREAST, surrounded by the pigmented skin of the AREOLA, and containing the outlets of the milk ducts. The skin of the areola contains many small elevated nodules beneath which lie the sebaceous glands. These glands are responsible for the lubrication of the nipple and help prevent cracking of the skin of the nipple and areola. A circular, smooth muscle band surrounds the base of the nipple, and lengthwise smooth muscle fibers branch out from this muscle ring to encircle and protect the milk ducts as they converge toward the nipple.

Frequently, changes in the nipple indicate some types of breast disease, including cancer. Awareness of these changes is important in the early diagnosis of any breast abnormality. See BREAST CANCER, PAGET'S DISEASE.

Nipple discharge can be a clear, serous fluid, bloody, green or brown, milky, or purulent (containing pus). Discharge from the nipple can indicate breast abnormalities that are not cancer, including: (1) papillomas (benign epithelial tumors) of the milk ducts; or (2) mammary dysplasia (also fibrocystic disease), which encompasses a wide variety of painful, benign breast changes. These can include masses, dramatic fluctuations in breast size during certain menstrual phases, CYSTS, glandular disorders, and abnormal growth of fibrous connective tissue (fibrosis).

In addition to the above conditions, nipple discharge can also be caused by hormonal abnormalities, use of ORAL CONTRACEPTIVES, ABSCESS, or ductal infection. Medical evaluation should be sought promptly in the event of any nipple changes or discharge.

In breast cancer, nipple retraction or crusting occurs in 2 to 3% of all cases, but nipple retraction may frequently be an important early sign. Other symptoms include nipple erosion, enlargement, itching, and discharge. Twenty-five percent of all breast cancers occur in the region of the nipple and/or areola.

Paget's disease is a rare cancer of the breast (about 1% of all cases) that involves infiltration of the disease through the milk ducts. The skin of the nipple is involved, but obvious nipple changes are often minimal. The first symptoms are often itching or burning of the nipple, with a superficial erosion or sore. Diagnosis is established by biopsy of the erosion. Though rare, Paget's disease is often diagnosed and treated as a skin irritation or bacterial infection, leading to a delay in detection.

Laboratory examination of nipple discharge may be helpful in the diagnosis of breast cancer on rare occasions.

nonstress test (NST)   A test that records the response of the fetal heart to fetal movement. It is usually the primary means of fetal evaluation when any condition is suspected that could place the FETUS at high risk for placental insufficiency.

An external fetal monitor is used with the mother lying on her side or back and slightly tilted to the side. Since the fetus is more active one to two hours after a meal, the NST is best performed during that interval. Fetal movements and heart rate are then monitored.

The frequency of fetal heart rate acceleration during the testing period, usually 20 to 45 minutes, will determine if the fetus is at risk. The test is performed once or twice weekly, depending on the reason for testing. If the test is negative, the PREGNANCY is allowed to continue and the test is repeated at an appropriate interval. If the test is positive, additional testing is performed.

nuchal cord   Description of the UMBILICAL CORD when it is wrapped around the neck of the FETUS.

nucleic acid   The genetic material of all living organisms, containing the blueprint for physical characteristics passed from parent to offspring. There are two types of nucleic acid, deoxyribonucleic acid (DNA) and ribonucleic acid (RNA). DNA constitutes the coded genetic information of all cellular organisms. RNA helps transform the genetic information into protein structures.

nulligravida   A woman who has never been pregnant.

nullipara   A woman who has never carried a PREGNANCY to the point where the FETUS is VIABLE (able to survive).

nurse midwife
    See MIDWIFE.

obesity   Body weight exceeding ideal standards by more than 20%, based on height and build. Obesity is almost always related to overeating and can affect a woman's self-esteem, attractiveness to others, enjoyment of sexual activities, and long-term health. Although all causes of obesity are not completely understood, researchers believe both biochemical and psychological factors play a role.

Obesity increases the risk of life-threatening diseases such as DIABETES, heart disease, gallbladder and kidney disorders, osteoarthritis, BREAST CANCER, and endometrial cancer. Researchers believe hormonal relationships may increase the risk of breast cancer in obese women since fat cells raise levels of female sex HORMONES. The risks of disease are increased for postmenopausal women. Obesity can impair FERTILITY in women of childbearing age by inducing persistent ESTROGEN stimulation, interfering with the ovary/pituitary feedback system necessary for OVULATION and conception to occur.

Correlations have been made between excessive WEIGHT GAIN DURING PREGNANCY and higher rates of CESAREAN DELIVERY as the function of uterine muscles is inhibited by excessive fatty tissue; the baby's descent and CERVIX dilation can also become impeded. Nonetheless, overweight women should avoid severe dieting during PREGNANCY in order to maintain what is deemed safe caloric intake (approximately 1,800 calories per day).

See also BREAST CANCER; DIABETES; DIET; WEIGHT GAIN.

obstetrician   A physician specializing in obstetrics, that is, childbirth (from PRENATAL CARE to DELIVERY, whether vaginal or cesarean) and the POSTPARTUM period.

See also BIRTH ATTENDANT; GYNECOLOGIST; MIDWIFE.

oligohydramnios
> See AMNIOTIC SAC; HYDRAMNIOS.

oligomenorrhea   Menstrual periods more than 35 days apart. This condition is especially common during the first few years after MENARCHE (the beginning of menstruation), and during MENOPAUSE. In both cases, it is probably related to hormonal imbalance and not to OVULATION; thus it is also called anovulatory bleeding. OBESITY, severe dieting, or stress can also cause infrequent menstruation. A consistent longer-than-normal cycle may be normal for some women, however, and is not always cause for alarm or treatment.
> See also MENOPAUSE; MENSTRUAL CYCLE; OVULATION.

oligospermia   Also *subfertility*. An abnormally low SPERM count in a SEMEN sample. This condition can be caused by previous infection such as mumps, poor nutrition, chemical or environmental toxins, HYPERTHERMIA (as in hot tubs or saunas), constriction by tight underwear, anatomical abnormalities such as undescended testicles (CRYPTORCHIDISM), blockage to the VAS DEFERENS, or a VARICOCELE (a VARICOSE VEIN in the scrotal sac). Alcohol or other drugs can also contribute to the problem. Sons of women who took DIETHYLSTILBESTROL (DES) during PREGNANCY often experience oligospermia.
> Treatment varies according to the cause. Nutritional supplements, particularly vitamins C and E, the B vitamins, and zinc may be helpful. In some cases, clomiphene nitrate (see FERTILITY PILL) may be prescribed; however, studies have not shown improved pregnancy rate. Varicocele can be treated surgically, resulting in 25 to 50% postoperative pregnancy rates. If none of these measures is effective, ARTIFICIAL INSEMINATION may be the only method available.
> See also GIFT (GAMETE INTRAFALLOPIAN TRANSFER); IN VITRO FERTILIZATION; INFERTILITY.

oogenesis   Production of primitive cells in the fetal OVARY that develop into eggs (oocytes).

oophorectomy   Surgical removal of one or both of the OVARIES. Removal of one ovary is termed *unilateral oophorectomy*; removal of both is *bilateral oophorectomy,* generally performed at the same time as HYSTERECTOMY and SALPINGECTOMY. Removal of the ovaries results in STERILITY and ESTROGEN depletion. Premenopausal women who undergo this procedure are thrust into MENOPAUSE, and experience hot flashes, MOOD SWINGS, and all the other symptoms of menopause. Bilateral oophorectomy is usually performed in premenopausal women who have ovarian cancer or serious PELVIC INFLAMMATORY DISEASE. Unilateral oophorectomy may be performed to remove a large benign ovarian CYST in women of childbearing age.

See also CYST (ovarian).

oophoritis   Infection or inflammation of the OVARIES.

ophthalmia neonatorum   Eye infection of the newborn, usually caused by GONORRHEA in the mother. The administration of medication soon after birth to prevent this infection is legally required in the United States. In the past, a silver nitrate solution was used; now, however, antibiotic ointment (erythromycin, tetracycline, or penicillin) is used since it is also effective against *Chlamydia trachomatis*.

oral contraceptive   Also *the Pill, birth control pill.* Taken regularly, oral contraceptives prevent conception by suppressing OVULATION and maintaining a type of mucus hostile to SPERM. Available since the 1960s, oral contraceptives now provide a significantly lower hormonal dose than their original formulation. It is estimated that 80 to 100 million women in the world use "the Pill" today.

The Pill's advantages include high effectiveness, convenience, and its regulating effects on the MENSTRUAL CYCLE. Disadvantages include side effects and/or conditions contraindicating use in some women (for example, PREGNANCY; BREASTFEEDING; known or suspected BREAST CANCER or tumor; genital bleeding of unknown cause; DIABETES; age over 40; heavy smoking; circulatory and vascular disorders, or a history of these disorders; impaired liver function; cystic fibrosis or SICKLE CELL ANEMIA). Because oral contraceptives affect the endocrine system, their effects are not limited to reproductive function; they have been associated with potentially life-threatening disorders of the liver and cardiovascular system. The Pill may also lose effectiveness when taken with other drugs such as antibiotics (ampicillin and tetracycline), barbiturates, and drugs to treat epilepsy or arthritis.

Minor but unpleasant side effects commonly include water retention, NAUSEA, leg cramps, bloating, WEIGHT GAIN, HEADACHE, vision changes, irritability, BREAST tenderness, skin changes, increase or loss of hair, changes in vaginal discharge, depression, and repeated YEAST

INFECTIONS. For some women, side effects may be alleviated with another kind of Pill.

The two principal types of oral contraceptive are the *combination pill* (both ESTROGEN and PROGESTERONE) and the *minipill* (progesterone only and slightly less effective). Both work by maintaining constant body levels of these two basic menstrual HORMONES. The combination Pill is taken once a day for 21 days and discontinued for 7. During the week the Pill is not taken, placebos ("dummy" pills with no active ingredients) are taken instead, causing HORMONE levels to drop and causing a lighter, more brief bleeding than menstruation to occur, with few or no cramps. Some women have no periods at all when "on the Pill," but a PREGNANCY TEST is advised for a woman missing more than one period. If not pregnant, she may require a prescription with less progesterone.

If a woman wants to become pregnant, she stops taking the Pill, but may not ovulate for several cycles thereafter. In most cases, this is usually corrected within six months. For the 2 to 3% of women for whom ovulation does not begin and for whom there is secretion from the breasts, medication may be required after disease is ruled out. Some clinicians believe this condition can be avoided by stopping the Pill for two cycles every two years, allowing for early detection of a suppressed natural cycle. Others believe cessation of the Pill for this reason is unwarranted.

See also CONTRACEPTION; CONTRAGESTIVE; ESTROGEN; PROGESTERONE.

oral sex   Also *oral-genital intercourse*. Intercourse involving the use of the mouth (lips, tongue) in sexual stimulation and pleasure. Oral sex may include one or both partners kissing, biting, sucking, licking, or exploring erogenous zones and genital organs, and tasting and swallowing sexual secretions. It may be performed in conjunction with or instead of vaginal, anal, or other kinds of sexual intercourse. Many SEXUALLY TRANSMITTED DISEASES (particularly AIDS, SYPHILIS, GONORRHEA, and HERPES) can be transmitted through participation in oral sexual activities.

See also COITUS; CUNNILINGUS; FELLATIO; SEXUAL RESPONSE.

orgasm   Also *climax, coming* (slang). The physical climax or peak of intense sexual pleasure. Orgasm is the sudden release of sexual tension in involuntary muscle contractions, forcing accumulated blood away from genital tissues. It is usually accompanied by feelings of acute pleasure and relief, clouded consciousness, and an increase in blood pressure and heart rate. In women, orgasm typically involves a series of rhythmic muscular contractions in the lower VAGINA and surrounding tissues; it may also involve the UTERUS. In men, the focus of orgasm is the PENIS and seminal vesicles involving contractions of the pelvic muscles and EJACULATION of SPERM. While men must reach orgasm to impregnate their partner, women can become pregnant without even experiencing arousal.

Female SEXUAL RESPONSE varies more widely than that of males. Sex researchers Masters and Johnson report that, on average, women take longer than men to reach climax (15 minutes compared to 3 minutes). Although a very individual experience, orgasms differ according to sexual stimulation. Some women experience more than one orgasm; such multiple orgasms may occur within only a few minutes. While penile thrusting alone is not enough to bring some women to orgasm, many experience climax most easily by stimulation of the CLITORIS in conjunction with ORAL SEX or vaginal intercourse. Pelvic discomfort can occur in some women when stimulation stops short of orgasm; for others, orgasm can relieve pelvic congestion associated with menstrual cramps. Women's ability to experience orgasm is not affected by age, but for men, the time between potential orgasms, or refractory period, increases with age.

For most women, feelings of mutual warmth and understanding with their partner are an important factor in achieving sexual gratification. Many women enjoy sexual activity without orgasm and some, lacking sensation in the lower parts of their bodies, find stimulation of other erogenous zones stimulating and satisfying. While orgasm is not linked to CERVICAL DILATATION in PREGNANCY, it can increase CONTRACTIONS during LABOR. The term frigidity has been used to describe the condition of a woman who never achieves orgasm during sex; female orgasmic dysfunction describes difficulty in achieving orgasm.

See also CLITORIS; SEXUAL RESPONSE.

orientation (in relation to newborn infant)   A newborn's ability to observe, fixate on, and follow complex visual stimuli that are appealing and attractive. The human face, especially the eyes, and bright shiny objects are most attractive to the newborn's line of vision. A newborn responds with bright, wide eyes, still limbs, and fixed staring as a way of becoming familiar with family, friends, and surroundings.

orifice   The entrance of any body cavity.

Ortolani's maneuver   A procedure performed by the clinician to assess hip stability when the legs of a newborn are of unequal length. With the baby on its back, the clinician realigns hip displacement by rotating the hip inward following downward pressure.

outpatient   A person receiving treatment from a health care facility without being hospitalized. Outpatient surgical and medical procedures can save considerable time and money. Some health plans, however, provide little or no coverage for outpatient procedures.

ovarian cyst
>   See CYST.

ovarian dysgenesis
>   See TURNER'S SYNDROME.

ovary   The female sex gland, or gonad, in which the ova or egg cells are formed and ESTROGEN and PROGESTERONE are produced. The ovaries direct sexual maturation, regulate the MENSTRUAL CYCLE, and enable PREGNANCY. Normally a woman has two ovaries located in the lower abdomen on either side of the UTERUS and just below the FALLOPIAN TUBES.

The ovaries contain several hundred thousand FOLLICLES at birth—no more are produced during a woman's life. After PUBERTY, approximately 20 follicles begin to ripen during each menstrual cycle, but typically only one matures completely to release an egg. Once the egg is free of the ovary and drawn into the adjacent fallopian tubes, the empty follicle secretes progesterone for two weeks as the *corpus luteum* before disintegrating. Should the egg become fertilized by a SPERM while in the fallopian tube and implanted in the UTERUS, progesterone production is assumed by the PLACENTA. If fertilization does not take place, the cycle of OVULATION begins again as a result of lower hormonal levels.

Typically, eggs are released by alternate ovaries at a rate of about one per month between the onset and cessation of menstruation. During pregnancy, the ovaries stop producing ova. In mature women each ovary has an almond-like size and shape. A special ligament attaching the ovaries to the uterus allows them to shift somewhat in position.

After MENOPAUSE the remaining egg follicles disintegrate and the ovary shrinks to about one-third its former size.

Every GYNECOLOGICAL EXAMINATION should include PALPATION (feeling) of the ovaries. Their comparative size can vary significantly. CYSTS and cancer are the most common ovarian disorders. Their normal function can also be altered by infection through SEXUALLY TRANSMITTED DISEASES, making conception more difficult. Surgical removal of both ovaries when more conservative treatments fail induces menopause and is called OOPHORECTOMY.

See also MENSTRUAL CYCLE; OVULATION.

overdue baby
See POSTDATE PREGNANCY; POSTMATURE INFANT.

ovulation   The process of producing an egg cell (ovum) from an OVARY approximately 14 days prior to the onset of menses (menstrual period). Ovulation occurs more or less monthly, except during PREGNANCY, from soon after the onset of menstruation until MENOPAUSE (or roughly from the ages of 14 to 55), and is necessary for pregnancy to occur. Sex HORMONE production is greatly increased at PUBERTY, and FSH (FOLLICLE-STIMULATING HORMONE) is stimulated by the PITUITARY GLAND to induce the growth and development of ovarian FOLLICLES. Each follicle contains an egg, and as it develops, produces ESTROGEN, which then stimulates the production of LH (LUTEINIZING HORMONE). Together, the two hormones suppress the growth of numerous follicles stimulated during the cycle except for one or two. When an egg cell is mature, it moves toward the ovary wall, which thins and eventually breaks, releasing the follicle. The follicle on the surface of the ovary then ruptures, releasing the egg. Some women experience pain, *mittelschmerz,* or bleeding during ovulation while others have no symptoms.

Following ovulation, the egg cell moves into a FALLOPIAN TUBE where it may be fertilized by a SPERM. It takes an egg about four days to move the length of the tube; unless fertilized by a sperm within one day of its release from the ovary, the egg will no longer be viable. Double ovulation occurs when two eggs are released during a single cycle; if both are fertilized, fraternal twins result. Approximately 40% of mothers who choose not to BREASTFEED resume menstruation within six weeks and 90% resume within 24 weeks following birth. Of these, approximately 50% ovulate during the first cycle.

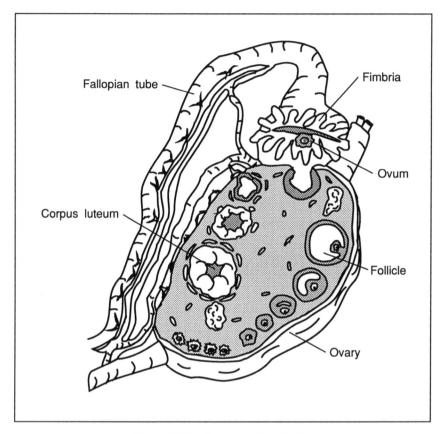

Figure O-1   Ovary and ovulation

Because the egg is viable for only a short time, women may better assess the likelihood of conception by using fertility awareness techniques to determine ovulation. See BASAL BODY TEMPERATURE (BBT) METHOD; RHYTHM METHOD; CERVICAL MUCUS METHOD (also ovulation method or Billings method).

Infection can destroy the normal function of the ovaries, making conception more difficult. Ovulation problems account for 15 to 20% of female INFERTILITY, and are most commonly treated by the drug Clomid.

See also FERTILITY PILL.

ovum   (Latin for "egg") The female reproductive cell or GAMETE, more commonly referred to as the egg, present in all animals that reproduce sexually. At birth, a girl has approximately 300,000 to 500,000 immature ova in her two ovaries. Beginning around PUBERTY she will retain only about 75,000 ova; of these, 400 to 500 will reach maturity during her reproductive lifetime. Following MENOPAUSE, she will have none. The human ovum is about 1/200 inch in diameter. The process of releasing the ovum from the OVARY is called OVULATION. The average ovum survives outside the ovary for about 24 hours before it degenerates. For conception to occur, the egg must be fertilized within 12 hours after its release from the ovary.

See also FERTILIZATION; OVARY; OVULATION.

oxygen in childbirth   Administration of oxygen to the mother during LABOR, or to the newborn. Oxygen is given to counteract hyperventilation, NAUSEA or other discomfort, and to relieve FETAL DISTRESS. Prior to birth, oxygen reaches the baby through the UMBILICAL CORD until the baby's lungs take over the breathing completely. The normal color of a newborn at birth is slightly bluish; this quickly changes to pink when oxygen enters the lungs. Hard, frequent CONTRACTIONS or a compressed umbilical cord can cause a baby to suffer oxygen deprivation and lead to brain damage. Oxygen may be given to a newborn, especially a PREMATURE INFANT and/or one suffering respiratory distress. The concentration of oxygen must be carefully monitored, however, since too much oxygen can damage the newborn retina and cause blindness.

See also OXYGEN TOXICITY; RETROLENTAL FIBROPLASIA.

oxygen toxicity   Excessive levels of oxygen therapy resulting in abnormal tissue change. Oxygen toxicity can cause RETROLENTAL FIBROPLASIA (RLF), or the formation of tissue behind the lens, and result in blindness, particularly in PREMATURE INFANTS.

oxytocin   A naturally occurring HORMONE, secreted by the PITUITARY GLAND, responsible for uterine CONTRACTIONS in ORGASM and childbirth, and secretion of breast milk. Oxytocin is stored and released by the pituitary gland in response to stimulation by the HYPOTHALAMUS. Its name derives from the Greek *"oxys,"* meaning "sharp, quick" and *"tokos,"* meaning "childbirth." In both its natural and synthetic form (brand names Pitocin and Syntocinon), oxytocin induces LABOR, strengthens uterine contractions during labor, and acts to expel the PLACENTA and to slow bleeding. A nursing INFANT also stimulates the release of oxytocin, causing cellular contractions in the milk ducts of the BREAST and release of milk. Oxytocin substitutes can be administered through inhalation or injection to accelerate labor. However, inappropriate use can result in violent contractions, uterine rupture, and severe damage to or death of the baby. The United States Food and Drug Administration (FDA) has ruled out its use in elective INDUCTION OF LABOR.

See also CONTRACTION STRESS TEST; FETAL MONITORING.

oxytocin challenge test (OCT)

See CONTRACTION STRESS TEST.

P

Paget's disease A rare cancer of the BREAST (about 1% of all cases) involving infiltration of the disease through the milk ducts. The first symptoms are often itching or burning of the NIPPLE, with a superficial erosion, crusting, or sore. Though the skin of the nipple is affected, other obvious nipple changes may be minimal. Diagnosis is established by a biopsy of the affected area. Though rare, Paget's disease is frequently diagnosed and treated as a skin irritation or bacterial infection, delaying the diagnosis of cancer.

Any nipple changes or discharge should be promptly assessed by a physician. In breast cancer, nipple retraction or crusting occurs in 2 to 3% of all cases, but nipple retraction may be an important early sign. Twenty-five percent of all breast cancers occur in the region of the nipple and/or AREOLA. See BREAST CANCER.

extramammary Paget's disease A cancer *in situ* (one that has not spread) of the anogenital region, particularly the VULVA. It involves reddish LESIONS interspersed with patches of white epithelial tissue, which microscopic examination shows to contain "Paget's" cells, large pale cancer cells (named for British surgeon, Sir James Paget). In about 5% of patients, this condition indicates the presence of cancer elsewhere in the body. The treatment is surgical excision of the affected tissue.

Extramammary Paget's disease is also known as *osteitis deformans,* a skeletal disease of older persons that causes the bones to thicken and soften. More common in men than women, it most often affects the PELVIS, hips, and skull. There is no known cure.

pain
See PELVIC PAIN.

pain relief
See ANALGESIC.

palpate To examine internal organs and structures by pressing the surface of the body with the fingers, to detect abnormalities such as BREAST lumps (see BREAST SELF-EXAMINATION). Palpation is one of the techniques used by clinicians in physical assessment; other techniques include *inspection, percussion* (tapping or thumping), and *auscultation* (listening to body sounds such as the heartbeat).

palpitation A heartbeat so forceful and/or fast that the "owner" is aware of it; the rhythm may or may not be irregular. It may indicate tachycardia but often is simply the result of emotional stress or anxiety. Palpitations are also associated with MENOPAUSE.

pancreas One of the ENDOCRINE GLANDS, located in the ABDOMEN, behind the stomach, responsible for the production of insulin and digestive juices. When inadequate insulin is produced, the body is unable to metabolize carbohydrates, proteins, and fat, and hyperglycemia (abnormally high levels of blood sugar) results.
See also DIABETES MELLITUS.

Pap smear Also *Papanicolaou smear, Pap test.* A screening test to detect cervical cancer, named for the Greek physician and cytologist who developed it, Dr. George N. Papanicolaou. Authorities recommend an annual Pap test for every woman beginning at age 18 and earlier for those who became sexually active prior to age 15. After three consecutive tests show normal findings, Pap smears can be done every two or three years, *if* the woman has only one sexual partner, has no history of HERPES VIRUS, and did not become sexually active prior to age 15. Any one of the foregoing factors puts women at higher than normal risk for cervical cancer.
A Pap test is relatively painless; the clinician scrapes a thin layer of cells from the surface of the CERVIX, using a wooden or plastic spatula. The cells are placed on a slide, stained, and examined under a microscope by a pathologist or laboratory technician with special training. Performed and interpreted carefully, the test can detect abnormal cells on the cervix, including any precancerous or malignant changes. It can also reveal common vaginal infections and help assess ESTROGEN levels. However, it does not detect vaginal, ovarian, or uter-

ine cancer. Any abnormal findings in a Pap test are usually followed up with a surgical biopsy to remove additional tissue for further examination.

Abnormalities detected by a Pap smear are most commonly classified as follows:

Class I   Negative; all cells normal.

Class II   Some abnormal cells, often caused by infection or inflammation; followup recommended after infection/ inflammation treated.

Class III More serious abnormality, usually indicating the need for biopsy.

Class IV   Positive; distinctly abnormal cells, possibly malignant and definitely requiring biopsy.

Class V   Malignant cells; biopsy essential for staging the cancer (classifying it according to size and location—whether it has spread from original site to other organs and tissues).

para A woman who has carried one or more pregnancies to the point of viability.

paracervical anesthesia Also *paracervical block.* A type of regional ANESTHESIA used for a DILATATION AND CURETTAGE (D & C) or for an ABORTION. It involves injecting an anesthetic agent through the VAGINA into the cervical ligaments and lower uterine walls. It is no longer used during LABOR because it can lower the mother's blood pressure, thereby interfering with the baby's supply of oxygen.

parametritis Also *pelvic cellulitis.* An infection involving the connective tissue of the broad ligament of the UTERUS. Generally spread through the lymphatic system of the uterus, it can also result from a cervical laceration (tear) that extends upward into the broad ligament. If untreated, it can develop into a potentially fatal peritonitis (infection of the peritoneum, the lining of the abdominal cavity). Symptoms of parametritis include marked high temperature (102 to 104 degrees Fahrenheit; 38.9 to 40 degrees Celsius), chills, lethargy, abdominal pain and tenderness, and tachycardia (rapid heartbeat).

parathyroid glands   Paired ENDOCRINE GLANDS (some persons have four; others have six) located on the back surface of the THYROID gland that secrete parathyroid HORMONE (PTH). This hormone regulates calcium levels in the blood; if levels drop below a certain point, PTH causes calcium to be released from the bone into the bloodstream. It also helps regulate phosphorus levels in the blood.

parent-infant attachment
    See ATTACHMENT.

parturition   Another term for childbirth.
    See LABOR.

passive acquired immunity   Transfer of the immunoglobulin IgG to the FETUS in utero, creating an immunity that protects the fetus against bacterial infection.

patient's rights   An individual's justifiable claims in relation to health care services, particularly when hospitalized. These rights include the right to the whole truth about one's condition, the tests and treatments recommended, and the prognosis (predicted outcome of the situation, both with and without treatment), the right to privacy and personal dignity, the right to participate in decisions about one's health, and the right of complete access to medical records, both during and after hospitalization. In response to consumer demands, the American Hospital Association formalized these rights in 1973 in "A Patient's Bill of Rights" (Table P-1).
    See also PREGNANT PATIENT'S RIGHTS.

pediatrician   A physician who cares for children from birth until adolescence. It is important to choose a pediatrician before giving birth and arrange for an initial evaluation of the newborn as soon as possible after birth. If the woman has experienced complications during PREGNANCY and expects to give birth to a high-risk infant, she may prefer a pediatrician with a specialty in NEONATOLOGY. In any case, it may be necessary to interview several pediatricians before finding the "right" one, someone who answers questions clearly and thoroughly, and who takes seriously parents' concerns about the baby. It is also important to ask whether the pediatrician ever sees children without appointments and how emergency situations are handled.

Table P-1   A Patient's Bill of Rights

---

1. The patient has the right to considerate and respectful care.

. . . .

2. The patient has the right to obtain from his physician complete current information concerning his diagnosis, treatment, and prognosis, in terms the patient can be reasonably expected to understand. When it is not medically advisable to give such information to the patient, the information should be made available to an appropriate person in his behalf. He has the right to know by name the physician responsible for coordinating his care.

. . . .

3. The patient has the right to receive from his physician information necessary to give informed consent prior to the start of any procedure and/or treatment. Except in emergencies, such information for informed consent should include but not necessarily be limited to the specific procedure and/or treatment, the medically significant risks involved, and the probable duration of incapacitation. Where medically significant alternatives for care or treatment exist, or when the patient requests information concerning medical alternatives, the patient has the right to such information. The patient also has the right to know the name of the person responsible for the procedures and/or treatment.

. . . .

4. The patient has the right to refuse treatment to the extent permitted by law and to be informed of the medical consequences of his action.

. . . .

5. The patient has the right to every consideration of his privacy concerning his own medical care program. Case discussion, consultation, examination, and treatment are confidential and should be conducted discreetly. Those not directly involved in this care must have the permission of the patient to be present.

. . . .

6. The patient has the right to expect that all communications and records pertaining to his care should be treated as confidential.

. . . .

7. The patient has the right to expect that within its capacity a hospital must make reasonable response to the request of a patient for services. The hospital must provide evaluation, service, and/or referral as indicated by the urgency of the case. When medically permissible, a patient may be transferred to another facility only after he has received complete information and explanation concerning the needs for and alternatives to such a transfer. The institution to which the patient is transferred must first have accepted the patient for transfer.

. . . .

Table P-1 A Patient's Bill of Rights (continued)

---

8. The patient has the right to obtain information as to any relationship of his hospital to other health care and educational institutions insofar as his care is concerned. The patient has the right to obtain information as to the existence of any professional relationships among individuals, by name, who are treating him.

. . . .

9. The patient has the right to be advised if the hospital proposes to engage in or perform human experimentation affecting his care or treatment. The patient has the right to refuse to participate in such research projects.

. . . .

10. The patient has the right to expect reasonable continuity of care. He has the right to know in advance what appointment times and physicians are available and where. The patient has the right to expect that the hospital will provide a mechanism whereby he is informed by his physician or a delegate of the physician of the patient's continuing health.

. . . .

11. The patient has the right to examine and receive an explanation of his bill regardless of source of payment.

. . . .

12. The patient has the right to know what hospital rules and regulations apply to his conduct as a patient.

. . . .

Source: American Hospital Association, 1973. Reprinted by permission.

---

pelvic cavity

See under PELVIS.

pelvic cellulitis

See PARAMETRITIS.

pelvic inflammatory disease (PID) Also *pelvic infection, salpingitis.*

Inflammation and/or infection of the FALLOPIAN TUBES, often involving the OVARIES and UTERUS as well. The term "pelvic inflammatory disease" has become a catch-all description for any infection or inflammation of the female reproductive organs, even though more specific terminology exists. Technically speaking, inflammation of the tubes is *salpingitis;* inflammation of the OVARY, *oophoritis;* inflammation of the CERVIX, CERVICITIS; and inflammation of the uterus, ENDOMETRITIS.

PID occurs in about 1% of women between ages 15 and 39; the incidence is highest in sexually active women between ages 15 and 24. Authorities estimate that PID is responsible for 15 to 40% of all INFERTILITY. It is more prevalent among women who have had multiple sexual partners, sexual activity before age 15, a history of PID, recent gynecologic surgery, or an INTRAUTERINE DEVICE (IUD). This condition usually involves a tubal infection that may or may not be accompanied by a pelvic ABSCESS.

PID is largely associated with organisms that cause SEXUALLY TRANSMITTED DISEASES: *Chlamydia trachomatis,* which causes CHLAMYDIA INFECTION; and *Neisseria gonorrhoeae,* which causes GONORRHEA. Other organisms responsible for some cases include *Mycoplasma hominis* and *Escherichia coli,* a bacterium present in the gastrointestinal tract, which may enter the pelvic area during MISCARRIAGE, therapeutic ABORTION, childbirth, or via an IUD.

PID can range from mild to life-threatening, and may be acute, subacute (not as severe), or chronic. Symptoms include sharp, cramping pain and tenderness in the lower abdomen, fever, chills, purulent (filled with pus) vaginal discharge, irregular bleeding, DYSURIA (difficult or painful urination), NAUSEA, and vomiting. Some of these symptoms mimic appendicitis and ECTOPIC PREGNANCY, both of which must be ruled out.

Diagnostic measures for PID include a pelvic examination, BLOOD TESTS, a gonorrhea culture, and a test for chlamydia. Additional procedures may include ULTRASOUND to detect and locate a pelvic abscess and LAPAROSCOPY to confirm the diagnosis and obtain culture specimens from the fimbria (the flared opening of the fallopian tubes).

In all but the most mild cases of PID, the woman is hospitalized for administration of intravenous antibiotics appropriate to the infectious organism. After treatment of the infection, microsurgery may be necessary to repair tubal damage if the woman wishes to become pregnant.

pelvic pain   Discomfort in the area of the female reproductive organs (UTERUS, OVARIES, FALLOPIAN TUBES, VAGINA) centered either in the ABDOMEN or in the lower back. Pelvic pain can be either acute or chronic and can range from mild to severe, depending on the cause. It can result from infection or inflammation such as PELVIC INFLAMMATORY DISEASE, from a CYST or tumor that displaces other organs, from

ECTOPIC PREGNANCY, ENDOMETRIOSIS or ENDOMETRITIS. Pelvic pain can also be caused by problems in the urinary tract (kidneys, BLADDER, ureters) such as kidney stones, or by inflammation of the gastroin-testinal tract (colon, intestines, bowel) such as colitis, diverticulitis, or appendicitis. In some cases, the source of pelvic pain is skeletal, such as osteoporosis, osteoarthritis, scoliosis, or a bone tumor.

If diagnostic tests have ruled out all possible sources of chronic pelvic pain, some clinicians recommend surgical removal of some or all of the pelvic organs. Others, however, suggest treatment in a pain clinic, available at many major hospitals, using biofeedback, physical therapy, heat, electrical stimulation, and other methods.

pelvic tilt　Also *pelvic rocking.* One of several exercises recom-mended during PREGNANCY and after childbirth to reduce back strain and improve abdominal muscle tone. The exercise can be performed lying on one's back on the floor, or while sitting in a chair or standing with one's back against the wall. It involves decreasing the curvature of the spine by pressing the spine against a flat surface (floor, chair, or wall) and tightening the buttocks and abdominal muscles while tuck-ing in the buttocks.

pelvimetry　Clinical measurement of the female PELVIS to determine whether vaginal DELIVERY is possible. Measurement can be estimated by the clinician during a pelvic examination; precise measurement must be done by X-RAY pelvimetry. Exposure to radiation, however, can harm the developing FETUS, particularly in the first TRIMESTER; therefore, X-ray pelvimetry is done only late in the PREGNANCY or even during LABOR when the clinician suspects that a narrow pelvis may prevent vaginal delivery, or if the baby is in a BREECH, FACE, or other ABNORMAL PRESENTATION.

The two most critical measurements in pelvimetry are often done at the first prenatal visit during the vaginal examination: the *diagonal conjugate* and the *pelvic outlet.* The *diagonal conjugate* is the distance from the underside of the pubic bone to the top of the sacrum (the bony back wall of the pelvis) where it meets the last vertebra. If this dis-tance is $12\frac{1}{2}$ centimeters (5 inches) or more, it means that the *pelvic inlet* (upper part of the pelvis) is large enough for an average size baby to pass through. The *pelvic outlet* is an arch-like opening formed by two bony columns on each side, called the *ischial spines* or *ischial tuberosities.* These structures are actually part of the hipbones. The pelvic outlet must be at least 10 centimeters (4 inches) to permit vaginal delivery.

When either the diagonal conjugate or the pelvic outlet are too small to accommodate the baby's passage, the condition is called CEPHALOPELVIC DISPROPORTION (CPD). In these instances, CESAREAN DELIVERY is performed.

pelvis   The hip girdle at the base of the spine, just above the thigh bones. It surrounds the *pelvic cavity,* the bottom portion of the abdominal cavity, and supports the internal reproductive organs (UTERUS, FALLOPIAN TUBES, OVARIES) as well as the urinary BLADDER and rectum. (Figure P-1)

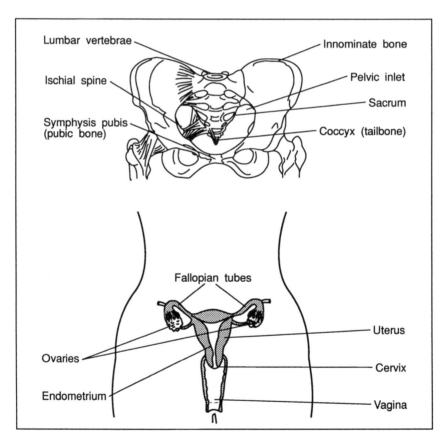

Figure P-1   Female pelvis and pelvic organs

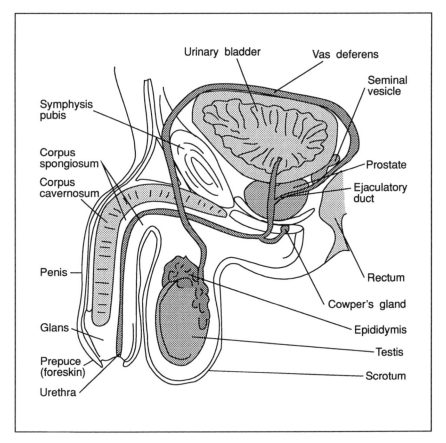

Figure P-2   Male Reproductive System

penis Also *phallus; dick, cock, prick* (slang). The male organ used for urination and copulation (sexual intercourse), consisting primarily of spongy erectile tissue which becomes engorged with blood during sexual excitement, stiffening the penis so that it can be inserted into the female VAGINA. The URETHRA is contained within the shaft of the penis, extending from the glans, the sensitive tip of the penis, to the urinary BLADDER. (Figure P-2) The outside of the penis is covered with loose skin, one fold of which is called the PREPUCE or foreskin. This fold of skin is surgically removed in some male infants (see CIRCUMCISION). Males who are not circumcised must retract the foreskin to remove SMEGMA, a waxy substance secreted by glands under the foreskin. At the tip of the glans is the urethral opening, through which both urine and SPERM are released.

During sexual arousal, the penis becomes erect, hard, and three to four inches longer than its length at rest. When the male reaches ORGASM, SEMEN or seminal fluid is ejaculated from the urethral opening. Semen contains sperm and other fluids secreted by the seminal vesicles, the prostate gland, and Cowper's glands. Sperm are produced in the TESTES, beginning at PUBERTY, and are stored in the ampulla, from which they are released into the ejaculatory duct. The seminal vesicle produces a yellow, viscous fluid rich in fructose, PROSTAGLAND-INS, and amino acids. During EJACULATION, this fluid mixes with sperm in the ejaculatory duct, providing a favorable environment for sperm MOTILITY and survival. The prostate gland secretes a thin, milky, alkaline fluid that helps protect sperm from the acidic environment of the vagina. Cowper's glands secrete a clear, thick mucus that helps lubricate the urethra and neutralizes the acid of the male urethra and the female vagina, thus boosting sperm motility.

percutaneous umbilical blood sampling (PUBS) An experimental prenatal procedure for obtaining a blood sample from the FETUS in order to detect genetic disorders, blood disorders such as HEMOPHILIA, and infections such as toxoplasmosis. It can also be used for intrauterine blood transfusion or administration of medication to the fetus in utero. The clinician uses ULTRASOUND to guide the syringe needle through the abdominal wall, UTERUS, and AMNIOTIC SAC to the UMBILICAL CORD. Once inserted, the syringe can be used to withdraw a small sample of blood or to infuse medication. The test takes from 30 minutes to an hour, and sometimes causes bleeding and/or cramping. Test results are generally available within hours. PUBS can be performed as early as the 18th week of PREGNANCY; however, it appears to increase the risk of MISCARRIAGE.

perinatal mortality rate The number of fetal and neonatal deaths per 1,000 live births in a given population during a year. Fetal death is death in utero at 20 weeks' or more GESTATION; neonatal death is death between birth and 28 days of life.

perinatology The medical specialty concerned with diagnosis and treatment of high-risk conditions in the pregnant woman and her baby. In any PREGNANCY at risk, the woman needs to be near a perinatal center if at all possible so that she and the baby have access to care by a perinatologist.

perineum   The area of tissue between the female anus and VAGINA, and between the male anus and SCROTUM. During childbirth, the female perineum is stretched significantly and may tear, requiring surgical repair, and involve painful healing. Some OBSTETRICIANS perform EPISIOTOMY to prevent such tearing (laceration); however, this practice is controversial and many authorities believe that episiotomy increases rather than decreases the possibility of serious laceration. Perineal massage during late PREGNANCY is believed by some clinicians to decrease the risk of laceration. See EPISIOTOMY.

Immediately after birth, the perineum is often swollen and tender. Ice packs can offer relief by numbing the tissue. These should be applied for no more than 20 minutes with at least a 10-minute interval before reapplication. Later on, perineal discomfort can be relieved by SITZ BATHS, heat lamps, or anesthetic ointments (such as Nupercainal) or sprays (such as Dermoplast). To avoid burns, these preparations should *not* be applied before using a heat lamp. Sitting may be very uncomfortable for a few days and some women find a rubber "doughnut" helpful during this time. It is important to carefully clean the perineum after urinating or having a bowel movement, remembering to cleanse from front to back to avoid contamination of the VULVA from the anus, and to apply a fresh perineal pad (also from front to back). When wiping with toilet tissue, a blotting motion will prove more comfortable.

periodic breathing   A condition commonly found in PREMATURE INFANTS, involving sporadic episodes of APNEA (interruptions of breathing), not associated with cyanosis (bluish coloration of the skin due to reduced oxygen in the blood), and lasting about 10 seconds.

periods of reactivity   Predictable patterns of newborn behavior during the first few hours after birth.

Pfannenstiel incision   Also *bikini incision.* A horizontal (transverse) incision about five inches long in the lower abdomen just above the pubic hair. It is used for HYSTERECTOMY, CESAREAN DELIVERY, or abdominal TUBAL LIGATION, resulting in a less noticeable scar than the longer, vertical incision once used exclusively.

phenotype   The total physical, biochemical, and physiologic makeup of a person as determined by genetics and environment.

phenylketonuria (PKU)   An inherited metabolic disorder occurring once in 12,000 live births worldwide, characterized by the inability to convert excess phenylalanine into tyrosine. As excess phenylalanine accumulates in the blood, it causes progressive, severe mental retardation. Fortunately, PKU can be detected by means of a simple urine and BLOOD TEST as soon as the INFANT begins to digest food. Most states in the United States require PKU testing on all newborns. PKU is also detectable by CHORIONIC VILLUS SAMPLING. PKU occurs most commonly among white northern European and U.S. populations. It is rare in African, Japanese, or Jewish people.

Treatment consists of a DIET low in phenylalanine; this diet may need to be continued into adolescence. In addition, any woman who was diagnosed with PKU as a newborn needs to return to the low phenylalanine diet *before* becoming pregnant and during pregnancy. She should also avoid all foods sweetened with ASPARTAME (Equal® or NutraSweet®). Otherwise, her baby may be born too small, with abnormally small head circumference or other malformation, and possible mental retardation.

phlebitis   Inflammation of a vein. When this inflammation also involves a blood clot, it is called *thrombophlebitis*.

See also THROMBUS; EMBOLUS.

phlegmasia   Also *phlegmasia alba dolens, milk leg*. Inflammation of one of the deep veins (femoral, popliteal [behind the knee], or tibial [in the calf of the leg]). Symptoms may include EDEMA (swelling) of the ankle and leg, fever, and chills. The leg may be painful, pale (hence the name "milk leg"), and cool to the touch. At one time, this condition was very common, particularly after difficult LABOR; today, however, it is rare. Treatment includes bed rest with the leg(s) elevated, support stockings, ANALGESICS, and perhaps anticoagulants to prevent the formation of blood clots.

phototherapy   Treatment of NEONATAL JAUNDICE by exposure to light.

physiologic anemia of infancy   A temporary drop in the newborn's hemoglobin levels during the first 6 to 12 weeks after birth. Levels then revert to normal without treatment.

physiologic jaundice   A common, harmless condition of the newborn resulting from the normal reduction of red blood cells, occurring 48 or more hours after DELIVERY. Bilirubin levels peak at the fifth to seventh day, and the jaundice disappears between the seventh and tenth days of life.
See also NEONATAL JAUNDICE.

pica   The persistent eating of substances not ordinarily considered edible, such as clay, laundry starch, raw flour, baking powder, or baking soda. Pica is usually associated with PREGNANCY among poor women, and is believed to be part of a folk tradition rather than an actual dietary deficiency. This practice can be harmful to any woman but presents a real danger to the pregnant woman and her baby by blocking iron absorption, causing severe ANEMIA.

pineal body   A small gland, shaped like a pine cone, located in the brain, that produces the HORMONE melatonin, believed to inhibit the function of the sex glands (OVARIES, TESTES). However, its action is incompletely understood. Studies suggest that prolonged exposure to sunlight, such as occurs in Scandinavian countries during June and July, inhibits production of melatonin, thereby increasing FERTILITY and reducing depression.

Pitocin   Also *pit.* A brand name for synthetic OXYTOCIN, used to strengthen uterine CONTRACTIONS.

pituitary gland   Also *hypophysis.* An ENDOCRINE GLAND, located below and connected to the HYPOTHALAMUS just below the base of the brain. The pituitary gland has two lobes, anterior and posterior, each of which secretes specific HORMONES with specific functions, including interactions with other hormones.
The anterior pituitary secretes the following hormones: *thyroid-stimulating hormone* (TSH), which causes the THYROID gland to secrete thyroid hormones; *adrenocorticotropic hormone* (ACTH), which causes the ADRENAL GLANDS to secrete sex hormones; *growth hormone* (GH) or *somatotropic hormone* (STH), which stimulates growth and metabolism in bones, muscles, and other organs; LUTEINIZING HORMONE (LH), which causes the ovarian FOLLICLE to form the corpus luteum; FOLLICLE-STIMULATING HORMONE (FSH), which targets the female OVARIES, stimulating the development of the ovarian FOLLI-

CLE or the male seminiferous tubules, stimulating the production of SPERM; and PROLACTIN (*luteotropic hormone* [LTH]), which helps maintain the corpus luteum, secretes PROGESTERONE, and stimulates LACTATION (milk secretion). During PREGNANCY, the anterior pituitary may double or even triple in size, largely in response to increased prolactin secretion (10 to 20 times higher at the end of pregnancy than in a nonpregnant state).

The posterior pituitary secretes *antidiuretic hormone* (ADH), or *vasopressin,* which acts on the kidneys, and OXYTOCIN, which stimulates uterine CONTRACTIONS, secretion of milk, and aids the movement of sperm in the FALLOPIAN TUBES.

placenta   Also *afterbirth*. A specialized organ that develops on the lining of the UTERUS around the implanted EMBRYO, and the means through which nutrients, secretions, and oxygen are exchanged between the mother and the developing FETUS. The placenta is connected to the fetus by the UMBILICAL CORD.

The maternal portion of the placenta develops from the ENDOMETRIUM where the embryo implants, and makes up about one-fifth of the total placenta; its surface is red and flesh-like. The fetal portion develops from the CHORION, and makes up about four-fifths of the placenta; its surface is covered by the amniotic membrane and is shiny and gray. Placental development begins at the third week of GESTATION, stimulated by PROGESTERONE, secreted by the corpus luteum, and continues until about 20 weeks, when it covers about one-half the interior surface of the uterus, usually the upper portion. If located lower in the uterus, near the INTERNAL OS, it is termed PLACENTA PREVIA.

Once developed, the placenta itself secretes HORMONES essential to the growth and survival of the fetus: ESTROGEN, progesterone, HUMAN CHORIONIC GONADOTROPIN (HCG), and chorionic somatomammotropin. Estrogen promotes growth of the uterine muscles and blood vessels; progesterone prevents uterine CONTRACTIONS that might cause spontaneous ABORTION. HCG and chorionic somatomammotropin contribute to fetal growth.

During the birth process, the placenta normally detaches or separates from the uterine lining, and is expelled during the third stage of LABOR, after the baby has been delivered. Some clinicians assist the delivery of the placenta by gently pulling on the umbilical cord (controlled cord traction) and by administration of OXYTOCIN to enhance contractions and help control bleeding. If the placenta does not detach completely from the uterine lining, it may be removed by external pressure on the mother's uterus or with instruments. The birth attendant needs to examine the placenta carefully to be sure that no fragments have been retained in the uterus; otherwise, HEMORRHAGE and/or infection can result.

placenta accreta   A rare condition (once in 2,000 births) in which the PLACENTA adheres directly to the lining of the UTERUS rather than to an underlying layer called the *decidua basalis*. To avoid severe HEMORRHAGE in removing the placenta, HYSTERECTOMY must be performed. Factors associated with placenta accreta include PLACENTA PREVIA, previous CESAREAN DELIVERY, a prior DILATATION AND CURETTAGE (D & C), and grand multiparity (having had six or more deliveries).

placenta previa   A condition in which the PLACENTA is located over or close to the INTERNAL OS (the opening where the CERVIX flares into the body of the UTERUS) instead of in the upper portion of the uterus. Placenta previa carries a major risk of HEMORRHAGE since it is in the area of cervical dilatation and EFFACEMENT and can obstruct the baby's passage through the BIRTH CANAL. Placenta previa and ABRUPTIO PLACENTAE are the two principal causes of hemorrhage during the third TRIMESTER.

When the placenta completely covers the os, it is called *total previa*. When it partially covers the os, it is termed *partial previa*. If it is only near enough to the os as to risk detachment during LABOR, it is called *low-lying* or *marginal*. Placenta previa occurs approximately once in 200 births, and only 20% of these occurrences are total. Among grand multiparas (women with six or more previous births), however, it may occur once in every 20 births. Placenta previa may also be responsible for at least 5% of spontaneous ABORTIONS. Once this condition has occurred with a pregnancy, it is likely to recur in subsequent pregnancies.

Symptoms of placenta previa include spotting during the first and second trimester, followed by sudden, painless, profuse bleeding during the third trimester. Diagnosis involves ULTRASOUND, since manual vaginal or rectal examination is CONTRAINDICATED, except in a surgical setting.

Placenta previa jeopardizes the baby due to the potential of premature birth, and jeopardizes the mother with the risk of life-threatening hemorrhage. Thus most clinicians recommend hospitalization if this condition is suspected, delaying DELIVERY until the baby is sufficiently mature to survive.

Total placenta previa requires CESAREAN DELIVERY, as does any type of previa that involves severe bleeding or FETAL DISTRESS. In other cases, vaginal delivery may be possible; however, it requires careful monitoring of both mother and baby.

polycythemia   An excessive increase in the number of total red blood cells in the circulation (hematocrit value greater than 65%), affecting from 2 to 17% of newborns. It occurs more commonly in small and full-term INFANTS than in preterm babies. Symptoms include rapid heartbeat, respiratory distress, hyperbilirubinemia, decrease in peripheral pulses, discoloration of hands and feet, decreased urine output, or seizures. Controversy surrounds the treatment of asymptomatic infants; however, many authorities believe that all infants with polycythemia benefit from EXCHANGE TRANSFUSIONS to restore normal values. During the exchange transfusion, blood is removed from the infant and replaced, millimeter for millimeter, with fresh plasma.

polydactyly   A CONGENITAL ABNORMALITY characterized by extra fingers or toes. This condition is more common in Black infants.

polygalactia   Excessive secretion of breast milk, particularly at weaning.
    See also BREASTFEEDING; LACTATION.

polyhydramnios   Another term for HYDRAMNIOS.

polymenorrhea   MENSTRUAL CYCLE with less than a 20-day interval between periods, usually related to a HORMONE imbalance. It can also be caused by a uterine FIBROID, or may simply be a normal cycle for some women.

polyp   A soft, vascular, usually benign (noncancerous) tumor, generally attached to normal tissue by a stalk or pedicle; it may be round or fingerlike. Polyps most often develop from MUCOUS MEMBRANE, particularly that lining the nasal passages, gastrointestinal tract, and PELVIS.

cervical polyp   A polyp that grows in the cervical canal, most commonly near the endocervix, the entrance to the body of the UTERUS. Polyps occasionally grow near the ectocervix, the lower end of the cervical canal where it opens into the VAGINA. Endocervical polyps are more likely to bleed than ectocervical polyps, causing bleeding between menstrual periods or staining in postmenopausal women. However, they may cause no symptoms at all and be detected only during pelvic examination. Polyps are common in women over age 20 who have borne several children. Though most polyps are not cancerous, their potential for malignant change makes it advisable to remove all polyps when detected and to have them biopsied. This is usually an OUTPATIENT surgical procedure and can sometimes be performed in the clinician's office.

endometrial polyp   Also *intrauterine polyp, uterine polyp.* A polyp that develops from the ENDOMETRIUM (the uterine lining) in women ages 29 to 59, with the highest incidence in women over age 50. Polyps may be single or multiple and may range in size from 1 centimeter to masses that fill or even distend the uterus; they can grow into and through the CERVIX, projecting into the vagina. Like cervical polyps, endometrial polyps can cause bleeding and cramping, but they may be asymptomatic. They are removed by DILATATION AND CURETTAGE (D&C) and biopsied to rule out cancer; if they recur, either a myomectomy (removal of the polyps or tumors) or a HYSTERECTOMY may be necessary.

Pomeroy method   The most commonly used surgical technique for TUBAL LIGATION. The clinician raises a small section of each tube and ties a SUTURE, creating a loop of tube, which is then cut off. When the suture has been absorbed several weeks later, the two stumps of the tube retract, leaving a space between them. This technique cannot be used with LAPAROSCOPY.

positive signs of pregnancy   Objective indications that confirm PREGNANCY, usually not present until the fourth month. They include a fetal heartbeat, discernible with a fetoscope (weeks 17 to 20); fetal movements (after about 20 weeks); and ULTRASOUND observation of the gestational sac (5 to 6 weeks), fetal parts, and fetal heart movement (10 weeks).

postdate pregnancy   A pregnancy that lasts longer than 42 weeks.

posterior presentation   Also *posterior position.* The most common ABNORMAL PRESENTATION for birth in which the baby is head first in the BIRTH CANAL but facing toward the mother's belly instead of her back. The normal birth position is *anterior,* or facing the mother's back. Most babies gradually rotate into an anterior presentation, making delivery much easier; however, this sometimes happens only when the head has reached the pelvic floor. Posterior presentation tends to prolong LABOR and increase the woman's discomfort. If the baby does not rotate completely, the clinician will attempt external rotation, either manually or with FORCEPS. Forceps delivery almost always involves a large EPISIOTOMY; thus external rotation of the baby is much more desirable.

postmature   An infant born more than two weeks beyond the full 40 weeks of PREGNANCY who exhibits characteristics of the *postmaturity syndrome.* Only about 5% of post-term babies show signs of postmaturity syndrome, which include: HYPOGLYCEMIA (low blood sugar); MECONIUM aspiration, related to intrauterine hypoxia (lack of oxygen); POLYCYTHEMIA; CONGENITAL ABNORMALITIES; seizures; and cold stress. These complications result from inadequate placental function, decreased reserves of oxygen and glucose, prolonged exposure to amniotic fluid, and the stress of LABOR. Their long-term effects are unclear, and authorities disagree on whether these complications affect weight gain and/or IQ scores.

If pregnancy persists beyond 40 weeks, it is important to assess how well the PLACENTA is working. This is done by weekly or twice weekly measurement of the amount of estriol (an ESTROGEN produced by the placenta) in the mother's urine or blood. If the level is steady, there should be no problem for the baby. This test may also be combined with a weekly NONSTRESS TEST to evaluate fetal well-being. If either test suggests a problem, an immediate cesarean is essential.

postpartal hemorrhage   Blood loss that exceeds 500 milliliters after DELIVERY. Hemorrhage occurring within the first 24 hours is called *early* or *immediate;* that which occurs after the first 24 hours is called *late* or *delayed* hemorrhage.

postpartum   Also *puerperium, postnatal period.* The adjustment period following the birth of the baby during which time the woman adjusts both physically and psychologically to the process of childbearing. It lasts about six weeks, beginning immediately after birth, until the woman's body has returned to a near pre-pregnant state.

Immediate postpartum care includes measurement of the mother's temperature, pulse, respirations, and blood pressure every six hours. Most hospitals permit women to walk to the bathroom soon after DELIVERY, depending on whether the delivery was vaginal or cesarean, and the type of ANESTHESIA used, if any. Some women find it difficult to urinate after delivery and may need intermittent catheterization. Breast engorgement occurs within the first two days after birth; those women who choose to BREASTFEED will experience uterine CONTRACTIONS (AFTERPAINS) for several days afterward. Those who choose not to breastfeed may find that the engorgement lasts for several days.

If all indications are normal, most hospitals will discharge women within the first 24 to 48 hours after the birth (3 to 4 days for women who have CESAREAN DELIVERY). Once at home, the woman can begin to resume normal activity but needs additional rest and extra fluids if she is breastfeeding. Most clinicians recommend that vaginal intercourse be delayed until after the six-week checkup. Some women, however, prefer not to wait that long; others wish to wait longer.

Some authorities refer to the POSTPARTUM period as "the fourth trimester." During this time, the uterus contracts and descends into the PELVIS; the VAGINA decreases in size. LOCHIA, a vaginal discharge similar to menstrual flow, continues for three to four weeks. The PERINEUM begins to heal and gastrointestinal and urinary function return to normal. After an immediate weight loss of 10 to 12 pounds, the woman's weight gradually returns to pre-pregnant levels, provided she has gained the average 25 to 30 pounds.

The six-week checkup consists of measuring weight, blood pressure, and hemoglobin, plus BREAST and pelvic examinations. If using a DIAPHRAGM for birth control, a new fitting is appropriate at this time since size often changes after childbirth.

The principal postpartum complications are bleeding and infection, usually indicated by persistent pain, an odorous vaginal discharge, or a fever.

See also DEPRESSION, POSTPARTUM; POSTPARTAL HEMORRHAGE; PUERPERAL FEVER.

post-term infant   A baby born more than 42 weeks following the last menstrual period, occurring in about 4% of all pregnancies. The baby may or may not be considered POSTMATURE.

post-term labor   Labor that occurs after 42 weeks' GESTATION.

precipitous birth   An unusually rapid progression of LABOR, without a physician or nurse-MIDWIFE in attendance.

precipitous labor   Extremely rapid LABOR, lasting less than three hours. Precipitous labor is associated with multiparity (having given birth many times), large PELVIS, a history of precipitous labor, and a small baby in a favorable position; if any of these are the causes, complications are unlikely. However, precipitous labor can also result from OXYTOCIN overdose, in which case the CERVIX may not be ripe (soft) and the tissues of the VAGINA and PERINEUM unable to stretch adequately. This can result in lacerations of these tissues and in uterine rupture. It also endangers the baby by increasing pressure in and on his or her head.

preeclampsia
    See ECLAMPSIA.

pregnancy   The term during which a woman's UTERUS harbors a fertilized egg (ZYGOTE) that develops first into an EMBRYO and then into a FETUS; pregnancy begins with conception and ends with birth (DELIVERY). A *full-term pregnancy* lasts approximately nine months (39 to 40 weeks) and is divided into three equal time periods called TRIMESTERS.
    During pregnancy, a woman's body undergoes enormous physiological changes, beginning almost immediately after conception. (Changes in the egg, embryo, and fetus are described under GESTATION). The first signs of pregnancy are subjective, felt only by the woman, and can be caused by other conditions (see PRESUMPTIVE SIGNS OF PREGNANCY). These signs include AMENORRHEA, NAUSEA and vomiting (see MORNING SICKNESS), urinary FREQUENCY, BREAST tenderness, sleepiness and fatigue, and QUICKENING. Not all women experience all these signs, however, nor is each pregnancy the same for a particular woman.
    All the signs of pregnancy are caused by hormonal changes. The first measurable change is the appearance of HUMAN CHORIONIC GO-

NADOTROPIN in the urine, occurring within five to seven days of conception; this is the basis of every PREGNANCY TEST. Next, levels of PROGESTERONE and ESTROGEN begin to rise. Blood supply to the PELVIS increases (see CHADWICK'S SIGN; HEGAR'S SIGN). Within three or four weeks after conception, the pregnancy can be detected by ULTRASOUND.

In the second trimester, objective or PROBABLE SIGNS OF PREGNANCY can be measured, including enlargement of the abdomen, and the changed shape and size of the uterus. The sound of the fetal heart, a POSITIVE SIGN OF PREGNANCY, can be heard at 17 to 20 weeks' gestation. Skin changes occur (see CHLOASMA; LINEA NIGRA; STRIAE GRAVIDARUM). CONSTIPATION and HEARTBURN may occur as the expanding uterus crowds the gastrointestinal organs. As the uterus expands upward, however, it relieves pressure on the urinary BLADDER, decreasing the need for frequent urination.

VARICOSE VEINS may appear in the legs, VULVA, and/or rectum (HEMORRHOIDS), resulting from pressure by the enlarging uterus. Overall blood volume increases 30 to 50% over the course of the nine months, and the heart rate accelerates in order to pump this increased volume, causing some women to feel PALPITATIONS. Backache, leg cramps, increased perspiration and salivation are common problems; abdominal skin begins to itch as it stretches. Figure P-3 shows the changes in posture and body contour as pregnancy progresses. EDEMA may also be a problem; hands and feet tend to swell toward the end of the day and need to be elevated periodically.

As the uterus and abdomen continue to expand, other organs are further displaced, sometimes causing shortness of breath. Urinary frequency returns in the later months of pregnancy as the baby "drops" into the pelvic cavity. Stretch marks multiply and fatigue increases. The baby grows more active, and may disrupt the mother's sleep.

To ensure the well-being of both mother and baby, PRENATAL CARE should begin as soon as pregnancy is diagnosed. This usually means regular visits to a clinic, physician, or nurse-MIDWIFE to ensure that the pregnancy is progressing normally. These visits also offer opportunities to ask questions of the clinician and report observations of the physiological and psychological changes occurring. Two of the most important components of prenatal care are DIET and EXERCISE. Most women can and do continue their normal pre-pregnant activities, including sexual intercourse, throughout pregnancy.

Table P-2 Danger Signs in Pregnancy

Danger sign	Possible cause
Sudden gush of fluid from vagina	Premature rupture of membranes
Vaginal bleeding	Abruptio placentae, placenta previa, lesions of cervix or vagina, "bloody show"
Abdominal pain	Preterm labor, abruptio placentae
Temperature above 38.8°C (101°F) and chills	Infection
Dizziness, blurring of vision, double vision, spots before eyes	Hypertension, preeclampsia
Persistent vomiting	Hyperemesis gravidarum
Severe headache	Hypertension
Edema of hands, face, legs, and feet	Preeclampsia
Muscular irritability, convulsions	Preeclampsia
Epigastric pain	Preeclampsia—ischemia in major abdominal vessels
Oliguria	Renal impairment, decreased fluid intake
Dysuria	Urinary tract infection
Absence of fetal movement	Maternal medication, obesity, fetal death

Source: From *Maternal Newborn Nursing,* Fourth Edition, by S. Olds, M. London, and P. Ladewig. © 1992 by Addison-Wesley Nursing. Reprinted by permission.

Even with good care, unexpected complications can occur, and it is important to recognize the signs of complications requiring **emergency attention.** See Table P-2. **If any of the following occur, it is important to seek immediate emergency attention:** vaginal BLEEDING;

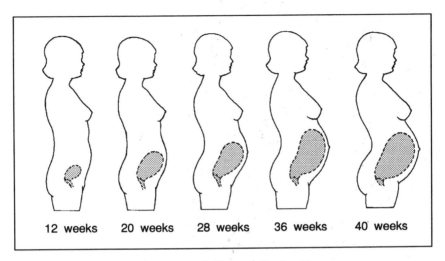

Figure P-3   Postural Changes During Pregnancy

(*From* Maternal Newborn Nursing, *Fourth Edition, by S. Olds, M. London, and P. Ladewig.* © *1992 by Addison-Wesley Nursing. Reprinted by permission.*)

severe or persistent abdominal pain; dimness or blurred vision; sudden puffiness or swelling of the face, eyelids, or fingers; chills and fever; intense persistent HEADACHE during the third trimester; absence of fetal movement for 24 hours or more after the fifth month; and RUPTURE OF THE MEMBRANES.

See also AMNIOTIC SAC; LABOR; PREGNANCY COUNSELING; PREGNANT PATIENT'S RIGHTS.

pregnancy counseling   Assisting a woman or couple in FAMILY PLANNING. This may be either *preconception* counseling, exploring the options related to whether and/or when to become pregnant, or *postconception* counseling related to an unplanned pregnancy.

BIRTH CONTROL and legalized ABORTION have made it possible for women and couples to plan their lives and to choose when and if they will become parents. Increasingly, couples are seeking advice before pregnancy to assess how children will affect their lifestyle and their relationship. This preconception counseling may or may not include GENETIC COUNSELING.

Postconception counseling assists the woman in evaluating the consequences of (1) continuing the pregnancy and keeping the child; (2) continuing the pregnancy and relinquishing the child to adoptive parents; or (3) terminating the pregnancy by abortion. Though every pregnant woman theoretically has these three choices, circumstances may make one or more of the choices unrealistic. When the pregnancy results from a RAPE, or when tests have shown that the FETUS is severely damaged, continuing the pregnancy might not be feasible. However, if a woman's personal beliefs oppose abortion, or if no abortion facility is available within her area and she is unable to travel, she may need help in evaluating her options as well as referral to appropriate community resources.

pregnancy-induced hypertension (PIH)
     See HYPERTENSION.

pregnancy, mask of
     See CHLOASMA.

pregnancy test   A test to detect PREGNANCY by measuring the levels of HUMAN CHORIONIC GONADOTROPIN (HCG) in either blood or urine. The do-it-yourself home test kits are done with a urine sample; they can be expensive, however, and can give false positive or false negative results. They can detect HCG as early as six days after CONCEPTION.

     BLOOD TESTS are the most accurate way to detect pregnancy. The Beta HCG test can detect pregnancy as early as nine days after implantation with 97 to 98% accuracy. Given four weeks after a woman's last period, the test is 100% accurate. Blood tests are preferable, not only because they are more accurate than URINE TESTS, but because they can determine whether the pregnancy is normal or ECTOPIC.

     Detecting the pregnancy early has several advantages: women who want to continue the pregnancy can begin prenatal self-care by eating a healthful diet and avoiding any potentially harmful substances (alcohol, tobacco, and other drugs); women who are considering ABORTION can seek counseling or early termination of the pregnancy while risk is minimal.

pregnant patient's rights   When childbirth moved from the home to the hospital during the early 20th century, it became a medical event managed by physicians and hospital staffs rather than a normal, family-centered, physiological event controlled by the laboring woman and supported by her partner and caregivers. During the 1960s and

(text continued on page 245)

Table P-3   Pregnant Patient's Bill of Rights

The Pregnant Patient has the right to participate in decisions involving her well-being and that of her unborn child, unless there is a clearcut medical emergency that prevents her participation. In addition to the rights set forth in the American Hospital Association's "Patient's Bill of Rights," the Pregnant Patient, because she represents *two* patients rather than one, should be recognized as having the additional rights listed below.

1. The Pregnant Patient has the right, prior to the administration of any drug or procedure, to be informed by the health professional caring for her of any potential direct or indirect effects, risks, or hazards to herself or her unborn or newborn infant which may result from the use of a drug or procedure prescribed for or administered to her during pregnancy, labor, birth, or lactation.

2. The Pregnant Patient has the right, prior to the proposed therapy, to be informed, not only of the benefits, risks, and hazards of the proposed therapy but also of known alternative therapy, such as available childbirth education classes which could help to prepare the Pregnant Patient physically and mentally to cope with the discomfort or stress of pregnancy and the experience of childbirth, thereby reducing or eliminating her need for drugs and obstetric intervention. She should be offered such information early in her pregnancy in order that she may make a reasoned decision.

3. The Pregnant Patient has the right, prior to the administration of any drug, to be informed by the health professional who is prescribing or administering the drug to her that any drug which she receives during pregnancy, labor, and birth, no matter how or when the drug is taken or administered, may adversely affect her unborn baby, directly or indirectly, and that there is no drug or chemical which has been proven safe for the unborn child.

4. The Pregnant Patient has the right if cesarean birth as anticipated, to be informed prior to the administration of any drug, and preferably prior to her hospitalization, that minimizing her and, in turn, her baby's intake of nonessential preoperative medicine will benefit her baby.

Table P-3   Pregnant Patient's Bill of Rights (continued)

5. The Pregnant Patient has the right, prior to the administration of a drug or procedure, to be informed of the areas of uncertainty if there is *no* properly controlled follow-up research which has established the safety of the drug or procedure with regard to its direct and/or indirect effects on the physiological, mental, and neurological development of the child exposed, via the mother, to the drug or procedure during pregnancy, labor, birth, or lactation—(this would apply to virtually all drugs and the vast majority of obstetric procedures).

6. The Pregnant Patient has the right, prior to the administration of any drug, to be informed of the brand name and generic name of the drug in order that she may advise the health professional of any past adverse reaction to the drug.

7. The Pregnant Patient has the right to determine for herself, without pressure from her attendant, whether she will accept the risks inherent in the proposed therapy or refuse a drug or procedure.

8. The Pregnant Patient has the right to know the name and qualifications of the individual administering a medication or procedure to her during labor or birth.

9. The Pregnant Patient has the right to be informed, prior to the administration of any procedure, whether that procedure is being administered to her for her or her baby's benefit (medically indicated) or as an elective procedure (for convenience, teaching purposes or research).

10. The Pregnant Patient has the right to be accompanied during the stress of labor and birth by someone she cares for, and to whom she looks for emotional comfort and encouragement.

11. The Pregnant Patient has the right after appropriate medical consultation to choose a position for labor and for birth which is least stressful to her baby and to herself.

12. The Obstetric Patient has the right to have her baby cared for at her bedside if her baby is normal, and to feed her baby according to her baby's needs rather than according to the hospital regimen.

13. The Obstetric Patient has the right to be informed in writing of the name of the person who actually delivered her baby and the professional qualifications of that person. This information should also be on the birth certificate.

Table P-3   Pregnant Patient's Bill of Rights (continued)

14. The Obstetric Patient has the right to be informed if there is any known or indicated aspect of her or her baby's care or condition which may cause her or her baby later difficulty or problems.

. . . .

15. The Obstetric Patient has the right to have her and her baby's hospital medical records complete, accurate, and legible and to have their records, including Nurses' Notes, retained by the hospital until the child reaches the age of majority, or to have the records offered to her before they are destroyed.

. . . .

16. The Obstetric Patient, both during and after her hospital stay, has the right to have access to her complete medical records, including Nurses' Notes, and to receive a copy upon payment of a reasonable fee and without incurring the expense of retaining an attorney.

. . . .

It is the obstetric patient and her baby, not the health professional, who must sustain any trauma or injury resulting from the use of a drug or obstetric procedure. The observation of the rights listed above will not only permit the obstetric patient to participate in the decisions involving her and her baby's health care, but will help to protect the health professional and the hospital against litigation arising from resentment or misunderstanding on the part of the mother.

. . . .

Prepared by Doris Haire, Chair, Committee on Health Law and Regulation, International Education Association, Inc., Rochester NY. Reprinted by permission.

early 1970s, childbearing couples began to demand a voice in where and how their children were born, favoring less technology and more education and psychological support. That grass roots movement eventually changed hospital and medical practice in many areas of the country and led to various expressions of patients' rights. Table P-3 shows one such statement.

premature infant   Also *preemie* (slang). Any baby born before 38 weeks' GESTATION; also defined as an INFANT with a BIRTH WEIGHT of less than 2,500 grams (about 5.5 pounds). Premature babies risk many complications that threaten their ability to survive. However, advances in medical knowledge and technology have enabled many tiny premature babies not only to survive but to thrive, providing they have access to special care. Most infants born after 35 weeks' gestation and/or weighing 2,500 grams or more have a good chance for survival including normal growth and development. Those who are born earlier or weigh less face greater risk of death or permanent impairment. These parameters apply to white infants; babies of other ethnic groups are normally smaller and may survive at lesser weights. Generally, however, babies weighing under 500 grams (1.1 pounds) have no chance of survival; those who weigh between 500 and 999 grams (1.1 to 2.2 pounds) have a poor chance; and those who weigh 1,000 to 2,499 grams (2.2 to 5.5 pounds) have a variable chance, ranging from poor to good, depending on their weight, their lung maturity, and the care they receive. See also APGAR SCORE.

In North America, prematurity is the leading cause of neonatal death, responsible for about 50% of such deaths. Eighty percent of these newborns die within the first 24 hours, despite improved pediatric care. Authorities believe that good PRENATAL CARE and good maternal health can help prevent much of the prematurity that occurs, even though more than half the cases of prematurity are due to unknown causes.

Women at higher-than-normal risk for premature labor and birth include those under age 20 or over age 40, those who smoke or use addictive drugs, those from lower socioeconomic groups (who are less likely to have adequate nutrition and early prenatal care), those women whose mothers were given DIETHYLSTILBESTROL, and those with MULTIPLE PREGNANCY.

premenstrual syndrome (PMS)   Also *premenstrual tension syndrome, congestive dysmenorrhea.* A group of symptoms experienced by some women a few days before their menstrual periods begin. These symptoms can include bloating, HEADACHE, irritability, depression, anxiety, hostility, sleep disorders, vertigo, acne, breast tenderness, CONSTIPATION, diarrhea, NAUSEA, vomiting, and craving for sweets.

prenatal care   Care of the expectant woman within the context of her support system—her partner and/or family—throughout her PREGNANCY. Unless the woman is in a high-risk category, this care can be supervised by a nurse-MIDWIFE. It consists primarily of monitoring the progress of the pregnancy, teaching the woman and her partner about the physiological and psychological changes that are occurring, and helping them to anticipate future changes as they prepare for the birth of their child. The goal of prenatal care is the birth of a healthy baby to a healthy mother who is part of a healthy family. It is designed to detect any sign of potential complications in the natural process, and to implement preventive or therapeutic measures wherever possible. Such problems as urinary tract infection (UTI), genital HERPES, HIV (AIDS), preeclampsia, and ECTOPIC PREGNANCY must be treated promptly to avoid life-threatening situations.

Choosing a caregiver for pregnancy and a facility for birth should be done with great care. It is important to consider the location of the facility, the convenience of the hours, the professional qualifications of the staff, the cost, and the overall approach of the caregiver to pregnancy and birth. Does the caregiver view pregnancy and birth as an illness or a natural life process? Does he or she take time to answer questions willingly and clearly? Is HOME BIRTH a possibility? What about ANESTHESIA? EPISIOTOMY? What do other patients say about the care?

The first prenatal visit is generally a long one, including a complete medical history, particularly any previous pregnancies; a complete physical examination, including BREAST and pelvic examinations; measurement of height, weight, blood pressure, temperature, pulse, respirations; and several laboratory tests. The laboratory tests include a CBC (complete blood count) and BLOOD TESTS for SYPHILIS, blood type (in the event transfusion is necessary), RH-FACTOR, and ANTIBODY levels; a test for GONORRHEA; a PAP SMEAR; and a URINE TEST and culture. African-American women need to be tested for SICKLE CELL ANEMIA and Jewish women for TAY-SACHS DISEASE.

When the examination and tests are completed, the clinician should provide information on DIET, EXERCISE, general hygiene, and sexual activity, and answers to any questions the woman or her partner may have. Childbirth preparation classes may be discussed at any time during the pregnancy, but usually the classes do not begin until the last TRIMESTER.

Subsequent visits generally will be brief, involving only a check of blood pressure, weight, and urine, plus external examination of the abdomen, listening to the fetal heartbeat, and measuring the expanding UTERUS. These visits occur monthly through 28 weeks, then every two weeks until 36 weeks, and weekly until DELIVERY.

See also DIET; HIGH-RISK PREGNANCY; PELVIMETRY; PREGNANT PATIENTS' RIGHTS; WEIGHT GAIN.

prep   Shaving of the pubic area, formerly a routine practice prior to DELIVERY but now controversial. Some clinicians believe that a skin prep makes postpartum surgical repair of the perineal area easier and prevents infection. Others believe that a prep is unnecessary. Women who do not want a prep can request that it be omitted; this should be discussed with the clinician early in the PREGNANCY.

prepared childbirth   Also *natural childbirth, childbirth education.* A philosophical approach to childbirth based on education about PREGNANCY, LABOR, and birth, as a means to a less anxious, more satisfying birth experience for the woman and her partner. There are many different variations on this approach, but principally three schools of thought: DICK-READ METHOD; Lamaze (See PSYCHOPROPHY-LACTIC METHOD), and BRADLEY METHOD. All involve the woman's part-ner or another labor coach and minimize the use of technology and medications. In choosing a method of childbirth preparation, it is important that the approach of the method not conflict seriously with the approach of the caregiver. Small classes are best: no more than ten couples and preferably only five or six. Hospital classes may not offer alternatives nor encourage women to take an active role in birth, but instead teach women and their partners how to be good consumers of the hospital's prescribed program. Some communities offer a wide range of classes to choose from; others may be limited. If suitable classes are not available, videos or books may provide a rea-sonable substitute.

See also NATURAL CHILDBIRTH.

prepuce   Also *foreskin.* A hood or sheath of skin, partially retract-able, covering the PENIS in men and the CLITORIS in women. CIRCUMCI-SION is a surgical removal of part of the prepuce, commonly performed in male infants for hygienic or religious purposes, but deemed unnec-essary by the American Academy of Pediatrics. Female circumcision is still performed in some developing countries as a rite of passage.

presentation   Description of which fetal body part is leading the way through the BIRTH CANAL and "presenting" at the introitus (outer opening of the VAGINA). The most common presentation is CEPHALIC (head first); BREECH and SHOULDER presentations are abnormal and thus termed malpresentations.

presenting part   During birth, the part of the baby that "presents" at the vaginal opening, normally the head. The rump or sometimes a foot is the presenting part in a BREECH PRESENTATION. In a SHOULDER PRESENTATION, the baby is lying crosswise in the UTERUS (TRANSVERSE LIE) and thus the shoulder is the presenting part.

presumptive signs of pregnancy   Symptoms that suggest the possibility of PREGNANCY, but do not confirm it. These include AMENORRHEA (absence of menstruation), QUICKENING (sensing the movement of the FETUS), and MORNING SICKNESS.

preterm labor   Labor that begins between 20 and 38 weeks of PREGNANCY.

primagravida   A women who is pregnant for the first time.

primipara   A woman who has given birth to her first baby after reaching the point of viability, whether or not that child is living or was alive at birth.

probable signs of pregnancy   Strong indications of pregnancy, including a positive PREGNANCY TEST, enlarging abdomen, positive GOODELL'S and HEGAR'S signs, and BRAXTON HICKS CONTRACTIONS.

progesterone   A HORMONE produced by the corpus luteum, the ADRENAL GLAND, and the PLACENTA, that stimulates the buildup of the ENDOMETRIUM (uterine lining) in preparation for IMPLANTATION of a fertilized egg. Once the egg is implanted, progesterone helps maintain the developing PREGNANCY. If no egg is implanted, the lining is sloughed off as menstrual flow and the decreased levels of progesterone and ESTROGEN initiate the cycle again. During pregnancy, progesterone prevents uterine CONTRACTIONS and stimulates BREAST development. At OVULATION, progesterone triggers a slight temperature rise (about one degree Fahrenheit). See BASAL BODY TEMPERATURE METHOD.

Synthetic progesterone, *progestin,* is used to control excessive anovulatory bleeding, in ENDOMETRIOSIS, and in some types of endometrial cancer. It is also combined with estrogen in ORAL CONTRACEPTIVES and in estrogen replacement therapy, where it is believed to reduce the possibility of estrogen-induced cancer.

One synthetic progesterone, medoxyprogesterone acetate (Depo-Provera), was approved by the U.S. Food and Drug Administration (FDA) in 1992 as a female contraceptive, administered by injection once every three months. This approval came despite the objections of many women's groups, including the National Women's Health Network, that remain concerned about its association with increased incidence of breast and uterine cancer in animals, and cervical cancer and irregular bleeding in humans. It is also used in many countries outside the United States.

Progestins should be avoided during pregnancy and by women with JAUNDICE or other liver disease, kidney disorders, or Addison's disease.

progestin   Also *progestogen*. Synthetic PROGESTERONE, used in ORAL CONTRACEPTIVES and other medications.

prognosis   A prediction of the likely outcome of a disease or disorder. A favorable prognosis suggests that recovery will be complete; a poor prognosis means that recovery may be limited or even impossible.

prolactin   Also *luteotrophin, luteotropic hormone, LTH*. A HORMONE produced by the anterior PITUITARY that stimulates and maintains LACTATION and inhibits the production of the pituitary HORMONES, LH (LUTEINIZING HORMONE) and FSH (FOLLICLE-STIMULATING HORMONE), which stimulate OVULATION. In this way, BREASTFEEDING acts as a kind of birth control, though not a totally reliable method. Lactation without giving birth is called GALACTORRHEA, and is caused by the lack of PIF (prolactin-inhibiting factor), a substance produced by the HYPOTHALAMUS.

prolapsed cord   An UMBILICAL CORD that drops in front of or beside the PRESENTING PART in the BIRTH CANAL. This jeopardizes the baby's oxygen supply when the cord is compressed. This condition seldom occurs with VERTEX (head-first presentations) if the head is engaged when the membranes rupture. When the head is not engaged, or the baby is very small or malpositioned (BREECH or SHOULDER PRESENTATIONS), however, the cord can slip into the VAGINA when the membranes rupture. Management of this problem depends on how far the CERVIX is dilated and how the baby is positioned. If the cervix is fully dilated, immediate DELIVERY can usually save the baby's life. If the cervix is only partially dilated and the baby is full-term, immediate CESAREAN DELIVERY is the only option. Even with prompt response, however, prolapsed cord proves fatal in more than 15% of cases.

prolapsed uterus Also *fallen uterus*. Relaxation of the pelvic muscles, which allows the uterus to collapse and protrude down into the VAGINA and even beyond the vaginal opening. This can result in serious irritation, discharge, and bleeding. Symptoms include a feeling of heaviness or pressure in the vagina, STRESS INCONTINENCE, and back pain. This problem often is associated with a prolapsed bladder or rectum (see CYSTOCELE; RECTOCELE). Treatment may be unnecessary in mild cases which may be relieved by KEGEL EXERCISES, and, in overweight women, by weight loss. More severe prolapse may require surgical correction.

prolonged labor LABOR that exceeds the medically established norms. The first stage of labor is divided into three phases: *latent, active, and transition. Prolonged latent labor* is defined as latent labor lasting more than 20 hours for a first baby and more than 14 hours for subsequent babies. *Prolonged active labor* is any labor resulting in less CERVICAL DILATATION than 1.2 centimeters per hour for a first baby and 1.5 centimeters per hour for subsequent babies. Labor is also considered prolonged if CONTRACTIONS stop at any point. The second stage of labor is considered prolonged when it exceeds two hours, and the third stage when it exceeds 15 to 30 minutes.

These standards are somewhat artificial and are established by physicians who seldom witness an entire course of labor in a single patient. Nurse-MIDWIVES and independent midwives tend to view labor as more of a continuous process without precise time limits. Prolonged labor can be tiring for the mother but is seldom dangerous; it can, however, endanger the baby, particularly if the problem is MAL-PRESENTATION or CEPHALOPELVIC DISPROPORTION. If neither of these factors is present, the clinician may perform AMNIOTOMY (rupture of membranes) to speed up the process, or administer OXYTOCIN to strengthen contractions. However, oxytocin carries its own risk and both mother and baby must be carefully monitored during its use.

See also INDUCTION OF LABOR.

prophylactic The clinical term for *preventive*. Having one's teeth cleaned by a dental hygienist, for example, is prophylactic care designed to prevent cavities.

It is also another name for a CONDOM, worn to prevent PREGNANCY and/or transmission of SEXUALLY TRANSMITTED DISEASES (STDs).

prostaglandins (PGs)   A group of complex fatty acids manufactured in many body tissues and highly concentrated in the female reproductive tract and PLACENTA during PREGNANCY. Not all their functions are clearly understood; however, some of them stimulate uterine CONTRACTIONS and thus have been used in ABORTION and in INDUCTION OF LABOR.

protein in urine
See ALBUMIN, URINARY.

pseudomenstruation   Blood-tinged vaginal discharge in the newborn female due to withdrawal of maternal HORMONES present during PREGNANCY. This condition occurs during the first week of life and disappears without treatment.

psychogenic   Originating in or caused by the mind, such as the appearance of disease symptoms without apparent physical cause. For example, a person may complain of HEADACHE or backache, and yet medical examination will not reveal any physical reason for the pain. Such symptoms can be related to brief emotional stress or a more severe psychological disorder such as depression.
See also PSYCHOSOMATIC.

psychoprophylactic method   Also *Lamaze method.* A leading method of PREPARED CHILDBIRTH, devised by a French physician, Fernand Lamaze. It includes education about the physiology of birth as well as exercises and breathing patterns to be used before and during LABOR and DELIVERY. The term "psychoprophylactic" was coined from words meaning "mind" and "preventive" and suggests that the mind can prevent or minimize painful sensations.

This method is taught in a series of classes which the woman and her labor partner attend, beginning in the seventh month of pregnancy. The partner's role is to offer physical and psychological support and encouragement, to time CONTRACTIONS, and to remind the woman which kind of breathing to use.
See also BRADLEY METHOD; DICK-READ METHOD.

psychosomatic   Describes a physical symptom or illness related to emotional factors in a way not clearly understood. The illness is real and apparent to the clinician, but may be triggered or made worse by psychological factors.

ptyalism   Excessive salivation, an infrequent but troublesome problem in PREGNANCY; its cause is unknown and effective treatments are limited. Astringent mouthwash, chewing gum, or hard candy may offer some relief.

puberty   The life stage at which individuals achieve sexual maturity. Female puberty begins at age 9 or 10; male puberty begins between ages 12 and 14. During this time girls experience a growth spurt and begin to develop BREASTS and pubic and underarm hair. Their body contours change as ESTROGEN stimulates the deposit of body fat on upper arms, buttocks, hips and thighs. Soon thereafter, they experience MENARCHE, the onset of menstruation. Male puberty also includes a growth spurt and changes in body contours. Increased levels of ANDROGENS increase muscularity in the upper torso and stimulate the growth of pubic hair, underarm hair, and sweat glands, leading to increased perspiration.

pubic lice   Also *crab lice, crabs, pediculosis pubis*. A tiny parasitic insect that infests pubic hair, underarm hair, and eyebrows. Generally spread by sexual contact, pubic lice can also be spread through infested bedding or clothing. The female louse lays her eggs at the base of hair shafts where they reproduce within seven to nine days. The usual symptom is intense itching unrelieved by scratching, which only serves to spread the infestation. Pubic lice should be treated with specially prepared over-the-counter preparations available as cream, lotion, or shampoo. All clothing and bedding should also be thoroughly washed.

pubococcygeous muscle
    See KEGEL EXERCISES.

pudendum
    See VULVA.

pudendal anesthesia
    See under ANESTHESIA.

puerperal fever   Also *childbed fever, postpartum infection, puerperal sepsis*. A POSTPARTUM infection of the reproductive tract, usually the ENDOMETRIUM. Its name reflects the most common sign of postpartum infection: elevated temperature (fever) of 38 degrees Centigrade (100.4 degrees Fahrenheit) or higher on any two of the first 10 postpartum days.

Puerperal fever was the leading cause of maternal mortality until the mid-19th century when Ignaz Semmelweis, an Austrian physician, surmised that the infection was spread by the unwashed hands of physicians, midwives, and medical students. Many of these clinicians went directly from working on cadavers in the anatomy laboratory to the bedsides of laboring women, without stopping to wash their hands. Small wonder that infections spread. Semmelweis ordered all persons who examined laboring women to disinfect their hands with chlorine solution, dramatically dropping the MATERNAL MORTALITY rate from 10% to 1% almost immediately. Despite this compelling evidence, however, his theory was not accepted for many years and outbreaks of puerperal fever continued in hospitals in the United States as late as 1968. Eventually, improved aseptic techniques and antibiotic therapies greatly reduced the number of deaths from puerperal fever.

Streptococcus is the most common infectious organism in puerperal fever and usually invades during LABOR. Treatment is determined by the kind of organism as isolated by laboratory analysis. In recent years, another severe, potentially fatal postpartum infection has been associated with *Staphylococcus aureus:* TOXIC SHOCK SYNDROME, originally associated with tampon use, although the mechanism remains unclear. Symptoms include high fever, vomiting, dizziness, diarrhea, a sunburn-like rash, and rapid drop in blood pressure. Prompt treatment with antibiotics is essential.

puerperal morbidity   A maternal temperature of 100.4 degrees Fahrenheit (38.0 degrees Celsius) or higher on any two of the first 10 days after DELIVERY, except for the first 24 hours. The temperature should be taken at least four times daily using an oral thermometer.

puerperium   The period of time after DELIVERY of the PLACENTA until complete involution of the UTERUS (return to its pre-pregnant size), usually about six weeks.

pyelonephritis   Inflammation of the kidney, most commonly the result of bacterial infection that has migrated upward from the URETHRA and ureters into the kidney. Unless it is treated, permanent damage to the kidney can occur, impairing its ability to rid the body of harmful wastes. It is common during PREGNANCY and in the POSTPARTUM period, particularly if a urinary CATHETER has been inserted. Pyelonephritis is an acute illness with chills, high fever, flank pain, NAUSEA and vomiting, plus pain and burning on urination. Antibiotics are the usual treatment, plus drinking six to eight glasses of water each day. It is important to empty the BLADDER frequently and wear cotton-crotch underwear so that air can circulate around the genital area. Women with any urinary tract infection should practice careful perineal hygiene, always wiping from front to back so that bacteria from the bowel are not carried into the urethra.

quickening The first movements of the FETUS, felt by the pregnant woman sometime between 16 and 18 weeks' GESTATION. This first flutter of life normally progresses into more active and noticeable movements in later PREGNANCY, and also can be felt by placing a hand on the lower abdomen. Movement of the fetus is supported by the amniotic fluid in which it floats. External pressure on the ABDOMEN or against the CERVIX causes the fetus to move away and then rebound to its original position, a passive movement called *ballottement*. After the 30th week of pregnancy, absence of fetal movements for more than 24 hours indicates fetal jeopardy and should be reported to the clinician at once.

See also FETAL MONITORING.

R

rabbit test   A test to determine PREGNANCY by injecting a woman's urine into an ear vein of a mature female virgin rabbit. Should the woman be pregnant, the hormonal substance HUMAN CHORIONIC GO-NADOTROPIN (HCG) induces ovulation in the rabbit within 16 to 48 hours. Also known as the Friedman test, this pregnancy assessment method was replaced by immunologic and other biologic tests in the 1960s.

radiation   A type of heat loss in the newborn, when body heat is transferred to cooler surfaces and objects not in direct contact with the INFANT. Because of their relative mass, body size, and limited amount of insulating fat, newborns lose about four times the body heat of a grown adult.
   See also EVAPORATION.

radioreceptor assay   A highly sensitive BLOOD TEST using radioio-dine to assess PREGNANCY. Developed in the 1970s, it works by detect-ing the pregnancy hormone HUMAN CHORIONIC GONADOTROPIN (HCG) in the bloodstream but can mistake very low levels and yield false negative results. Another such test is the *radioimmunoassay* which also detects pregnancy by relying on the competition of HCG to be measured with radioactively labeled HCG. Both can be performed in about an hour and achieve a positive result in more than 99% of pregnant women, but they should be repeated after a week to ensure accuracy.

rape   Any sexual contact against a person's will. Although legal defi-nitions vary by state in the United States, rape is an act of violence, not of sexual desire, and women and children are its principal victims. The term *sexual assault* is also used to describe physically forced or coerced acts of sexual aggression including anal, vaginal, and oral intercourse. Force may constitute anything from the use of weapons to the threat of withdrawn economic support. Of reported rapes, approximately half are committed by a friend or relative of the woman attacked *(acquaintance rape, date rape),* and half occur in her own home. It is estimated that these statistics are low because a woman is less likely to report a rape under such circumstances. It has been proven that the majority of rapes are planned, involve threat of weapons or force, and are usually committed by married men with regular sexual partners. It is a crime motivated by power, control, and anger, not sexual desire. Incidence of rape in the United States, particularly acquaintance rape, is increasing. Current estimates suggest that one in three women will be raped during her lifetime.

Societal myths can influence a culture's understanding of rape (for example, rapists are sex-crazed lunatics, victims must have somehow "asked for it," and are responsible for the rape), but rape is a community responsibility and education has begun to alter views. Fear of rape works to control women in society by limiting their choices and activities as they may feel a need for protection and to be on constant alert. Unfortunately, many rapists have not been held accountable for their actions and the legal process for the woman often victimizes her a second time. The work of rape awareness groups, however, has helped to address issues of treatment, law enforcement, and community responsibility regarding rape. Survivors are now better able to secure medical care and pursue legal action against their attackers. DNA "fingerprinting," or identification based on blood and semen samples, is one more recent method helping to correctly identify rapists. Hair or tissue of her assailant found on the woman's clothes or body may also help in identification.

Rape puts a woman at risk for immediate injury, SEXUALLY TRANSMITTED DISEASES (STDs), and PREGNANCY. She may interrupt the possibility of conception by taking the MORNING-AFTER PILL within 72 hours after the assault or by using a *menstrual extraction kit* at the time of her next period; she may also choose a therapeutic ABORTION. Antibiotics are usually administered to prevent STDs, but an INTRAUTERINE DEVICE (IUD) should be avoided as a birth control method after a rape because of increased infection rates from transmitted bacteria.

Rape survivors often experience serious traumatic reaction (*rape trauma syndrome*), including extreme depression, anger, phobias, sexual dysfunction, and blame, as a result of attack. Once immediate medical care is assured, a woman needs to seek rape counseling to resolve post-traumatic stress, either at a hospital, rape crisis center, or other community resource where professional help may be available. The rights of rape survivors include nonjudgmental support by health care providers, respect and confidentiality, the need to answer only relevant questions regarding the rape, information regarding all proposed treatments and their potential risks, and legal advice.

See also CONTRAGESTIVE; SEXUALLY TRANSMITTED DISEASE (STD).

reciprocal inhibition   An approach to deep relaxation technique based on the principle that it is impossible to feel relaxed and tense at the same time. Relaxation exercises decreasing pain and anxiety in PREGNANCY and childbirth are guided by this premise and include breathing techniques, muscle relaxation, and imagery.

recommended dietary allowance (RDA)   Officially recommended allowances of specific vitamins, minerals, and other nutrients by the U.S. federal government. Although nutritional requirements vary according to the individual, the human body requires approximately 40 nutrients and most are provided by a well-balanced DIET. RDAs typically exceed daily requirements for most people because they are set above the estimated average. Therefore, a daily diet falling short of the RDA does not necessarily mean it is insufficient, but it does increase the risk of inadequate intake. Maternal and fetal development requires increases of essential recommended nutrients; deficiencies can significantly affect cell and organ development.

rectocele   Also *proctocele*. Intrusion of the rectum into the VAGINA due to weakened pelvic muscles that normally hold it in place, resulting in bulging of the posterior vaginal wall. After one or more difficult births or surgery, or during old age, some women experience uterine prolapse or "falling" of the UTERUS into the vagina accompanied by rectocele and CYSTOCELE, or falling of the BLADDER. Rectocele is usually painful during bowel movement pressure and some women with the condition insert a finger into their vagina to hold back the rectal wall when they defecate. Rectocele may also reflect a congenital weakness. It often can be corrected with minor reconstructive surgery.

regional anesthesia
See under ANESTHESIA.

relaxin   A water-soluble protein secreted primarily from the corpus luteum that inhibits activity in the UTERUS and induces softening of the CERVIX. It is detectable in a pregnant woman's serum at the time of her first missed menstrual period. *Porcine relaxin* is the hormone extracted from the corpus luteum of the female pig and used as a cervical softening or "ripening" agent. Some trials have indicated its use results in lower CESAREAN DELIVERY rates while others offer no practical evidence to prove beneficial uterine effects. Although approximately 25% of women experience labor during ripening with relaxin administration, researchers say it requires further study before being adopted as clinical practice.

See also INDUCTION OF LABOR.

remission   Temporary or permanent abatement or disappearance of a chronic or malignant disease. As a term, remission is most commonly used in cases of serious illness that tend to recur and advance such as cancer and multiple sclerosis. Remission may occur spontaneously or with treatment and, in some cases, becomes permanent.

respiratory distress syndrome (RDS)   An acute respiratory disease in the newborn due to immaturity of the lungs.

See also HYALINE MEMBRANE DISEASE.

retroflexed uterus   A tilting or bending backward of the UTERUS whereby the cervical neck touches the body of the uterus. The condition is often considered normal and may not be problematic.

See also RETROVERTED UTERUS; UTERUS.

retrolental fibroplasia   A potentially blinding eye condition in PREMATURE INFANTS caused by excessive levels of OXYGEN administered within the first few days of life. Retrolental fibroplasia results when excessive levels of oxygen lead to the formation of vascular tissue behind the lens, abnormal development of the retina, and slowed eye growth. Infants with RESPIRATORY DISTRESS SYNDROME may initially require high oxygen levels, but they should be carefully monitored to prevent toxicity.

See also OXYGEN IN CHILDBIRTH; OXYGEN TOXICITY.

retroverted uterus   Also *tipped uterus, tipped womb.* Normally, the UTERUS is positioned at a right angle to the VAGINA, but stretched ligaments resulting from PREGNANCY, congenital inheritance, or history of infection could cause the uterus to be pulled back so far as to be adjacent to the vagina. Of those 25 to 30% of women developing a retroverted uterus, not all experience adverse effects or require treatment. Symptoms can include dull backache or pain during vaginal intercourse.

Formerly, uterine suspension surgery was conducted to correct a retroverted uterus. Today treatment typically consists of adjusting the vaginal position with a specially designed ring. Women with this condition who find conception difficult are advised to try alternatives to "missionary" style intercourse.

See also RETROFLEXED UTERUS; UTERUS.

Rh factor   A specific ANTIGEN, or bodily substance inducing the production of ANTIBODIES, found in the blood of persons whose blood is considered Rh-positive. Without the Rh factor, the blood is considered Rh-negative. Should an Rh-negative woman and an Rh-positive man conceive an Rh-positive baby, her body may produce antibodies to attack Rh-positive blood in the FETUS, resulting in *Rh incompatibility.* The Rh factor is present in 85% of the population and Rh incompatibility occurs in approximately 0.5% of pregnancies. Consequences for Rh-positive infants include STILLBIRTH, ANEMIA, and severe sickness requiring transfusion with Rh-negative blood. Methods of fetal and intrauterine transfusion have been developed whereby Rh-negative blood can be injected directly into the mother's ABDOMEN or UMBILICAL CORD to reduce risk. Early birth is another option, but it carries its own risks.

The preventive vaccine for Rh incompatibility is RhOGAM. If administered within several days of DELIVERY or ABORTION to an Rh-negative woman who has previously conceived, it blocks the formation of Rh antibodies in future pregnancies. All women continuing a pregnancy should undergo Rh factor BLOOD TESTS if there is a chance the father is Rh-negative or a transfusion may have caused the formation of antibodies in the woman's blood. Should the results prove positive, antibody levels must be checked regularly by means of an indirect COOMBS' TEST of the mother's blood, and ULTRASOUND scanning to determine fetal condition. Most Rh-negative women do not experience difficult pregnancy, but 10 to 15% do become sensitized thereafter. Of these, RhoGAM eliminates risk in 90% of subsequent pregnancies, but it must be administered again following birth or termination of the pregnancy.

See also COOMBS' TEST; RhoGAM.

RhoGAM Rh immunoglobulin administered to prevent maternal sensitivity to the Rh blood antigen and to prevent future fetal complication. It is injected within 72 hours of birth in those Rh-negative women delivering Rh-positive babies so that ANTIBODY production is obstructed in the mother at the time of placental separation and fetal blood absorption. It is also given maternally at 28 weeks' GESTATION to prevent HEMORRHAGE. Should the mother become sensitized, the production of positive Rh blood cells with subsequent pregnancies may cause her immune system to attack the FETUS and induce MISCARRIAGE or result in ANEMIA or retardation. RhoGAM is also injected if maternal sensitization cannot be assessed, and with every ABORTION, ECTOPIC PREGNANCY, and AMNIOCENTESIS in the nonsensitized Rh-negative woman conceiving with a partner who has Rh-positive or unknown blood type.

See also COOMBS' TEST; RH FACTOR.

rhythm method Also *natural family planning, rhythm system, calendar method.* A method of FERTILITY awareness based on observing natural bodily cycles. The rhythm method of birth control is based on abstinence from sexual intercourse during a woman's monthly fertile period, or OVULATION. Menstruation indicates the beginning of a cycle. Once a woman identifies her longest and shortest cycles over eight months, ovulation is assessed at 18 days before the completion of the shortest cycle and 11 days from the end of the longest. Because the ovulatory cycle varies greatly in women (generally calculated at approximately 14 days before the next menstrual period), the rhythm method is unreliable as a means of CONTRACEPTION. Use of the method may, however, aid in conception when ARTIFICIAL INSEMINATION or IN VITRO FERTILIZATION are to be performed.

See also OVULATION.

ripe cervix
See INDUCTION OF LABOR.

risk factors Any indications suggesting the possibility of negative outcome of PREGNANCY in the mother or unborn child. Risk factors include: maternal age under 15 or over 35; maternal disease such as DIABETES, heart disease, or SEXUALLY TRANSMITTED DISEASE, history of prolonged labor, abnormal fetal presentation, or multiple birth; societal conditions such as poverty, poor nutrition, and difficulty in communication; congenital or inherited conditions, OBESITY, and problems related to use of tobacco, ALCOHOL, or other DRUGS.

High-risk conditions are identified through prenatal screening and assessment, including personal medical history and regular physical exams. Clinicians estimate the implications of the risk factors and implement appropriate interventions for mother and FETUS in conjunction with client education and counseling.

rubella   Also *German measles, three-day measles*. A preventable virus that can cause MISCARRIAGE, STILLBIRTH, or permanent major birth defects when a woman contracts the virus during the first 12 weeks of PREGNANCY. Because the FETUS has no ANTIBODIES against rubella, when the virus is transmitted from the mother, it multiplies quickly, causing eye and ear disorders, brain damage, and abnormalities of the heart and other organs.

An effective vaccine against rubella has been available since 1969, and is commonly given to babies at one year of age, or given with measles and mumps vaccines at 15 months. Women who intend to become pregnant who have not been vaccinated against rubella should have the vaccine at least four months before conception takes place; otherwise, the vaccination itself can transmit the virus to the fetus.

See also TORCH SYNDROME.

Rubin test   Also *carbon dioxide test, tubal insufflation test*. An INFERTILITY test that involves injection of carbon dioxide through the CERVIX and UTERUS to detect blockage of the FALLOPIAN TUBES. This pressure test has been known to clear small blockages of scar tissue and mucus. Although carbon dioxide is readily absorbed by the body, disadvantages of the Rubin test include such side effects as shoulder pain, cramping, and NAUSEA, as well as its failure to indicate precisely which tubes are open and whether the gas escaped by other means. This relatively simple, low-risk procedure has been superseded by X-RAY technology and is now considered obsolete.

rugae   Ridges of MUCOUS MEMBRANE that crisscross the vaginal wall and permit it to stretch during fetal descent.

rupture of membranes (ROM)   Breaking of the amniotic membranes that contain the fluid surrounding the FETUS throughout PREG-

NANCY. It involves the expulsion of varying amounts of fluid and usually indicates the onset of LABOR within 24 hours. ROM is typically brought about by an intense CONTRACTION of the UTERUS once the amniotic membranes begin to bulge through the CERVIX. Some dangers associated with large amounts of fluid being produced include UMBILICAL CORD expulsion and infection of the exposed uterus. Smaller amounts of fluid may be mistaken for urinary or other discharge and should be checked.

Premature ROM (PROM) entails the spontaneous rupture or leakage of the membranes before labor and 37 weeks after the LAST MENSTRUAL PERIOD. It most often occurs in women 35 and older, and in those with cervical damage or abnormality and low weight gain. Dangers include the possibility of infection, improper fetal and umbilical cord presentation, and increased risk of fetal and maternal death.

See also AMNIONITIS; AMNIOTOMY.

S

saddle block anesthesia
See under ANESTHESIA.

safe period
See NATURAL FAMILY PLANNING.

safe sex   A misleading term that developed during the early stage of the AIDS epidemic to describe sexual intercourse in which the penetrating male wears a CONDOM. Since the HIV virus that causes AIDS is still not completely understood, however, it cannot be said with certainty that wearing a condom makes sex "safe." It is possible that condoms may not offer total protection against HIV, and that wearing a condom only makes sex "safer" than unprotected sex.

saline abortion
See under AMNIOINFUSION.

salpingectomy   Surgical procedure to remove one or both FALLOPIAN TUBES, most commonly performed in conjunction with OOPHORECTOMY and/or HYSTERECTOMY. Removal of one tube is called *unilateral salpingectomy;* removal of both is called *bilateral salpingectomy.* ECTOPIC PREGNANCY (pregnancy outside the UTERUS, usually in a fallopian tube) is the primary reason for salpingectomy.

salpingitis   Inflammation and/or infection of the FALLOPIAN TUBES, most frequently caused by GONORRHEA or bacteria that invade during childbirth, ABORTION, or other gynecologic procedure.
See also PELVIC INFLAMMATORY DISEASE.

sanitary napkin   Also *sanitary pad, Kotex®*. An absorbent pad, worn externally to soak up menstrual flow. The first such products were developed during World War I by Kimberly-Clark, a manufacturer of surgical supplies, and were called Kotex®, which has become the generic term for all sanitary napkins, much as Kleenex® has been adopted as the generic name for all disposable facial tissues. Until sanitary napkins were available, women used pieces of cloth or paper to absorb menstrual flow.

sauna; hot tub
See HYPERTHERMIA.

scarf sign   A neurologic reflex elicited in the newborn by drawing the baby's arm across its chest and noting the position of the elbow in the midline of the body. In a baby of 30 or fewer weeks' GESTATION, there is no resistance and the elbow easily crosses the midline. At 36 to 40 weeks' gestation, however, there is sufficient resistance to prevent the elbow from crossing the midline. Beyond 40 weeks' gestation, the resistance is great enough to keep the elbow from moving past the nipple area of the chest.

Schultze's mechanism   Also *shiny Schultz.* DELIVERY of the PLACENTA in which the shiny fetal surface presents first, as opposed to *dirty Duncan,* placental delivery in which the maternal (rough) surface presents first.

scopolamine   Also *twilight sleep.* An amnestic (causing amnesia) drug formerly used during LABOR and DELIVERY. Generally scopolamine was given with other drugs, narcotics, and/or barbiturates to help women forget labor pains. Scopolamine, however, can cause wildly irrational behavior and hallucinations so it is seldom used during childbirth today. More recently, a low-dose scopolamine patch has been developed to curb motion sickness in nonpregnant adults.

scrotum   The wrinkled sac that holds the male TESTES, located behind the PENIS.

sebaceous cyst
See CYST.

secondary sex characteristics   The   physical   characteristics   other than GENITALS that identify an individual as male or female: body build, voice, facial hair in men, and so on. Development of these characteristics is regulated by the sex HORMONES (ESTROGEN in females, ANDROGENS in males).

See also PUBERTY.

self-help   A concept that has gained increasing acceptance since the late 1960s, involving personal responsibility for one's own health and well-being. The self-help movement grew in large part from the women's movement and the rebellion against all male-dominated patriarchal systems, particularly gynecology and obstetrics. Women began to assert their right to have a voice in their own care and their children's birth. Many groups founded self-help clinics to offer routine gynecologic care, including breast and pelvic examination, simple laboratory tests, BIRTH CONTROL devices and procedures, and, perhaps most important, the exchange of information among women and their caregivers: physicians, nurse-practitioners, and other nurses. The self-help movement has also led to the formation of many support groups for persons with particular health problems or issues. One such group is Resolve, Inc., a national network of couples dealing with the issues of INFERTILITY.

self-quieting ability   Newborns' ability to comfort themselves by sucking their fist or responding to external stimuli, such as the movement of bright-colored objects. Babies with neurologic impairment do not have this ability and need more frequent comforting from caregivers.

semen   Also *seminal fluid*. Fluid containing SPERM and other secretions, ejaculated from the male at ORGASM.

See also SPERM.

sepsis neonatorum   Infection in the newborn during the first month of life.

septic abortion   A MISCARRIAGE resulting from pelvic infection or an elective ABORTION that results in infection and/or HEMORRHAGE.

See also INTRAUTERINE DEVICE; PELVIC INFLAMMATORY DISEASE.

serologic test, serum
See BLOOD TEST.

sex chromosomes   The X and Y chromosomes, which determine an individual's gender.

sexual desire
See LIBIDO.

sexual response   A physiological and psychological process of achieving sexual satisfaction, developing after PUBERTY in both males and females. This response was studied under laboratory conditions during the 1960s by researchers William Masters and Virginia Johnson, who described the response as having four phases: *excitement* (foreplay), *plateau* (penetration and coital movements), ORGASM (climax), and *resolution* (relaxation). The sequence is the same for men and women; however, women take longer than men to reach orgasm. On an average, men reach orgasm after three minutes of uninterrupted sex, whereas women take about 15 minutes.

The *excitement phase* can be triggered by many different stimuli, including sights, sounds, scents, colors, images, music, thoughts, and fantasies. Direct stimulation of the erogenous areas of the body (BREASTS, NIPPLES, and GENITALS) can produce sexual excitement, characterized by increased heart and respiratory rate. Erectile tissue (female nipples and CLITORIS; male PENIS) becomes congested with blood (vasocongestion) and enlarged. Women begin to secrete vaginal fluid; men experience ERECTION.

The *plateau phase* involves further vasocongestion, increased heart and respiratory rate, and increased muscle tension. The clitoris withdraws under the PREPUCE and the vaginal opening swells to grip the entering penis. The male TESTES become engorged and retract to the base of the penis.

The plateau phase climaxes with orgasm, an intense release of muscle tension and congestion. The male's seminal vesicles contract, forcing the SEMEN into the URETHRA where it is ejaculated by the penis. The female VAGINA contracts and relaxes.

Resolution follows orgasm. Blood leaves the erectile tissues, vasocongestion diminishes, and the body returns to its pre-excitement state. Females can experience additional orgasms soon thereafter; however, males usually need a period of recovery (refractory period) ranging from a few minutes to hours before an additional orgasm is possible.

See also EJACULATION; ORGASM.

sexually transmitted disease (STD)   Also *venereal disease, VD.* Infections spread primarily by sexual contact, usually vaginal or anal intercourse but also oral-genital contact, and by passage of a baby through the BIRTH CANAL of its infected mother. The most common STDs are CHLAMYDIA, GONORRHEA, SYPHILIS, CONDYLOMA, HERPES, TRICHOMONAS, CHANCHROID, GRANULOMA, scabies, louse infestation, and AIDS. In addition to these diseases, HEPATITIS and other infections may be transmitted by oral-anal sexual contact, especially in HOMOSEXUAL males. Except for AIDS and herpes, most STDs can be successfully treated. Nevertheless, they can permanently impair FERTILITY and may seriously jeopardize a developing FETUS. Table S-1 summarizes STDs and their treatment during PREGNANCY.

The incidence of STDs has risen dramatically over the past three decades, due to increased sexual activity and replacement of the CONDOM (a barrier method that protects against STD transmission) by ORAL CONTRACEPTIVES as a means of birth control for many couples. While oral contraceptives protect against pregnancy, they do *not* offer protection against STDs.

Sheehan's syndrome   Also *postpartum pituitary necrosis.* Destruction of the mother's anterior lobe of the PITUITARY GLAND after POSTPARTUM blood loss and subsequent hypotension (low blood pressure). Symptoms may begin with failure to lactate (secrete breast milk) and progress to AMENORRHEA (failure to menstruate); it can also take years for symptoms to appear. If the essential HORMONES are replaced, a woman can become pregnant again. PREGNANCY can improve the condition since it stimulates the growth of the pituitary.

shortness of breath   Feeling breathless, a sensation of not being able to take in enough oxygen. In the third TRIMESTER, this shortness of breath is caused by the expanding UTERUS pressing upward against the DIAPHRAGM and crowding the lungs. Deep breathing (from the ABDOMEN) becomes difficult. This does not mean, however, that the mother or the baby is being deprived of oxygen. To minimize shortness of breath, it is important to maintain good posture while seated, and to

(text continued on page 271)

*Table S-1   Sexually Transmitted Diseases
and Their Treatment During Pregnancy*

Disease	Organism	Diagnosis	Treatment during pregnancy
Vulvovaginal candidiasis	*Candida albicans*	Wet-mount hyphae	Miconazole
Bacterial vaginosis	Anaerobic normal flora	Wet-mount clue cells	Clindamycin
Trichomoniasis	Trichomonads	Wet-mount trichomonads	None
Syphilis	*Treponema pallidum*	Dark-field examination VDRL or RPR	Benzathine Penicillin G
Herpes genitalis	Herpes simplex virus	Herpes culture	None
Chlamydia	*Chlamydia trachomatis*	Chlamydia culture	Erythromycin base
Gonorrhea	*Neisseria gonorrhoeae*	Gonorrhea culture	Ceftriaxone and Erythromycin base
Acquired immune deficiency syndrome (AIDS)	Human immunodeficiency virus	ELISA test	Varies
Condyloma acuminata	Human papilloma virus	Virapap biopsy Pap smear	Cryotherapy Trichloracectic acid
Pediculosis pubis	*Phthirus*	Microscopic identification of lice or nits	Permethrin 1% creme rinse
Scabies	*Sarcoptes scabiei*	Confirmation of symptoms or scraping of furrows	Crotamiton 10% lotion

Source: Adapted from *Maternal Newborn Nursing,* Fourth Edition, by S. Olds, M. London, and P. Ladewig. © 1992 by Addison-Wesley Nursing. Reprinted by permission.

sleep with the head elevated. Breathing becomes easier after LIGHTEN-ING, when the FETUS moves down into the PELVIS two to three weeks before birth in preparation for DELIVERY.

shoulder presentation   A baby positioned for birth with the shoulder as the PRESENTING PART (leading the way into the BIRTH CANAL). This occurs when the baby is horizontal in the UTERUS, rather than vertical with its head down in the PELVIS. Shoulder presentation occurs approximately once in every 200 deliveries and is usually discernible by observation of the mother's ABDOMEN. Vaginal delivery in this position is almost impossible and carries the potential risk of PROLAPSED CORD, injury from attempted VERSION (turning), extraction (with FORCEPS or a VACUUM EXTRACTOR), and compromised OXYGEN. CESAREAN DELIVERY is generally the only option.

show   Also *bloody show.* Blood-tinged or pinkish discharge that appears a few days or hours before LABOR begins.
See also MUCUS PLUG.

sickle cell anemia   A recessive genetic disorder that primarily affects Black people, both men and women. It is present in less than 1% of African Americans; however, an additional 12% carry the sickle cell trait. If both parents have the gene for sickle cell trait, their child has a 25% chance of having sickle cell anemia. This makes it important for all black people to be tested for sickle cell trait.

This anemia is characterized by red blood cells that are sickle-shaped (crescent-shaped) and thus unable to pass through small blood vessels. The sickle-shaped cells accumulate and form *thrombi* (clots) and *infarcts* (clumps of tissue that died from lack of oxygen). Because they are predisposed to blood clots, women with sickle cell anemia should never take ORAL CONTRACEPTIVES, nor should they have a saline ABORTION. See AMNIOINFUSION.

Symptoms of sickle cell anemia include painful joints, acute abdominal pain, and leg ulcers. Pregnant women with sickle cell anemia face higher risk of nephritis (kidney infection), urinary tract infection, HEMATURIA, congestive heart failure, and acute renal failure. Thus, women with sickle cell anemia may wish to avoid PREGNANCY or at least seek GENETIC COUNSELING.
See also FETAL MONITORING.

silver nitrate   A metallic compound used in a very diluted form to destroy infectious organisms. At one time it was widely used in the eyes of newborns to prevent blindness caused by gonococcal infection; now, however, most hospitals use antibiotic ointment for this purpose. Many clinicians advise delaying the administration of eyedrops a few minutes or hours so the baby can see the parents during the first interval after birth. After silver nitrate drops are administered, the eyes must be carefully rinsed with water to prevent irritation.

simian line   A single crease in the palm of the hand often found in children with DOWN SYNDROME.

Sims-Huhner test   Also *postcoital examination, Huhner test.* An analysis of the cervical mucus to determine its receptivity to SPERM, part of a clinical work-up for infertile couples. It is performed four to six hours after intercourse. The clinician aspirates mucus from both the INTERNAL OS and the EXTERNAL OS by means of a small plastic catheter attached to a syringe. The mucus is measured and examined under a microscope for texture and structure, and to determine the number of active sperm as well as the number with poor or no MOTILITY. It does not take the place of semen analysis.
    See also SPERM.

Sims position   Also *left lateral position.* Lying on the left side, a LABOR position preferable to lying on one's back (DORSAL LITHOTOMY). The side-lying position avoids compressing the VENA CAVA during uterine CONTRACTIONS, permitting more oxygen to reach the baby.

single room maternity care (SRMC)
    See BIRTHING ROOM.

sitz bath   A small tub filled with six inches of warm water, used for soaking the GENITAL area without immersing the entire body. Sitz baths can help relieve the discomfort of HEMORRHOIDS, EPISIOTOMY stitches, and VAGINITIS.

skin changes   Alterations in the texture, pigmentation, and general condition of the skin related to shifts in hormonal levels and DIET. High levels of ESTROGEN during PREGNANCY or the use of ORAL CONTRACEPTIVES can cause acne, CHLOASMA, or the LINEA NIGRA.

Decreased estrogen levels during and after MENOPAUSE reduce the skin's elasticity and flexibility. The function of oil and sweat glands is slowed, often causing dry, flaky skin with more apparent wrinkles.

sleep patterns Cycles of sleeping and waking. During PREGNANCY, normal sleep patterns may be disrupted by fetal movements, difficulty in finding a comfortable position, URINARY FREQUENCY, or psychological stressors such as financial problems. This problem is more common during the third TRIMESTER when the weighty UTERUS makes movement difficult and the long-awaited birth comes closer to being a reality. Sometimes a warm, noncaffeinated beverage at bedtime and/or a backrub helps induce more restful sleep. Relaxation techniques can also be helpful.

During the third trimester, dreams, both pleasant and unpleasant, grow more vivid and sometimes deeply disturbing. Researchers believe, however, that dreams and fantasies are a way of helping pregnant women work through their concerns and fear. Dreams about losing or forgetting things, including the baby, may reflect a woman's fear of not being ready or able to be a mother. Dreams about the baby's appearance can represent concerns about the child's health or his future. It is important to remember that dreams are not reality, but only a means of better understanding oneself.

small for gestational age (SGA) Inadequate weight or growth for GESTATIONAL AGE, or BIRTH WEIGHT below the tenth percentile.

smegma A waxy secretion of sebaceous glands under the PREPUCE (hood or foreskin) of the PENIS and CLITORIS. Uncircumcised men need to retract the foreskin regularly to remove the accumulated smegma; otherwise they risk irritation and possibly infection.

smoking, tobacco Habitual smoking of cigarettes, cigars, and pipes, recognized as a health hazard for all people, but particularly for pregnant women and their developing babies. Smoking increases the risk of MISCARRIAGE, low BIRTH WEIGHT, and maternal HYPERTENSION (high blood pressure) which in turn increases the risk of preeclampsia. Nicotine is passed on to the baby through breast-milk and as secondhand smoke, leading to pediatric asthma and other respiratory problems. Smoking increases the risk of heart attack and stroke for women who take ORAL CONTRACEPTIVES, particularly after age 30.

sound A slender rod used to measure the length of the UTERUS prior to fitting an INTRAUTERINE DEVICE or performing an endometrial biopsy or other gynecologic procedure. In the nonpregnant woman, the uterus usually sounds to a depth of 6 to 8 cenimeters (2 to 4 inches).

speculum *Specula,* plural. A metal or plastic device used to examine the inside of the VAGINA and the CERVIX. Consisting of two blades, the speculum is inserted into the vagina with the blades closed, then rotated to the proper position by the clinician. Once rotated, the blades are opened and locked in place, holding the vaginal walls apart so the clinician can examine the walls and the cervix. Specula are available in a range of sizes including a tiny one for infants.
See also GYNECOLOGIC EXAMINATION.

sperm Also *spermatozoan (spermatozoa* plural) The male reproductive cell or GAMETE. At PUBERTY, rising levels of ANDROGENS stimulate the production of sperm, called *spermatogenesis,* in the TESTES. The first cells (spermatogonia) develop for about three months before they are ejaculated as mature sperm.
Each sperm is a microscopic wormlike organism with an oval head containing the CHROMOSOMES, and a tail that propels it forward, a quality called MOTILITY. It is about $7/100$ millimeter ($1/600$ inch) long overall; 90% of the length is in the tail. FERTILITY, the ability of the sperm to fertilize an egg, depends on the size, shape, motility, and quantity of the sperm produced. See EJACULATION; ORGASM; PENIS; SEXUAL RESPONSE.

semen analysis Couples seeking treatment for INFERTILITY undergo a battery of tests, one of the most important of which is a *semen analysis* of the man. This test analyzes the semen ejaculated to determine the volume, number of sperm, the sperm motility, and structure. The semen specimen is collected after two to three days of abstinence, placed in a clean dry container, and delivered to the laboratory for evaluation within two to three hours of EJACULATION. To achieve fertility, sperm must meet the minimum criteria in Table S-2. A man's sperm count may vary by as much as 20% from sample to sample; thus, a minimum of two separate semen analyses at least 74 days apart is recommended.
In about 4% of cases, semen analysis reveals that men are producing ANTIBODIES against their own sperm. To overcome this problem,

Table S-2   Normal Semen Analysis

Total volume	2 to 6 ml
Total sperm count	20 million per ml
Liquefaction	Complete in one hour
Motility	50% or greater
Normal shape	60% or greater

a technique known as sperm-washing (extracting the sperm from the semen) can be used, after which the sperm are inserted directly into the UTERUS. If a woman's cervical mucus contains antibodies that attack her husband's sperm, using CONDOMS for several months may reduce antibody production sufficiently to achieve conception. If not, steroid therapy to suppress antibody production may be tried, or insertion of the sperm directly into the uterus.

sperm bank   A tissue bank that collects, stores, tests, and sells frozen SPERM to be used for ARTIFICIAL INSEMINATION in cases where the husband is unable to father children or when a single woman or LESBIAN couple want to have a baby. The American Fertility Society recommends that all sperm donors be tested for AIDS and that their sperm be held for three months before use, until they have had a second negative AIDS test. Freezing sperm may destroy its MOTILITY; only one-fourth to one-half of frozen sperm can move when thawed.

spermatogenesis   Production of SPERM cells in the TESTES.

spermicide   A BIRTH CONTROL preparation that works by killing SPERM inside the VAGINA, most often used, in the form of jelly, foam, or cream, with a DIAPHRAGM or CERVICAL CAP. Creams and jellies are not as effective as foam alone and have a high failure rate. Used with a diaphragm, they are more effective than foam used by itself. All of these preparations should be inserted no more than 15 minutes before intercourse, and the applicator thoroughly washed after each use. Most spermicides also offer some protection against the organisms that cause AIDS, GONORRHEA, SYPHILIS, TRICHOMONAS, and YEAST INFEC-

TIONS; CONDOMS offer the best protection against the transmission of AIDS and other SEXUALLY TRANSMITTED DISEASES.

spina bifida
See NEURAL TUBE DEFECTS.

spinal anesthesia
See under ANESTHESIA.

spinal block
See under ANESTHESIA.

sphincter   A ringlike muscle that contracts to close a body orifice, such as the *anal sphincter,* which contracts to prevent the passage of feces.

spinnbarkeit
See CERVICAL MUCUS METHOD.

Stein-Leventhal syndrome   Also *polycystic ovaries.* A disorder involving the formation of numerous small CYSTS on both OVARIES, developed from egg FOLLICLES unable to release the eggs, and characterized by AMENORRHEA or OLIGOMENORRHEA, HIRSUTISM (excess body and facial hair), and OBESITY. Definitive diagnosis requires CULDOSCOPY or LAPAROSCOPY.

Stein-Leventhal syndrome is named for the two physicians who first described it in 1935, Irving Stein and Michael Leventhal. It is caused by overproduction of male HORMONES by the ADRENAL GLANDS and by the follicle capsule that forms on the ovary. Treatment consists of a combination ORAL CONTRACEPTIVE (ESTROGEN-PROGESTERONE) or medroxyprogesterone. If conception is desired, clomiphene or another FERTILITY PILL may induce OVULATION. If HORMONE THERAPY does not correct the problem, surgery may restore ovarian function and FERTILITY; the procedure is called *bilateral wedge resection,* and consists of removing a section or wedge of the cystic tissue from each ovary.

sterility   The condition of a male unable to impregnate a female, or a female unable to conceive.

See also INFERTILITY.

sterilization   To make a person incapable of reproduction. Sterilization can be an elective form of BIRTH CONTROL, as in TUBAL LIGATION or VASECTOMY, or the result of accident (radiation exposure) or illness (mumps in adolescent males sometimes causes STERILITY).

stillbirth   Also *intrauterine fetal death (IUFD)*. The DELIVERY of a dead FETUS, usually of 20 or more weeks' GESTATION, occurring once in every 1,000 births. Many fetal deaths result from unknown causes; others are associated with PREGNANCY-INDUCED HYPERTENSION (PIH), ABRUPTIO PLACENTAE, PLACENTA PREVIA, DIABETES, infection, CONGENITAL ABNORMALITIES, and Rh incompatibility. Symptoms include the cessation (stopping) of fetal movement and absence of fetal heart tones. Most women will experience spontaneous LABOR within two weeks of FETAL DEATH. If labor does not begin spontaneously within that time, the clinician will likely induce it since the mother is at risk for disseminated intravascular coagulation (DIC), a condition in which multiple tiny blood clots form in the mother's circulatory system.

stretch marks
> See STRIAE GRAVIDARUM.

stirrups   Metal footrests on a medical examination table that support a woman's feet when she is in the DORSAL LITHOTOMY POSITION.

striae gravidarum   Stretch marks; shiny, pink lines that appear on the ABDOMEN, BREASTS, thighs, and buttocks of women during and after PREGNANCY, caused by stretching of the skin.

stress incontinence   Also *urinary stress incontinence*. Inability to retain urine when sneezing, coughing, laughing, or performing any other activity that increases pressure on the BLADDER. This leakage of urine results from relaxation of the muscles of the pelvic floor, especially the pubococcygeous muscle. This muscle normally holds the URETHRA closed near the neck of the bladder; when weakened, however, it allows the bladder to leak urine. Weakening of this muscle can result from the stresses of LABOR and DELIVERY, particularly of large babies, and from many pregnancies. The pubococcygeous muscle can sometimes be strengthened by KEGEL EXERCISES, helping to relieve mild stress incontinence. If stress incontinence becomes severe and chronic, surgical correction may be required.

subconjunctival hemorrhage Bleeding on the sclera (the white part) of the newborn's eye, generally caused by changes in vascular tension or ocular pressure during birth. The condition disappears spontaneously in a few weeks without treatment.

subinvolution Failure of an organ to return to its normal size after functional enlargement, such as failure of the UTERUS to return to its pre-pregnant size after DELIVERY. Subinvolution of the uterus is most often caused by retained placental fragments or infection. Symptoms include irregular or excessive bleeding; vaginal discharge remains red rather than changing gradually to pinkish and then yellowish/whitish (see LOCHIA). Backache signals the presence of infection. Treatment consists of oral Methergine for 24 to 48 hours, plus antibiotics. If these medications prove ineffective, DILATATION AND CURETTAGE (D&C) may be necessary.

suction
See VACUUM ASPIRATION.

suppository Medication in a small, cone-shaped form that is solid at room temperature but melts readily at body temperature, designed for insertion into the VAGINA, rectum, or URETHRA. Rectal suppositories made of glycerin and sodium stearate are often used to relieve temporary CONSTIPATION.

surfactant
See HYALINE MEMBRANE DISEASE.

surrogate mother A woman who agrees to be impregnated with the SPERM of the male partner of an infertile woman, to carry the PREGNANCY to term, and to relinquish the baby to the biological father and his partner. In most cases, the surrogate mother is paid a fee for this service by the biological father and his partner; however, there have been isolated cases where a mother or a sister of an infertile woman has performed this service as an act of love. Commercial surrogacy has been declared illegal in some states; many persons oppose it on moral or legal grounds as well.

suture A surgical stitch, used to close an incision or accidental wound.

swollen feet, hands
    See EDEMA.

symphysis pubis   The section of pubic bone that lies directly beneath the MONS PUBIS.

syndactyly   A congenital malformation that involves webbing between two or more of the fingers or toes (digits), or complete fusion of two or more digits.

syndrome   A cluster of symptoms and/or signs that typify a particular disease or disorder. For example, DOWN SYNDROME is characterized by mental retardation, stunted growth, poor muscle tone, slanted eyes, and a flat nose.

syphilis   Also *bad blood, lues, pox*. One of the most common SEXUALLY TRANSMITTED DISEASES, caused by a spirochete, *Treponema pallidum*. Transmitted through vaginal, anal, or oral-genital intercourse, syphilis can be fatal if it remains untreated. It can also be transmitted from a pregnant woman to her FETUS at any time during PREGNANCY.
    Syphilis has three stages, the first of which can be divided into *primary* and *secondary*: *Primary early* syphilis involves blisters or CHANCRES where the organism entered the body, usually on the genital area; these appear within ten days to three months after exposure and disappear within one to five weeks without treatment. Painless swelling of the lymph nodes may also occur, particularly in men. *Secondary* syphilis is a recurrence of the first infection, spread to many parts of the body, appearing approximately six weeks after the first chancre develops. Symptoms may include fever, skin rash, sore throat, joint pain, hair loss, and eye inflammation. After a time, usually several months, the symptoms disappear and the disease enters a *latent* stage, detectable only by a BLOOD TEST. The latent stage can last 10 to 15 years during which time it is infectious only to the fetus of an infected woman. In the primary and secondary stages, however, it is highly infectious, even though no symptoms may be evident. *Late* (tertiary) syphilis involves the heart, blood vessels, brain, and spinal cord, resulting in memory deterioration, inability to concentrate, HEADACHES, insomnia, and general behavioral deterioration. Though the disease can still be treated at this stage, the damage to the central nervous system is permanent.

Syphilis can be successfully treated with penicillin or other antibiotics; however, diagnosis is not always easy since the symptoms can mimic many other disorders. Any sores on the GENITALS should be examined immediately and tested for syphilis. More than 200 different blood tests for syphilis exist, the most widely used of which are the VDRL (Venereal Disease Research Laboratory test, developed by the VDRL of the U.S. Public Health Service) and the RPR (Rapid Plasma Reagin). Once diagnosed and treated, persons with syphilis must be followed up and re-tested to be sure that the disease has been eradicated. Follow-up tests are performed one month after treatment, then every three months for a year. Sexual intercourse must be avoided for one month after treatment.

T

Tay-Sachs disease   Tay-Sachs is an inherited, fatal condition involving an enzyme deficiency (hexosaminidase A). Although rare, this recessive-gene disorder is more common in Jewish people of Eastern or Central European descent; as many as 1 in 30 persons may carry the disorder (see BIRTH DEFECTS). Hexosaminidase A is essential to the normal functioning of the nervous system and the METABOLISM of lipids, or fatty substances. Infants born with Tay-Sachs may appear normal, but by six months their growth slows, and paralysis, blindness, and severe mental and physical retardation progress until early death by the age of two to four years. There is no known cure.

BLOOD TESTS determining levels of hexosaminidase A are available for parents at risk for the recessive trait. AMNIOCENTESIS can reveal Tay-Sachs in the developing FETUS.

See also GAUCHER'S DISEASE.

telangiectatic nevi   Also *stork bites*. A skin condition in newborns characterized by pink or red spots in localized areas. They are common birth marks caused by dilation of capillaries (tiny blood vessels), and appear mainly on the back of the neck, around the eyes, mouth, and nose. They are harmless and typically fade by the age of two.

teratogen   Any nongenetic cause of fetal malformation, abnormality, or spontaneous ABORTION. Such factors include substances and processes that directly and indirectly affect GESTATION and development, including ALCOHOL and other DRUGS, chemicals, excessive heat (such as fever, hot tubs, or saunas), viruses, X-RAYS and other ionizing radiation, as well as maternal age and health. The FETUS is most vulnerable to toxins, environmental hazards, and other teratogens during the period of organ differentiation (between 3 and 12 weeks' gestation).

term   Also *full-term*. A baby born at the end of a PREGNANCY lasting from 38 to 42 weeks. Babies born before 38 weeks are referred to as preterm; those born after 42 weeks as POST-TERM.

See also GESTATION; TRIMESTER.

testes   Also *testicles, testis* (singular). The male sex glands or GO-NADS responsible for the secretion of TESTOSTERONE and other male SEX HORMONES, and production of SPERM. There are two testes located behind the PENIS, one suspended in each side of the SCROTUM. As opposed to the female OVARIES, they produce sperm only after PUBERTY, generating millions daily. The testes are approximately 3.5 centimeters (1.5 inches) long and 2.5 centimeters (1 inch) wide, and are divided into about 250 different chambers, each consisting of *seminiferous tubules* where sperm develop. These tubules then join at a compactly coiled duct called the *epididymis* where they are stored and continue to develop. The presence of scar tissue resulting from infection can obstruct the epididymis and cause STERILITY. When testes fail to descend into the scrotum from the abdomen the resulting condition is known as CRYPTORCHIDISM.

See also ANDROGENS; CRYPTORCHIDISM; SCROTUM; SPERM; SPERMA-TOGENESIS; TESTOSTERONE; VARICOCELE.

testosterone   The primary and most potent ANDROGEN, or male sex HORMONE produced by the TESTES. Like ESTROGEN, testosterone is present in both men and women and has been shown to affect sexual drive in both. It is stimulated by the PITUITARY hormones. Only small amounts of testosterone are present in women and prepubescent boys. During male PUBERTY, the testosterone level increases and is responsible for the production and maturation of sperm and the production of seminal fluid, as well as the development of male SECONDARY SEX CHARACTERISTICS such as body hair distribution, vocal chord enlargement, and increased bone and muscle mass. Testosterone affects male reproductive system structure and function by enabling EJACULATION. It is also thought to affect the central nervous system by producing aggressiveness as well as sexual drive. Although testosterone production is thought to slow with age, its action is constant, unlike the cyclic effects of specifically female hormones.

See also EJACULATION; SPERMATOGENESIS.

thermal neutral zone (TNZ)   An environment of minimized heat loss or expenditure. For newborns, this refers to their ability to maintain internal thermal balance between heat loss and generation within a specific temperature range through low metabolic and oxygen consumption rates. The TNZ for an unclothed, full-term newborn can range from 89.6 to 93.2 degrees Fahrenheit and is a higher temperature range than the TNZ of an adult. Factors affecting the TNZ of a newborn include size, age, presence of subcutaneous fat, and the location of blood vessels close to the skin. A flexed posture can reduce heat loss in the INFANT by reducing the area of body surface exposed to the air. Preterm babies require a higher environmental temperature to reach their TNZ than do larger, better insulated NEONATES. Once the temperature goes below or beyond an infant's TNZ, it either generates heat through increased metabolism and oxygen use or cools off through oxygen consumption.

See also CONVECTION; EVAPORATION; RADIATION.

thermatic sterilization   Also *thermatic male sterilization* or *TMS*. A heat-based method allegedly inducing temporary male STERILITY. It has been known since antiquity that heat impairs the activity of SPERM. Several birth control methods are based on this principle, but research has not determined whether heat impairs FERTILITY by slowing or killing sperm. Little research exists to support the effectiveness/reliability of this method.

thromboembolism
See EMBOLUS.

thrombophlebitis
See PHLEBITIS.

thrombus   A *blood clot*. One or more blood clots occurring within a blood vessel are known as *thrombi* and abnormal vascular clotting as *thrombosis*. Although not completely understood, a thrombus can occur spontaneously and can prove fatal if it prevents oxygen from reaching vital organs. In PREGNANCY, superficial clotting is more common after DELIVERY than during GESTATION; by walking the same day or the next day after giving birth, a woman can help prevent thrombus in the legs. Factors such as old age, poor circulation, inactivity, heart failure, infection, and ESTROGEN therapy, including ORAL CONTRACEPTIVES, may increase the risk of thrombus. *Anticoagulants* such as *heparin* or *Coumadin* can be administered to reduce this risk, but since they interfere with the clotting mechanism of the blood they should only be administered with caution, and never when there is risk of HEMORRHAGE.

See also EMBOLUS.

thrush   An oral YEAST INFECTION occurring most commonly in INFANTS, caused by the fungus *Candida albicans*. This microscopic organism is common in the mouth, rectum, VAGINA, and on the skin of healthy people. However, if a woman with a yeast infection gives birth, the baby will be at risk for thrush. Thrush is characterized by visible white plaques in and around the mouth and can be treated orally with a preparation of nystatin (Mycostatin).

thyroid   An ENDOCRINE GLAND located in the front of the neck. The two lobes of the thyroid gland encircle the trachea, or windpipe, and release two HORMONES (thyroxine and triiodothyronine) essential to normal growth and METABOLISM. It secretes these hormones only when stimulated by the presence of iodine.

Women are five times more likely than men to experience thyroid problems involving overproduction (hyperthyroidism) or underproduction (hypothyroidism) of hormones. Because most cases occur during PUBERTY, PREGNANCY, and MENOPAUSE, researchers believe there may be a connection between thyroid and ovarian function. FERTILITY problems linked to hypothyroidism include increased production of ESTROGEN and PROLACTIN, the growth hormone stimulating milk production. Women with an enlarged thyroid gland, or *goiter*, may also experience menstrual irregularity and impaired fertility. In most cases, hormonal supplements and regulatory drugs can be administered to either raise or suppress irregular levels, or, in more extreme cases, the gland may be surgically removed. Thyroid deficiency in older children and adults is known as *myxedema* and can delay menstruation in girls, cause heavy menstrual bleeding and ANEMIA post-puberty, and prevent pregnancy. It is also associated with weakness, fatigue, depression, HEADACHE, cold intolerance, dry and puffy yellow skin, thin and brittle nails, thin and coarse hair, and EDEMA (swelling caused by fluid retention).

In pregnant women, the thyroid gland is more active and increases in size to meet metabolic needs. The increase in size may also be linked to emotional stress at this time. Thyroid function generally returns to pre-pregnant levels within a few weeks of birth, but one study has shown a relation between pregnancy and decreased thyroid activity with each successive birth. When indicated, antithyroid drugs must be administered with caution as they can cause thyroid deficiency in the FETUS and result in goiter, dwarfism, and mental retardation.

tipped uterus
> See RETROVERTED UTERUS.

tonic neck reflex Also *fencing position.* A neurologic response in the newborn elicited when the head is turned to one side, involving extension of the arm and leg on the side to which the infant has turned, and the flexing of those limbs opposite. The tonic neck reflex is often more noticeable in the legs than in the arms and usually disappears by three months of age, when more symmetrical positioning is achieved. Absence or persistence of the reflex may indicate an impaired or damaged nervous system.

TORCH An acronym for the group of infections posing severe risks and problems for the developing FETUS, including *toxoplasmosis, rubella, cytomegalovirus,* and *herpes virus.* It is a term used by health professionals to quickly assess potential risk in the pregnant woman.

Toxoplasmosis is harmless to adults but can seriously affect a fetus when transmitted to a previously uninfected pregnant woman through poorly cooked meat or contact with the feces of infected cats (through the litter box or by gardening in an area where cats defecate). In some areas of North America, as many as 85% of women are at risk of infection. Incubation is approximately ten days and an infected woman may or may not exhibit symptoms. It is diagnosed by an ANTIBODY test and it can be treated with the drugs sulfadiazine and pyrimethamine if diagnosed within 20 weeks of conception. Otherwise, therapeutic ABORTION is generally advised due to severe fetal damage. Risks include STILLBIRTH, neonatal death, and severe CONGENITAL ABNORMALITIES such as brain damage, blindness, deafness, convulsions, and coma.

RUBELLA, or *German measles,* affects both pregnant and nonpregnant women equally, but exposure to the fetus and newborn can result in MISCARRIAGE, stillbirth, malformation, mental retardation, cerebral palsy, congenital heart disease, INTRAUTERINE GROWTH RETARDATION

(IUGR), and cataracts. Vaccine is strongly recommended for all children and nonpregnant young women considering PREGNANCY. Immunity can be assessed through a BLOOD TEST, but women given the vaccine are advised to wait four months before conceiving as the vaccine can lead to fetal damage. Gammaglobulin, a blood protein containing antibodies, may be administered to prevent infection in pregnant women exposed to rubella. A pregnant woman infected with rubella may be asymptomatic or exhibit signs such as rash, and muscular and joint pain. Therapeutic abortion may become an option if a woman is exposed and infected within her first TRIMESTER, since this is the time of greatest risk for the fetus. Infected INFANTS may remain contagious for months and should be isolated after birth. Problems developing after birth include increased likelihood of DIABETES, hearing loss, glaucoma, and progressive encephalitis.

Cytomegalovirus (also *cytomegalic inclusion disease [CID]*) is a type of HERPES VIRUS causing inherited and acquired infection and is the most prevalent in the TORCH group. It can be transmitted in previously unexposed pregnant women through the PLACENTA or BIRTH CANAL. About 50% of adults carry antibodies for the virus. This virus can be passed through kissing, sexual intercourse, and BREASTFEEDING. It is often asymptomatic in children and pregnant women but can prove fatal to the fetus. A chronic and persistent infection, CMV may continue over many years, harbored by the CERVIX, becoming pronounced after birth.

No treatment for maternal or neonatal CMV exists but tests can indicate the presence of antibodies. Of those infants exposed, 10% develop serious conditions including mental retardation and hearing impairment. Authorities believe that CMV may be the most common cause of mental retardation.

Herpes simplex virus type II (HSV-II) causes painful LESIONS in the genital area that may also develop in the cervix and ascend the birth canal to affect the fetus. The risk of spontaneous abortion or stillbirth increases 20 to 50% with infection in the first trimester; chances of PRETERM LABOR increase with infection after 20 weeks of pregnancy. More than half of all babies exposed to the herpes virus through birth develop some form of the infection; 70% of these will die if left untreated and more than 80% of survivors will experience permanent brain, nerve, and/or eye damage. Consequently, CESAREAN DELIVERY may be advised in the presence of ruptured membranes in the mother. Fetal symptoms for herpes virus include fever, JAUNDICE, seizures, poor appetite, and skin lesions. Vidaribine has proved helpful in reducing serious side effects from neonatal herpes; however, no conclusive treatment for herpes virus type II currently exists.

See also HERPES VIRUS.

toxemia of pregnancy
See ECLAMPSIA.

toxic shock syndrome (TSS)   A rare but potentially serious disease associated with the use of tampons. Although reported in men, children, and postmenopausal women, TSS primarily affects women under 25 years of age. It is characterized by the rapid development of symptoms such as high fever, diarrhea, dizziness, a peeling rash of the hands and feet, sudden drop in blood pressure, shock, and coma during a menstrual period when tampons are in use. TSS is an infection and its connection to tampons was first reported in the late 1970s. Manufacturers have since altered their products and included warnings in packaging; incidence of the disease among menstruating women has dropped as a result. Because the relationship of TSS to tampon use remains unclear, menstruating women are advised to avoid "super" absorbent tampon products, to change tampons frequently, and to alternate tampon use with external pads at night and during light menstrual flow. DIAPHRAGMS and CONTRACEPTIVE SPONGES left in place for more than a day may also increase risk for the disease. Early diagnosis and intervention are important to prevent death; treatment often requires hospitalization.

transition
See LABOR.

transverse diameter   Defined as the largest diameter of the pelvic inlet, or rounded upper limits of the PELVIS. It is one measurement to help determine pelvic shape, capacity, and type.

See also PELVIMETRY.

transverse lie   A crosswise or horizontal position of the FETUS in the UTERUS, as opposed to the normal vertical, head-down position for birth. The condition occurs about once per 300 to 400 deliveries and is associated with difficult and problematic LABOR, uterine rupture, and increased risk of a PROLAPSED UMBILICAL CORD in the fetus. If the fetus proves immovable from this position, CONTRACTIONS are strong, membranes have broken, and amniotic fluid is scant, CESAREAN DELIVERY may be necessary.

trichomonas vaginalis   A protozoal organism causing the vaginal infection *trichomonas* or *trichomoniasis*. Although primarily transmitted sexually, the organism can survive at room temperature in a moist environment and spread through contact with sheets, towels, and toilet seats. Symptoms include itching; burning; redness; swelling of the vulva; and profuse, smelly, frothy white to yellow-green discharge. In women, trichomonas can affect the urinary tract, causing CYSTITIS, and painful or difficult urination. Although symptoms may eventually disappear in chronically infected women, and infected men usually prove asymptomatic, intercourse should be avoided until both partners are cured.

Trichomonas does not ascend into the UTERUS or FALLOPIAN TUBES, nor does it affect FERTILITY. However, it may be severe enough to be detected through a PAP SMEAR. Testing should always be done for the presence of other SEXUALLY TRANSMITTED DISEASES, as trichomonas tends to be associated with venereal warts and YEAST INFECTION. Tight pants, tampons, vaginal sprays, and intercourse without a condom should be avoided. See CONDYLOMA ACUMINATA.

Treatment for trichomonas vaginalis requires the administration of the fungicidal drug metronidazole (Flagyl) over a seven-day period or in one 2-gram (.07 ounce) dose for both sexual partners to prevent reinfection. This drug should *not* be used by women in the first TRIMESTER of PREGNANCY or while BREASTFEEDING because of possible harm to the baby. Some argue pregnant women should not take it at all. Alcohol should also be avoided since it interacts with the drug to cause painful and severe side effects, including NAUSEA, tremors, allergic reaction, and a lowered white blood cell count. Therefore, caution during treatment is indicated and white blood cell levels should be continually assessed. There is *no* safe treatment for trichomonas in early pregnancy; some authorities believe that this caution applies throughout pregnancy.

trimester   One of the three stages of the nine months of PREGNANCY. The *first trimester* includes the first day of the LAST MENSTRUAL PERIOD until the 12th week of GESTATION. The *second trimester* refers to the 12th to 28th week of pregnancy, and the *third trimester* the 28th week until the time of DELIVERY. Each trimester is approximately three months long. The term described as the *fourth trimester* includes the six-week period following birth and is used to emphasize the importance of POSTPARTUM maternal care and adjustment.

See also GESTATION; PREGNANCY.

trisomy   A genetic abnormality indicated by the presence of one or more CHROMOSOMES in addition to a normal pair. Any condition caused by the presence of an extra chromosome is known as *trisomy syndrome*. A trisomy occurring in a specific pair is indicated by the number or letter assigned to that pair (for example, *trisomy 13* describes an extra chromosome on the thirteenth chromosomal pair). Effects vary according to the pair involved and include DOWN SYNDROME, the most common of the syndromes, as well as a range of other physical, mental, skeletal, muscular, nervous, and heart deformities and disorders.

tubal insufflation

See RUBIN TEST.

tubal ligation   Also *tubal sterilization, tying the tubes*. The deliberate and highly successful STERILIZATION procedure of surgically blocking both FALLOPIAN TUBES, and thereby preventing the union of egg and SPERM. Historically, tubal ligation has been the most commonly used method to sterilize Western women since the 1880s. This procedure may be performed through the VAGINA (CULDOSCOPY), or through one of several types of abdominal incision (see LAPAROSCOPY; LAPAROTOMY). Originally, the tubes were cut off, pinched shut, and then tied to prevent conception. More recent developments include cauterization (burning the tubes shut), the use of laser surgery, or placement of metal or plastic clips or bands around each tube.

Tubal ligation is often performed at the request of women or couples following the birth of their last desired child. Vaginal tubal ligation, or CULDOSCOPY, cannot be performed until six to eight weeks after birth because vaginal tissues are too congested.

Abdominal tubal ligation via laparotomy is now usually delayed until six to eight weeks after birth to allow the mother's body to recover from the stress of LABOR. It requires general anesthetic, a hospital stay, and a full recovery period of six weeks. In this procedure, a 4- to 5-inch horizontal or vertical incision is made just above the pubic hair and the tubes either sutured, crushed, cauterized, or clipped. It has the advantage of allowing the surgeon better access to the tubes and more successful rates of closure in the presence of scar tissue.

Minilaparatomy, or "minilap," is simpler, less expensive, and can generally be done on an outpatient basis. Postpartal tubal ligation via laparoscopy ("Band-Aid" surgery) is often done one to three days after birth under general ANESTHESIA.

Other means of tubal ligation include *hysteroscopy,* or operation through the uterus. Most recently, the use of chemicals in the uterus such as silver nitrate and zinc chloride and silicone plugs to block the tubes have been developed; however, not all are clinically sanctioned.

As with any surgery, infection is the primary risk in tubal ligation. Symptoms of infection include: any fever, severe or persistent pain (unrelieved by ANALGESIC or lasting longer than 12 hours), moderate to heavy bleeding either from the incision or the vagina, chest pain, shortness of breath, feeling faint, or pus draining from the incisions.

Tubal ligation may be followed by irregularities in the MENSTRUAL CYCLE, but it is unclear whether this results from the surgery itself or from the discontinued method of CONTRACEPTION used prior to the surgery (ORAL CONTRACEPTIVES, IUD). CONTRAINDICATIONS for tubal ligation include PREGNANCY, pelvic infection, abnormalities of the tubes or uterus, serious heart or lung conditions, and OBESITY. Although considered permanent, tubal ligation may sometimes be surgically reversed, with a procedure called *tuberoplasty.* Success is limited and highly variable; even when it does work, the risk for tubal or ECTOPIC PREGNANCY increases. Consequently, women should only have a tubal ligation if they are sure they want no more children.

See also ECTOPIC PREGNANCY; LAPAROSCOPY; LAPAROTOMY.

tubal pregnancy
    See ECTOPIC PREGNANCY.

Turner's syndrome   Also *ovarian dysgenesis, monosomy X.* A female BIRTH DEFECT characterized by the absence of OVARIES, related to having only one X chromosome instead of the normal pair of X chromosomes. Turner's syndrome thus is a *monosomy,* or shortage of a chromosome (either complete or partial). It is relatively rare, occurring once in 3,000 live female births. In general, it involves short stature, an underdeveloped reproductive system, webbed neck, puffy feet, absence of OVARIES and toenails, broad chest, organ malformation, and impaired perception, but without marked mental defects. Although not always readily diagnosed until PUBERTY, when BREAST development and menstruation fail to occur, Turner's syndrome is the most common genetic defect responsible for female INFERTILITY. Treatments include HORMONE therapy, but STERILITY is irreversible.

twins

See MULTIPLE PREGNANCY.

U

ultrasound Also *sonography, B-scan*. A painless, nonradiating diagnostic technique using sound echoes to produce pictures of soft-tissue structures inside the body, including the developing FETUS. It has no known harmful effects to either mother or fetus; routine ultrasonic screening is not recommended, however, because its long-term effects are not fully understood. High frequency sound waves (2.5 million to 10 million cycles per second) scan the mother's abdomen and pelvic area via either a transducer applied to the abdomen or an endovaginal transducer inserted into the VAGINA. As the sound waves meet structures of varying density or thickness, they echo, and those echoes are recorded on an oscilloscope screen (similar to a television screen). The recording is called a sonogram, and it can provide such valuable information as the size of the UTERUS, the size and position of a developing fetus, the presence of multiple fetuses, and evidence of some structural abnormalities. Ultrasound also can detect ECTOPIC PREGNANCY (PREGNANCY outside the uterus, usually in the FALLOPIAN TUBES), and discriminate between CYSTS and solid tumors of the OVARIES and BREAST. It has been used to locate INTRAUTERINE DEVICES (IUDs) that have slipped out of place, pelvic ABSCESSES, and cystic or solid masses. Ultrasound is also useful in guiding needle aspiration for AMNIOCENTESIS and other diagnostic and surgical procedures involving the PELVIS.

Ultrasound can be performed using either real-time or a combination of real-time and static scanners. Real-time ultrasound produces continuous, rapid, fixed images that give the impression of motion, and help clinicians assess such function as fetal breathing, movement, urination, and heartbeat. Static scanners produce a still picture.

There are two categories of ultrasound: level I and level II. Minimal training is required to perform level I ultrasound, used to assess GESTATIONAL AGE, number of fetuses, FETAL DEATH, and the status of the PLACENTA. Level II ultrasound must be performed by a highly trained

sonographic technician who understands assessment of specific CON-
GENITAL ABNORMALITIES and disorders.

umbilical cord   The mother-baby connection; a smooth, flexible,
rope-like organ linking the fetal abdomen with the PLACENTA, which is
attached to the wall of the UTERUS. At birth of a full-term INFANT, the
average cord is 2 centimeters (0.08 inch) across and about 55 centimeters (22 inches) long, but can range from 5 to 200 centimeters (2 to 80
inches). The umbilical cord transports oxygen and nutrients to the
FETUS, and carbon dioxide and other waste products from the fetus. It
contains one large vein and two smaller arteries within a special pro-
tective substance called *Wharton's jelly.* This substance, plus the high
blood volume pulsating through the cord vessels, prevents compression of the cord during PREGNANCY. Blood containing oxygen and
nutrients flows from the placenta to the fetus through the umbilical
vein. After circulating throughout the fetus, it returns to the placenta
through the umbilical arteries, carrying carbon dioxide and other
waste products which are then emptied into the mother's bloodstream
via the placenta.

Fetal movement can cause the umbilical cord to appear twisted
or spiraled. However, a true knot rarely occurs unless the cord is quite
long. The normal delivery sequence is baby, cord, placenta. On occa-
sion the cord is delivered ahead of or alongside the baby, a serious
complication called PROLAPSED CORD. Another complication is cord
strangulation or NUCHAL CORD, in which the cord becomes wrapped
around the baby's neck. ABNORMAL PRESENTATIONS, such as BREECH and
SHOULDER PRESENTATION, increase the risk of such complications. During CONTRACTIONS, *cord compression* can arise. As the uterus contracts, the cord can be compressed or squeezed, halting the flow of
blood and thus shutting off the baby's supply of OXYGEN.

Within seconds after birth, the baby normally begins to breathe
oxygen from the air, making the cord unnecessary. At birth, fetal circulation changes, allowing blood to pass from the right side of the heart
through the lungs, and from the lungs to the left side of the heart. Once
the baby starts to breathe, the cord is clamped about 5 centimeters (2
inches) from where it joins the *umbilicus* or *navel*, and cut with sterile
scissors. A sterile tape ligature or clamp is applied about 2 centimeters
($^3/_4$ inch) from the abdomen. The cord stump is cleaned with alcohol
and kept dry until it drops off, usually within a week or two.

See also HERNIA, UMBILICAL.

urea   A concentrated nitrogen solution, produced by protein and amino acid metabolism, and excreted in the urine. It is sometimes used in second-TRIMESTER ABORTIONS, usually in addition to PROSTAGLAND-INS.

See also AMNIOINFUSION.

ureaplasma   Also *mycoplasma*. A SEXUALLY TRANSMITTED DISEASE (STD) that causes ENDOMETRITIS (inflammation of the ENDOMETRIUM or uterine lining) and can lead to spontaneous ABORTION. It can also cause formation of SPERM ANTIBODIES in men leading to INFERTILITY problems. The complete name of the organism is *Ureaplasma urealyticum,* and it seems to cause some cases of URETHRITIS in both men and women, and CERVICITIS in women.

urethra   In women, a canal ranging in length from 2.5 centimeters (1¼ inches) to 5.25 centimeters (2½ inches) long, through which urine is excreted to the outside. The upper end of the urethra, *the internal urinary meatus,* opens into the BLADDER; the lower end, the *external urinary meatus* or *urethral orifice,* opens into the vestibule between the CLITORIS and the VAGINA. The urethra and the neck of the bladder are surrounded by muscle fibers which remain contracted through the action of the sympathetic nervous system. The SPHINCTER muscle of the bladder neck can be voluntarily relaxed for urination. Problems with bladder control (see STRESS INCONTINENCE) can develop when urethral or perineal muscles lose their elasticity, due to repeated stretching during PREGNANCY and birth or to a postmenopausal decrease in ESTROGEN.

Inflammation and infection of the urethra, URETHRITIS, is one of the most common disorders affecting women. It often occurs simultaneously with a bladder infection and is treated in the same manner.

See also CYSTITIS.

urethritis   Inflammation and/or infection of the URETHRA, a commonly occurring disorder in women, usually accompanied by a BLAD-DER infection and treated with the same medications (see also CYSTITIS). If no bladder infection exists, the urethritis may be associated with GONORRHEA, TRICHOMONAS, or some other vaginal infection. Thus it is important to identify the causative organism and take the appropriate medication to eliminate it (see URINE TEST). Urethritis can also be caused by irritation or injury from sexual intercourse, by irritation from the rim of a DIAPHRAGM, by scratching, or by wiping from back to front after bowel movements, thus contaminating the urethra with bacteria from the intestinal tract.

Symptoms of urethritis include pain, a burning sensation during urination, urinary FREQUENCY, and a discharge, sometimes tinged with blood. Both a gonorrhea culture and a urine culture are almost always indicated for urethritis, to identify the specific bacteria involved. *Chlamydia trachomatis,* which can also cause nonspecific VAGINITIS, is often responsible (see CHLAMYDIA), as is *Ureaplasma urealyticum* (see CHLAMYDIA; UREAPLASMA).

Treatment is the same as for cystitis. When no particular organism can be identified, the condition is called *nonspecific urethritis (NSU)* or *nongonococcal urethritis (NGU),* especially in men. Nonspecific urethritis is often sexually transmitted, even though the gonococcal organism is not responsible. Women may have almost no symptoms other than a thin, usually clear discharge in the urine and slight discomfort when urinating (DYSURIA). Symptoms appear two to three weeks after exposure. Unless urethritis is detected and treated, it can worsen and lead to complications (see below). Therefore, the partner of a person diagnosed with NGU should also be treated for the infection. Ordinarily a broad-spectrum antibiotic such as tetracycline will be effective; however, this drug should *not* be used during PREGNANCY since it will discolor the teeth of the baby.

Untreated urethritis can cause serious complications such as PELVIC INFLAMMATORY DISEASE and INFERTILITY in women, and epididymitis, a painful inflammation of the TESTES, in men. Except for NGU, however, urethritis is much less common in men (see under PENIS). Also, urethritis appears to be related to pneumonia and eye infections in babies born to infected women, and is suspected as a factor in infections leading to STILLBIRTH.

urethrocele   A ballooning of the URETHRA into the VAGINA caused by relaxation of the pelvic muscles that normally hold the urethra in place. It is usually accompanied by CYSTOCELE and is treated in the same manner.

urinalysis
    See URINE TEST.

urinary frequency
>See FREQUENCY, URINARY.

urinary incontinence
>See STRESS INCONTINENCE.

urine test A diagnostic test performed on a urine specimen (sample) to determine the presence of blood, protein, sugar, ALBUMIN, bacteria, and/or other substances in the urine. (For urine tests used to diagnose PREGNANCY, see PREGNANCY TEST). A *dipstick urine test,* often done as an office procedure, consists of dipping a strip of chemically treated paper into a urine specimen. The strip changes color according to the contents of the urine, such as the presence of blood (hematuria), protein (albumin), bilirubin, sugar, and acetone (ketones). These substances can indicate such disorders as DIABETES, kidney or BLADDER infection or, occasionally, contamination of the specimen by menstrual blood or vaginal discharge washed from the VULVA. In a pregnant woman, the presence of albumin may signal preeclampsia.

Urinalysis is more complex but can also be performed as an office procedure, though it is more commonly done in a laboratory. It measures both the concentration and acidity of the urine and, through spinning the specimen in a centrifuge, collects solid particles for microscopic examination. This can reveal white blood cells and bacteria (infection) as well as red blood cells, epithelial cells, and any abnormal cell formations (which might reveal kidney disease). If bacteria are found, a *urine culture* may be done. This means part of the sample is put in a nutrient, usually a jelly, and heated (incubated) to make the bacteria multiply rapidly. The specific organisms can then be more readily identified, and their sensitivity to various antibiotics can be determined.

Other more complicated urine tests include the measurement of HORMONE levels, which can require analysis of a woman's entire urinary output over a full day (sometimes called a *24-hour test.)*

uterine synechiae Also *uterine adhesions.*
>See ASHERMAN'S SYNDROME.

uterus Also *womb.* A hollow, muscular, pear-shaped organ that lies in the female pelvic cavity behind the BLADDER and in front of the rectum. Three layers of smooth muscle make up its thick walls. The

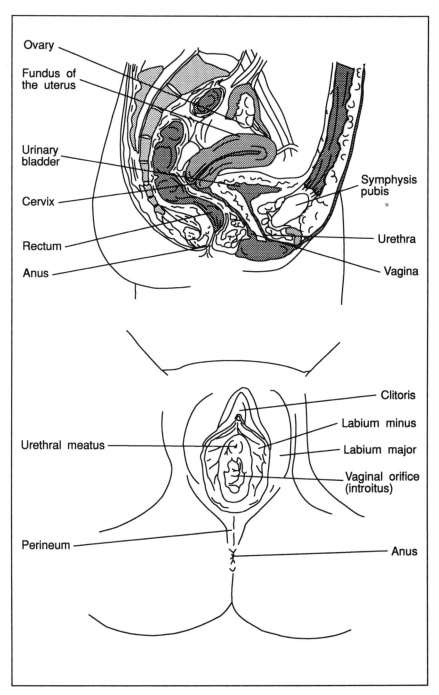

Figure U-1   Female Reproductive System

dome-shaped top of the uterus is called the *fundus* and the narrow neck at the bottom is called the CERVIX; the body of the uterus (everything but the cervix) is called the *corpus* (Latin for "body"). In adult women who have not borne children, the uterine corpus is about 8 to 9 centimeters (3 to $3\frac{1}{2}$ inches) long and 5 centimeters (2 inches) at its widest point. Its thick walls almost touch each other. PREGNANCY dramatically increases the size of the uterus to 30 centimeters (12 inches) long. After menopause, the uterus atrophies (shrinks) so that cervix and corpus are about equal in length.

The muscular walls of the uterus, about 1 to 1.24 centimeters ($\frac{1}{2}$ to $1\frac{1}{4}$ inches) thick, called the *myometrium,* make up almost 90% of its size. The outside walls are covered with the *peritoneum,* the membrane that lines the entire pelvic and abdominal cavity. The inside walls are lined with ENDOMETRIUM, which varies in thickness during each MENSTRUAL CYCLE. Initially, the endometrium is built up in preparation for pregnancy and, when no egg is fertilized, it is shed as menstrual flow, along with blood from its blood vessels.

The uterus has three openings: two near the fundus (where the FALLOPIAN TUBES enter on either side) and one at the bottom where the cervix opens into the VAGINA.

The uterine cervix is anchored, but the corpus is free to move backward and forward. In a standing position, a woman's uterus normally tilts forward where corpus and cervix meet, a position called *anteverted.* However, in about one-fourth of women, the uterus is tilted back (see RETROVERTED UTERUS). Uterine anomalies include *septate uterus,* in which a wall of varying thickness divides all or part of the corpus into two more or less separate compartments; *bicornate uterus,* in which the uterus is divided into two smaller, horn-shaped bodies, each connected to one fallopian tube but sharing a single (although sometimes septate or divided) cervix; and *double uterus* in which there are two separate small bodies, each with its own cervix. These congenital (present from birth) structural anomalies are all relatively rare, and can interfere with pregnancy and DELIVERY, depending on the extent of abnormality.

The principal function of the uterus is to provide a safe environment for the FETUS to grow and develop until mature enough to be born, an average of 38 to 42 weeks. Three sets of strong, supple ligaments support the uterus, nourished by a rich network of blood vessels. As the fetus grows—or in the case of MULTIPLE PREGNANCY, two or more fetuses grow—the muscular walls stretch to accommodate it. By the end of pregnancy, the organ has grown from pear-size to 30 centimeters (12 inches) long and from 50 grams (2 ounces) to 900 grams (2 pounds).

LABOR begins when the uterine muscles are stimulated to contract, probably by the hormone OXYTOCIN. These uterine CONTRACTIONS push the baby down toward the cervix and force the cervix to open sufficiently to allow the baby to pass through the vagina. The process of labor is not without discomfort; thus contractions have earned the name of labor pains. Nearly all pain originating in the uterus is perceived as a CRAMP, even though it may range in duration and severity from the shedding of endometrial tissue during menstruation to the contractions of labor. Following birth, the uterine muscles and ligaments return to their normal size and the excess tissues are absorbed into the bloodstream and eventually excreted in the urine. At the end of the first POSTPARTUM week, the uterus weighs 500 grams (1 pound) and after six weeks, 50 grams (2 ounces). Sometimes pregnancy weakens the muscles and ligaments sufficiently to cause the uterus to begin to sag from its normal position. See PROLAPSED UTERUS.

The uterus can be affected by a number of disorders and diseases (see also under CERVIX). Benign growths such as FIBROIDS or POLYPS are very common. More serious conditions include PELVIC INFLAMMATORY DISEASE, and endometrial cancer. Two of the most frequently performed surgical procedures are scraping of the uterine lining for biopsy and/or treatment and removal of the uterus. See DILATATION AND CURETTAGE; HYSTERECTOMY.

V

vacuum aspiration Also *vacuum curettage*. Removal of tissue from the UTERUS using suction. This procedure is performed to obtain diagnostic specimens of tissue, to remove menstrual flow (menstrual extraction), and to terminate pregnancies in the first TRIMESTER (ABORTION). It can be performed in a physician's office without ANESTHESIA and with less risk of infection than a surgical DILATATION AND CURETTAGE (D & C). The clinician inserts a SPECULUM into the VAGINA, holding the CERVIX in place with a clamp, and passes a slim plastic tube (vacurette) through the cervix into the uterus. The vacurette is connected to a syringe or to a vacuum pump, which, when activated, creates suction, removing fragments of tissue from the ENDOMETRIUM (uterine lining). Normally the procedure takes no more than five minutes, and involves only mild cramping.

When used to terminate a PREGNANCY of more than six weeks, vacuum aspiration is usually preceded by CERVICAL DILATATION, either with LAMINARIA, or other means. When cervical dilatation is necessary, many clinicians administer a local ANESTHETIC. The procedure can take up to 10 minutes; mild to moderate CRAMPS may occur, sometimes with NAUSEA. There is little postoperative bleeding although minimal staining may continue up to two weeks. Many clinicians prescribe PROPHYLACTIC antibiotics to minimize the risk of infection. All recommend that sexual intercourse, douches, and the use of tampons be avoided for at least a week and preferably two weeks. Heavy bleeding during the first menstrual period following vacuum aspiration abortion is not uncommon.

vacuum extractor A device used in DELIVERY as an alternative to FORCEPS. It consists of a suction cup, placed on the fetal head, connected to a pump that maintains suction and exerts traction (pulling) during PROLONGED LABOR. Although it has gained wide acceptance in Europe, the United Kingdom, Australia, and South Africa, the vacuum extractor is still not widely used in the United States. Its advantage over forceps is that it takes no additional space in the already crowded BIRTH CANAL; disadvantages include lack of precision, distortion of the fetal scalp into a CAPUT SUCCEDANEUM, and the danger of damage to tissues underlying the fetal scalp. Skilled use of the vacuum extractor requires special training, and many clinicians seem to prefer CESAREAN DELIVERY in difficult or prolonged labor. Use of the vacuum extractor is contraindicated in BREECH, BROW, or FACE PRESENTATIONS, in CEPH-ALOPELVIC DISPROPORTION (CPD), when the membranes have not ruptured, or when the head is not engaged in the PELVIS.

vagina   The muscular, membranous tube that connects the external GENITALS of the female with the UTERUS. It is the organ of sexual intercourse, and the exit route from the uterus, through which menstrual flow and babies emerge. Thus the vagina is often referred to as the BIRTH CANAL. At the upper end of the vagina is a cup-like area called the *fornix* into which the CERVIX protrudes. When a woman lies on her back after intercourse, semen pools in the fornix, increasing the chance of conception. At the lower end of the vagina is the opening to the outside, called the *introitus.* In young girls, the introitus may be partially or totally obstructed by the *hymen.* The SPHINCTER muscle near the introitus is what enables women to wear tampons and what contracts rhythmically during ORGASM.

The walls of the vagina are very thin, and lined with pinkish MUCOUS MEMBRANE. In premenopausal women, this membrane continually secretes slight amounts of acidic mucus, keeping the walls moist. Douches, antibiotics, or vaginal sprays can interrupt this process and cause irritation. The vaginal walls are covered with ridges, called *rugae,* which allow the vagina to stretch during childbirth.

The vagina has few nerve endings and thus is relatively insensitive. Although this insensitivity may limit sexual sensation, it also minimizes the discomfort of labor when these tissues are extremely stretched.

The most common vaginal disorder is infection, particularly YEAST INFECTION and TRICHOMONAS, plus the more serious SEXUALLY TRANSMITTED DISEASES. Vaginal cancer is rare, except in daughters of women who were given DIETHYLSTILBESTROL (DES).

vaginal discharge   Also *leukorrhea.* A thin, whitish discharge from the CERVIX or VAGINA, composed of mucus, sloughed off vaginal cells, and normal vaginal bacteria. This discharge normally precedes the menstrual period, and becomes heavier and increasingly acidic during PREGNANCY, promoting the growth of *Candida albicans.* This puts the pregnant woman at risk for YEAST INFECTIONS. To prevent these infections, women should wear cotton or cotton-crotch underwear and avoid nylon panty hose or tight pants. Any change in the vaginal discharge—becoming smelly, thick, yellow, or greenish—usually means an infection and should be reported to the clinician.

See also CERVICITIS; VAGINITIS; YEAST INFECTIONS.

vaginismus   An involuntary spasm of the muscles surrounding the VAGINA, making intercourse and vaginal examination painful or even impossible. Though a slight degree of vaginismus is not uncommon during a woman's first few sexual experiences, the condition does not persist unless serious psychological or physical causes exist. Memories of RAPE or molestation may trigger vaginismus; chronic VAGINITIS, vaginal dryness, or imperforate hymen (membrane inside the vagina that completely occludes the opening) may also be related. Treatment depends on the underlying cause, but may include teaching the woman to dilate her own vaginal muscles, using her fingers or a series of vaginal dilators.

vaginitis   Inflammation and/or infection of the VAGINA, resulting in severe itching and burning of the VULVA and, sometimes, a vaginal discharge. Some vaginal infections are caused by an overgrowth of normal vaginal bacteria, caused by medications such as antibiotics or ORAL CONTRACEPTIVES, or by hormonal changes such as those related to PREGNANCY.

The most common types of vaginitis are caused by a yeastlike fungus called *Candida albicans* or *Monilia,* and an organism called *Trichomonas vaginalis* (see YEAST INFECTION; TRICHOMONAS). These infections can occur simultaneously. Other causes of vaginitis include HEMOPHILUS VAGINALIS, HERPES VIRUS, GONORRHEA, and CHLAMYDIA.

Treatment of vaginitis depends on the cause. Antibiotics, antiviral, and antifungal drugs are effective for some cases, and may need to be administered to the sexual partner of the infected woman to prevent re-infection. Self-care measures that may be helpful include:

Keep the genital area clean and dry.

Wear all-cotton underwear.

Wipe from front to back after bowel movements.

Avoid clothing that is tight in the thighs or crotch.

Avoid "deodorant" soaps, sprays, tampons, and sanitary pads.

Take shallow SITZ BATHS in plain water.

See also VULVITIS; WET SMEAR.

varicocele A VARICOSE VEIN in the male TESTES, causing blood to pool in the SCROTUM. Varicocele is a leading cause of INFERTILITY, diagnosed in one-third of men in infertility clinics. Diagnosis is simple: the man stands and bears down, straining the abdominal muscles, while the clinician observes the testes. Varicocele causes swelling in the scrotum, usually on the left side, which clinicians describe as feeling like a bag of worms. Abnormal SPERM count, MOTILITY, and morphology (shape) are often associated with varicocele and are often resolved after surgical correction of the problem (varicocelectomy). Postoperative pregnancy rates of 25 to 50% have been reported.

varicose vein Also *varicosity*. A permanent swelling or bulge in a VEIN, caused by pressure that weakens the vessel wall. Varicose veins are three times more common in women than in men, and generally are found in leg veins. They also occur in the rectal area as HEMORRHOIDS, in the female VULVA, and in the male SCROTUM. See VARICOCELE.

PREGNANCY contributes to the development of varicose veins, due in part to the high levels of ESTROGEN, and also to the weight of the expanding UTERUS exerting pressure on femoral veins and the VENA CAVA. This pressure can be relieved by lying on one's left side, by sitting with the feet elevated periodically, and by regular walking or swimming. Tight boots, garters, and girdles should be avoided; support hose, however, may prove helpful in preventing varicose veins. Eating a high-fiber DIET helps avoid CONSTIPATION and straining during bowel movements, thereby helping to prevent HEMORRHOIDS.

Some varicosities disappear after pregnancy. Others may persist, particularly during subsequent pregnancies. Varicose veins should not be treated during pregnancy, either by injection or by surgery, because of risk to the FETUS.

vas deferens Also *vasa deferentia* (plural). One of two tubes leading from each TESTIS to the male URETHRA (see PENIS), through which

SPERM are carried. Unless these tubes are functioning, a man is INFERTILE. Surgical interruption of both vasa deferentia is called VASECTOMY, and is the primary method of male STERILIZATION.

vasectomy   Surgical STERILIZATION of the male, achieved by clipping each VAS DEFERENS, the tubes that transport SPERM from each TESTIS to the URETHRA within the PENIS. Used for more than 300 years, this operation may be performed either by a urologist or a general surgeon as an OUTPATIENT procedure, either in a clinic, physician's office, or outpatient department of a hospital. It is performed under local ANESTHETIC, requires only one or two absorbable SUTURES, and takes no more than 20 minutes. Postoperative pain is mild to moderate for a day or two. Clinicians recommend avoiding strenuous physical activity and sexual intercourse for at least a week.

Vasectomy does not provide immediate sterility, however, since some sperm are stored in the upper part of the vas deferens and in the seminal vesicles. Emptying this stored sperm requires from 15 to 20 EJACULATIONS, so couples need to use an alternate form of birth control, such as a CONDOM, until three successive tests of the male ejaculate indicate that no active sperm are present.

Vasectomy has been believed to be a rather benign procedure with few complications. However, some research suggests a possible association of vasectomy and early prostate cancer; further studies need to be done before results can be considered conclusive.

Sterilization by means of vasectomy should be considered permanent, although in some cases, surgical reversal has been achieved. The procedure is called *vasotomy* and is much more complicated and costly than vasectomy.

VDRL test   One of the most widely used BLOOD TESTS to detect SYPHILIS, developed by the Venereal Disease Research Laboratory of the U.S. Public Health Service.

vegan   A "pure" vegetarian, one who eats no meat, fish, chicken, eggs, or dairy products—in other words, no foods from animal sources. Pregnant women who are vegans must carefully monitor their DIET to ensure that they are getting sufficient calories, protein, and calcium requirements. Dietary supplements of vitamins B12 and D, plus calcium, will need to be added.

vein   A thin-walled blood vessel that returns blood to the heart; part of a network of such vessels. Even though veins are often surrounded by muscles, they are not muscular enough to achieve the pumping action of arteries. However, when the surrounding muscles contract, blood is forced toward the heart. In addition, many veins have one-way valves that prevent blood from flowing away from the heart. The most common problems associated with veins are VARICOSE VEINS and PHLEBITIS.

vena cava   The major blood vessel that returns deoxygenated blood from the lower part of the body to the heart. When a pregnant woman lies on her back, the expanding UTERUS presses on the inferior vena cava, reducing the blood flow to the heart which can causes a drop in blood pressure.
> See also VENA CAVAL SYNDROME.

vena caval syndrome   Also *supine hypotensive syndrome.* A group of symptoms related to lowered blood pressure caused by a pregnant woman's lying on her back, thereby compressing the VENA CAVA. The symptoms include dizziness, pallor, and clamminess, and can be relieved by lying on the left side.

venereal disease
> See SEXUALLY TRANSMITTED DISEASE.

vernix caseosa   A waxy, cheeselike substance that protects the fetal skin in utero.

version   Turning the FETUS within the UTERUS, either by manual manipulation from the outside *(external version)* or by reaching up into the uterus with a hand or with instruments after the CERVIX is fully dilated *(internal version).* Sometimes it is possible to turn a BREECH baby into the normal VERTEX presentation and so avoid a CESAREAN DELIVERY.

vertex   The top or crown of the fetal head; also the term for the normal head-first PRESENTATION of the FETUS in the BIRTH CANAL.

vestibule   The space enclosed within the LABIA minora (inner lips); the opening to the VAGINA (introitus) and to the URETHRA are within the vaginal vestibule, as are the openings of the two *Bartholin's glands.*

viable Capable of surviving. The term is generally associated with
PREMATURE INFANTS; those of less than 24 weeks' GESTATION or weighing less than 500 grams are rarely able to survive.

vitamins Chemical nutrients essential to good health. There are two
principal types of vitamins: *fat-soluble* and *water-soluble*. The fat-soluble vitamins include A, D, E, and K, and are generally stored in the
body. The water-soluble vitamins, those in the B-vitamin group and C,
are generally excreted in the urine, except for vitamin B_{12}, so adequate
amounts must be included in the daily DIET. During PREGNANCY, the
concentration of water-soluble vitamins in the maternal serum (the
liquid component of blood) decreases, whereas high concentrations
are found in the FETUS.

Much remains to be learned about vitamins and how much of
each one the body needs. However, it is known that overdoses of
certain vitamins, particularly the fat-soluble ones, can be toxic. Thus
it is important for a pregnant woman *not* to self-prescribe megavita-
mins but to follow carefully the recommendations of her caregiver.
Usually FOLIC ACID and iron are the only nutritional supplements recommended during pregnancy; however, some clinicians recommend a
daily multivitamin supplement during pregnancy.

vomiting
See MORNING SICKNESS; NAUSEA.

vulva Also *pudendum, external genitalia*. The external GENITALS of
the female, including the MONS PUBIS (also mons veneris), LABIA majora and minora, CLITORIS, VESTIBULE, the opening of the URETHRA,
introitus (vaginal opening), and hymen, (see also PERINEUM). The
vulva is affected by several disorders, the most serious of which are
cancer and SEXUALLY TRANSMITTED DISEASE.
See also SEXUALLY TRANSMITTED DISEASE; VULVITIS.

vulvitis Inflammation or infection of the VULVA, often caused by a
contact dermatitis. The dermatitis may be related to soap or detergent,
douches, vaginal foam or spray, SANITARY NAPKINS, CONDOMS, or clothing, especially synthetic fabrics that do not "breathe." Allergy to antibiotics or other medications can also cause vulvitis. Infections causing
vulvitis include PUBIC LICE ("crabs"), HERPES, and other SEXUALLY
TRANSMITTED DISEASES. Symptoms may include burning, itching, red-

dish inflammation, labial swelling, or blisters that break and then form a crust.

Treatment consists of identifying the cause and eliminating it, and SITZ BATHS or cool compresses to relieve itching and inflammation. Antihistamines or cortisone creams also help relieve itching. Wearing all-cotton underwear (or no underwear) and loose clothing minimizes irritation and aids healing. Any discharge should be analyzed for the presence of infectious organisms, and LESIONS should be examined to rule out cancer.

warts, vulvo-vaginal, anal
See CONDYLOMA ACUMINATA.

water retention
See EDEMA.

weight gain during pregnancy   Weight gain is expected and necessary during PREGNANCY; a pregnant woman is, in fact, "eating for two." Eating a well-balanced DIET with adequate calories for both mother and baby is important throughout pregnancy and LACTATION. The average weight gain ranges from 25 to 30 pounds; the optimal weight gain for each individual woman, however, varies according to her height, bone structure, and pre-pregnant nutritional state. Based on pre-pregnant weight, the following parameters offer general guidelines for weight gain:

Underweight woman:	28 to 36 pounds
Normal-weight woman:	24 to 32 pounds
Overweight woman:	16 to 24 pounds

The pattern of weight gain is also important. During the first TRIMESTER, a gain of two to five pounds is ideal, followed by an average gain of slightly less than one pound per week in the second and third trimesters. Weight gain in the second trimester primarily represents an increase in blood volume; enlargement of BREASTS, UTERUS, and other body tissue and fluid; plus deposits of maternal fat. During the third trimester, the weight gain reflects the growth of the FETUS and PLACENTA and an increase in the volume of amniotic fluid. Inadequate or excessive weight gain (less than 2.2 pounds or more than 6.6

pounds per month) should be promptly evaluated and nutritional counseling considered. Sudden, dramatic increases in weight should also be investigated since fluid retention is probably the reason and may indicate serious problems.

See also ECLAMPSIA; HYDRAMNIOS; HYPERTENSION.

wet smear   Also *vaginal fluid wet preparation, vaginal fluid KOH preparation.* A test of vaginal discharge to identify the cause of vaginal infection, generally done in the clinician's office. A small specimen of the discharge is placed on a glass slide, and two drops of either a sterile saline solution or potassium hydroxide are added to stain the specimen. The clinician then examines the slide under the microscope to determine whether the organism is TRICHOMONAS, *Candida (Monilia) albicans,* or *Hemophilus vaginalis.* GONORRHEA cannot be ruled out with this test, however.

See also TRICHOMONAS; VAGINITIS; YEAST INFECTION.

Wharton's jelly
See UMBILICAL CORD.

withdrawal
See COITUS INTERRUPTUS.

womb
See UTERUS.

X

X-ray A photograph taken with electromagnetic radiation, used to show internal soft tissues (as in a MAMMOGRAM or chest X-ray) and bony structures (as in dental X-rays or studies of a fractured leg). Because of the potential harm to the FETUS, especially during the early weeks of development, X-rays should be avoided during PREGNANCY unless the benefit clearly outweighs the risk. Research indicates that severe damage to the baby occurs only at high doses (50 to 250 rads) and no damage occurs when the dose is lower than 10 rads. Most modern diagnostic X-ray equipment involves no more than 5 rads and most X-rays are done with the woman's abdomen and pelvis shielded with a lead apron. Any time an X-ray must be performed during pregnancy, it is essential to inform the technician about the pregnancy. It should be done in a licensed facility, using up-to-date equipment to ensure minimum exposure to radiation.

See also MAMMOGRAM.

Y

yeast infection Also *Candida albicans, Monilia albicans, moniliasis, candidiasis, fungus, vaginal thrush, vaginal mycosis, mycotic vaginitis*. The most common form of VAGINITIS, caused by a yeastlike fungus called *Candida (Monilia) albicans*. The primary symptoms include severe vaginal and vulvar itching; pain and burning on urination; painful intercourse; and a thick, white, cheesy vaginal discharge. The male sex partner may notice irritation of the PENIS. *Candida* is part of the normal vaginal environment and only causes problems when it multiples rapidly. High ESTROGEN levels, such as during PREGNANCY or use of ORAL CONTRACEPTIVES, can cause such an increase in the organism as can DIABETES, antibiotic therapy, fecal contamination, or transmission from a sex partner. Between 15 and 25% of pregnant women are troubled with yeast infection.

Treatment consists of local application of miconazole nitrate cream (Monistat) or nystatin (Mycostatin) in SUPPOSITORY form for at least 10 days, and perhaps longer. Some women have found that eating yogurt helps reduce the incidence of yeast infections by suppressing the growth of fungi in the intestinal tract. The yogurt must be the natural, unpasteurized type found in health-food stores, containing live lactobacilli which help break down the sugar of the cervical discharge into lactic acid and inhibit the growth of organisms that thrive on sugar.

If both partners are using miconazole cream, sexual intercourse is permitted since it will help spread the cream throughout the VAGINA. If other treatment methods are used, however, abstinence is recommended until both partners are healed.

Z

zona pellucida   A thick, transparent, elastic capsule that develops around the cell membrane of an OVUM. Its function is unknown.

zygote   Also *fertilized egg*. The single cell that is formed from the union of a male germ cell (GAMETE), or SPERM, with a female germ cell (oocyte), or OVUM, before it begins the process of cell division. After the zygote implants in the uterine lining, it is referred to as an EMBRYO for the first eight weeks of GESTATION, and thereafter as a FETUS.

zygote intrafallopian transfer (ZIFT)
   See under EMBRYO TRANSFER.

Bibliography

Ammer, Christine. *The A-to-Z of Women's Health: A Concise Encyclopedia.* Alameda CA: Hunter House, 1989.

Boston Women's Health Collective. *The New Our Bodies, Ourselves: A Book By and For Women.* New York: Touchstone Press, Simon & Schuster, 1992.

Detmer, William M., Stephen J. McPhee, Diana Nicoll, and Tony M. Chou. *Pocket Guide to Diagnostic Tests.* New York: Appleton & Lange/Prentice Hall, Simon & Schuster, 1992.

Dorris, Michael. *The Broken Cord.* New York: Harper Perennial/Harper Collins, 1989.

Eisenberg, Arlene, Heide E. Murkoff, and Sandee E. Hathaway. *What to Expect When You're Expecting,* 2nd edition. New York: Workman Publishing, 1991.

Enkin, Murray, Mark J.N.C Keirse, and Iain Chalmers. *A Guide to Effective Care in Pregnancy and Childbirth.* New York: Oxford University Press, 1989.

Fitzgerald, Paul. *Handbook of Clinical Endocrinology.* New York: Appleton & Lange/Prentice Hall, Simon & Schuster, 1992.

Flaskerud, Jacquelyn Haak, and Peter J. Ungvarski. *HIV/AIDS: A Guide to Nursing Care,* 2nd edition. Philadelphia: W.B. Saunders, 1992.

Hales, Dianne and Timothy R. B. Johnson. *Intensive Caring: New Hope for High Risk Pregnancy.* New York: Crown Publishers, 1990.

Huggins, Kathleen. *The Nursing Mother's Companion.* Boston: Harvard Common Press, 1990.

Jones, Carl. *Alternative Birth: The Complete Guide.* Los Angeles: Jeremy P. Tarcher, 1991.

Kahn, Ada P. and Linda Hughey Holt, M.D. *The A-to-Z of Women's Sexuality: A Concise Encyclopedia.* Alameda CA: Hunter House, 1992.

Love, Susan M. with Karen Lindsey. *Dr. Susan Love's Breast Book.* Reading MA: Addison-Wesley, 1991.

Olds, Sally, Marcia London, and Patricia Ladewig. *Maternal-Newborn Nursing: A Family-Centered Approach.* Redwood City CA: Addison-Wesley Nursing, a Division of Benjamin-Cummings, 1992.

Pernoll, Martin L., ed. *Current Obstetric & Gynecologic Diagnosis & Treatment,* 7th edition. New York: Appleton & Lange/Prentice Hall, Simon & Schuster, 1991.

Simkin, Penny. *The Birth Partner: Everything You Need to Know to Help a Woman Through Childbirth.* Boston: Harvard Common Press, 1989.

Tanagho, Emil A. and Jack W. McAninch. *Smith's General Urology,* 13th edition. New York: Appleton & Lange/Prentice Hall, Simon & Schuster, 1992.

Tierney, Lawrence M. Jr., Stephen J. McPhee, Maxine A. Papadakis, and Steven A. Schroeder, eds. *Current Medical Diagnosis and Treatment 1993.* New York: Appleton & Lange/Prentice Hall, Simon & Schuster, 1993.

Resources

Catalogs

ICEA Bookmarks
ICEA Bookcenter
P.O. Box 20048
Minneapolis MN 55420

(800) 624-4934

Imprints
Birth & Life Bookstore
7001 Alonzo Avenue NW
P.O. Box 70625
Seattle WA 98107-0625

(206) 789-4444

Organizations

Abortion

National Abortion Federation
1436 U Street NW, Suite 103
Washington DC 20009

(202) 667-5881
Hotline: (800) 772-9100
(9:30 AM–5:30 PM Eastern time)

AIDS

AIDS National Hotline
Centers for Disease Control

(800) 342-2437
(24 hours)

Project Inform Hotline

Local/International (415) 558-9051
California (800) 334-7422
USA (800) 822-7422

Birth Control

Planned Parenthood Federation of America
810 Seventh Avenue
New York NY 10019

(212) 541-7800

Breast Cancer

Breast Cancer Advisory Center
11426 Rockville Pike, Suite 406
Rockville MD 20859   (301) 984-1020

Breast Cancer Action
1280 Columbus Avenue, Suite 204
San Francisco CA 94133   (415) 922-8279

Cancer Information Service of the
National Cancer Institute   (800) 4-CANCER

Women's Cancer Resource Center
3023 Shattuck
Berkeley CA 94705   (510) 548-9272

Y-Me Breast Cancer Support Group
18220 Harwood Avenue
Homewood IL 60430   Hotline: (800) 221-2141
                        (9:00 AM–5:00 PM weekdays, Central time)
            (708) 799-8228 in Chicago and for emergencies (24 hours)

Childbirth Education

Academy of Certified Childbirth Educators
2001 E. Prairie Circle, Suite 1
Olathe KS 66062   (913) 782-5116

American College of Nurse-Midwives
1522 K Street NW, Suite 1120
Washington DC 20005   (202) 347-5445

ASPO/Lamaze
1101 Connecticut NW, Suite 700
Washington DC 20036   (800) 368-4404
                            (9:00 AM–5:00 PM Eastern time)
                                                       (202) 857-1128

Association for Childbirth at Home International (ACHI)
P.O. Box 430
Glendale CA 91209   (213) 667-0839

Cesareans/Support Education and Concern (C/SEC)
22 Forest Road
Framingham MA 01701 (508) 877-8266

Informed Homebirth, Inc.
P.O. Box 3675
Ann Arbor MI 48106 (313) 662-6857

Intensive Caring Unlimited (ICU)
910 Bent Lane
Philadelphia PA 19118 (215) 233-6994

International Association of Parents and Professionals for Safe Alternatives in Childbirth (NAPSAC)
Route 1, Box 646
Marble Hill MO 63764 (314) 238-2010

International Cesarean Awareness Network (I-CAN)
(formerly the Cesarean Prevention Movement)
P.O. Box 152
Syracuse NY 13210 (315) 424-1942

International Childbirth Education Association (ICEA)
P.O. Box 20048
Minneapolis MN 55240 (612) 854-8660
(800) 624-4934 book orders only

La Leche League International, Inc.
Box 1209
9616 Minneapolis Avenue
Franklin Park IL 60131 (708) 455-7730

Maternity Center Association
48 East 92nd Street
New York NY 10128 (212) 369-7300

Midwives Alliance of North America
1411 North Main
Newton KS 67114

National Association of Childbearing Centers (NACC)
3123 Gottschall Road
Perkiomenville PA 18074 (215) 234-8068
Send $1.00 check or cash for a list of birth centers in your area.

Traditional Childbearing Group
P.O. Box 190784
Roxbury MA 02119   (617) 541-0086
(Midwives of African descent whose services include
home birth, childbirth classes, and counseling)

DES (Diethylstilbestrol)

DES Action USA
1615 Broadway
Oakland CA 94612   (510) 465-4011

Diabetes

American Diabetes Association
1660 Duke Street
Alexandria VA 22314   (800) 232-3472
                    (703) 549-1500 in Virginia and Metropolitan DC
                           (8:30 AM–5:00 PM Eastern time)

Down Syndrome

National Down Syndrome Congress
1605 Chantilly Drive, Suite 250
Atlanta GA 30324   (404) 633-1555

National Down Syndrome Society
666 Broadway
New York NY 10012   Hotline: (800) 221-4602
                           (212) 460-9330 in New York
                        (9:00 AM–5:00 PM Eastern time)

Endometriosis

The Endometriosis Association
8585 North 76th Place
Milwaukee WI 53223   (800) 992-3636 in the U.S.
                                     (800) 426-2363 in Canada

Grief and Loss

Compassionate Friends
P.O. Box 3696
Oak Brook IL 60522-3696   (708) 990-0010

Infertility

Resolve, Inc.
1310 Broadway
Somerville MA 02144-1731   (617) 623-0744

Lesbian Issues

National Lesbian and Gay Health Foundation
P.O. Box 65472
Washington DC 20035   (202) 797-3708

Sexually Transmitted Diseases (See also AIDS)

VD National Hotline   (800) 227-8922
                 (8:00 AM–11:00 PM weekdays, Eastern time)

Subject Index

This index is included to guide readers to the main entries on a larger subject. Only the main entries are listed; if an entry consists only of a cross-reference—for example, Adolescence, see PUBERTY—it is not listed in this index. Since entries are in alphabetical order, no page numbers are included. The subject headings listed are:

abortion
age, childbearing
birth control and sterilization
breastfeeding
cancer
diagnostic tests and procedures
drugs and medications
heredity and birth defects
hormones
infertility
labor and delivery
menstruation
newborn
nutrition
postpartum
pregnancy/prenatal care
sexuality
sexually transmitted disease

Abortion

abortion
amnioinfusion
contragestive
dilatation and curettage (D & C)
dilatation and evacuation (D & E)
hysterotomy
laminaria
rape
septic abortion
vacuum aspiration

Age, childbearing

adolescent pregnancy
age, childbearing
high-risk pregnancy
menarche
puberty
secondary sex characteristics

Birth control and sterilization

abortion
barrier methods
basal body temperature
cervical cap
cervical mucus method
coitus interruptus
condom
contraception
contraceptive sponge
contragestive
diaphragm
douching
family planning
hysterectomy
intrauterine device (IUD)
laparoscopy
laparotomy
male contraceptive
natural family planning
oral contraceptive
Pomeroy method
prophylactic
rhythm method
spermicide
sterilization
thermatic sterilization
tubal ligation
ultrasound
vasectomy

Breastfeeding

agalactia
alcohol use

areola
breast
breastfeeding
contraction, uterine
demand feeding
diet
drug use
galactocele
lactation
La Leche League
letdown reflex
mastalgia
mastitis
nipple

Cancer

breast cancer
breast self-examination
cervix
choriocarcinoma
cytology
endometrium
hysterectomy
mammogram
mastectomy
oophorectomy
ovary
Paget's disease

Diagnostic tests and procedures

acrosin test
alpha-fetoprotein test
blood test
breast self-examination
chorionic villus sampling
Coombs' test
culdocentesis
culdoscopy
curettage
cytology
dilatation and curettage (D & C)
early pregnancy test
fetal blood sampling

fetal heart rate
fetal monitoring
fetoscopy
gram stain
gynecologic examination
hysterosalpingography
karyotyping
laparoscopy
magnetic resonance imaging (MRI)
mammogram
palpate
Pap smear
pregnancy test
rabbit test
Rubin test
Sims-Huhner test
sound
speculum
syndrome
ultrasound
urine test
vacuum aspiration
wet smear

Drugs and medications

analgesic
anesthesia
contraindication
Demerol
diethylstilbestrol (DES)
diuretic
drug use
hormone therapy
oral contraceptives
pitocin
progesterone
scopolamine
silver nitrate
suppository
teratogens
vitamins

Heredity and birth defects

adrenogenital syndrome
alpha-fetoprotein test
amniocentesis
androgen insensitivity syndrome
birth defects
chorionic villus sampling
chromosome
congenital abnormalities
cryptorchidism
diethylstilbestrol (DES)
Down syndrome
epispadias
erythroblastosis fetalis
fetal alcohol syndrome (FAS)
folic acid
Gaucher's disease
genetic counseling
genetics
gestation
hemophilia
hermaphroditism
inborn error of metabolism
karyotyping
Klinefelter's syndrome
muscular dystrophy
neural tube defects
nucleic acid
phenylketonuria (PKU)
polydactyly
rubella
sickle cell anemia
simian line
syndactyly
Tay-Sachs disease
telangiectasia
Turner's syndrome

Hormones

adrenal glands
adrenogenital syndrome
androgen
diabetes

diethylstilbestrol (DES)
endocrine glands
estrogen
fertility pill
follicle-stimulating hormone (FSH)
hirsutism
infertility
hormones
hormone therapy
human chorionic gonadotropin (HCG)
human menopausal gonadotropin (HMG)
human placental lactogen (HPL)
hypothalamus
luteinizing hormone
oral contraceptives
oxytocin
parathyroid glands
pineal body
pituitary
progesterone
progestin
prolactin
prostaglandins
relaxin
Stein-Leventhal syndrome
testosterone
thyroid
Turner's syndrome

Infertility

acrosin test
artificial insemination
azoospermia
cryptorchidism
donor egg
ejaculation
embryo transfer
endometriosis
fertility
fertility pill
gamete intrafallopian transfer (GIFT)
habitual miscarriage
hydrosalpinx
hysterosalpingography

infertility
in vitro fertilization
laparoscopy
luteinized unruptured follicle
miscarriage
motility, sperm
oligospermia
pelvic inflammatory disease
Rubin test
semen
Sims-Huhner test
sperm
sperm bank
Stein-Leventhal syndrome
sterility
surrogate mother
ureaplasma

Labor and delivery

abdominal effleurage
abnormal presentation
acceleration
acme
afterpains
amniotic fluid embolism
amniotic sac
amniotomy
analgesia
anemia
anesthesia
attachment
back labor
birth attendant
birth canal
birth center
birthing bed
birthing chair
birthing room
birthing stool
birth weight
brachial palsy
Bradley method
Braxton Hicks contractions
breech presentation

brow presentation
cesarean delivery
cephalhematoma
cephalic presentation
cephalopelvic disproportion
cervical dilatation
contraction, uterine
crowning
deceleration
delivery
Demerol
Dick-Read method
dry labor
dystocia
eclampsia
effacement
engagement
episiotomy
face presentation
false labor
fetal bradycardia
fetal monitoring
fetoscopy
fetus
forceps
home birth
induction of labor
LDRP (labor, delivery, recovery, postpartum rooms)
Leboyer method
meconium
midwife
molding
mucus plug
nuchal cord
obstetrician
oxygen, in childbirth
oxytocin
pelvimetry
perinatology
Pitocin
placenta
posterior presentation
postmature
postpartum hemorrhage
precipitous birth

precipitous labor
premature
prep
presenting part
prepared childbirth
prolapsed cord
prolonged labor
psychoprophylactic method
Schultze's mechanism
scopolamine
shoulder presentation
show
Sims position
single room maternity care
stillbirth
transition
umbilical cord
uterus
vacuum extractor
version

Menstruation

amenorrhea
amenorrhea-galactorrhea syndrome
cramp
dysmenorrhea
emmenagogue
menarche
menopause
menorrhagia
menstrual cycle
oligomenorrhea
ovary
ovum
ovulation
polymenorrhea
premenstrual syndrome
sanitary napkin
toxic shock syndrome

Newborn

acrocyanosis
Apgar score

attachment
birth weight
brachial palsy
Brazelton's neonatal behavioral assessment
breastfeeding
brown adipose tissue (BAT)
caput succedaneum
cardiopulmonary adaptation
circumcision
cold stress
conduction
convection
ductus arteriosus
ductus venosus
Epstein's pearls
Erb's Duchenne palsy
erythema toxicum
exchange transfusion
fontanelle
forceps
Harlequin sign
hemolytic disease of the newborn
hyaline membrane disease
intrauterine growth retardation (IUGR)
large for gestational age (LGA)
macrosomia
milia
Moro reflex
mottling
neonatal jaundice
neonate
neonatology
neural tube defects
nevus flammeus
nevus vasculosus
newborn screening tests
ophthalmia neonatorum
orientation
Ortolani's maneuver
oxygen toxicity
pediatrician
perinatology
periodic breathing
phototherapy
physiologic anemia of infancy

physiologic jaundice
polydactyly
postmature
premature
pseudomenstruation
radiation
respiratory distress syndrome
retrolental fibroplasia
scarf sign
self-quieting ability
sepsis neonatorum
small for gestational age (SGA)
subconjunctival hemorrhage
syndactyly
telangiectic nevi
thermal neutral zone
thrush
tonic neck reflex
umbilical cord
umbilical hernia
vacuum extractor

Nutrition

anemia
calcium
diabetes
diet
folic acid
lacto-ovovegetarian
lactose intolerance
lacto-vegetarian
obesity
recommended dietary allowance (RDA)
vegan
vitamins
weight gain during pregnancy

Postpartum

afterpains
agalactia
Apgar score
atony, uterine
breastfeeding

catheter, urinary
contraction, uterine
demand feeding
depression, postpartum
drug use
grief
involution, uterine
Kegel exercises
lactation
lochia
parametritis
pelvic tilt
perinatology
phlegmasia
polygalactia
postpartal hemorrhage
postpartum
puerperal fever
puerperium
Sheehan's syndrome
sitz bath
subinvolution
uterus

Pregnancy/prenatal care

abruptio placentae
active acquired immunity
adolescent pregnancy
age, childbearing
albumin, urinary
alcohol use
amniocentesis
amnion
amnionitis
amniotic sac
antibody
antigen
apnea
areola
attitude, fetal
artificial insemination
baseline rate
baseline variability
battering

biophysical profile
birth attendant
birth canal
birthing chair
birthing room
birthing stool
bladder
bleeding, vaginal
Bradley method
Braxton-Hicks contractions
breastfeeding
breech presentation
brow presentation
cephalic presentation
cervix
cesarean delivery
Chadwick's sign
chloasma
chorion
chorionic villus sampling
chromosome
congenital abnormalities
constipation
contraction stress test
contraction, uterine
couvade syndrome
cystitis
cystocele
diabetes
Dick-Read method
diet
drug use
duration
eclampsia
ectopic pregnancy
edema
embryo
embryo transfer
engagement
episiotomy
exercise
face presentation
false labor
false pregnancy
fertility

fertility pill
fertilization
fetal blood sampling
fetus genetic counseling
frequency, urinary
gestation
gestational age
Goodell's sign
gravida
grief
habitual miscarriage
hair loss
Hegar's sign
hematuria
hemorrhage, vaginal
hemorrhoids
high-risk pregnancy
home birth
hydramnios
hypertension
implantation
incompetent cervix
itching
lanugo
Leboyer method
Leopold's maneuvers
lightening
linea nigra
LMP (last menstrual period)
McDonald's sign
measles
meconium
metabolism
midwife
mitleiden
morning sickness
mucus plug
multigravida
multipara
multiple pregnancy
Nagele's rule
natural childbirth
nausea
nonstress test
nuchal cord

nullipara
obstetrician
palpitation
passive acquired immunity
pediatrician
pelvic tilt
pelvis
pelvimetry
perineum
phlebitis
pica
Pitocin
placenta
placenta accreta
placenta previa
postdate pregnancy
posterior presentation
positive signs of pregnancy
pregnancy
pregnancy counseling
pregnancy tests
pregnant patient's rights
prenatal care
prepared childbirth
presumptive signs of pregnancy
primagravida
primipara
probable signs of pregnancy
psychoprophylactic method
ptyalism
pyleonephritis
quickening
rabbit test
rape
rectocele
Rh factor
Rhogam
risk factors
rubella
rupture of membranes (ROM)
shoulder presentation
show
skin changes
smoking
stillbirth

striae gravidarum
superfecundation
superfetation
teratogen
test-tube baby
thrombus
TORCH
transverse diameter
transverse lie
trimester
umbilical cord
urethra
urethritis
uterus
varicose veins
vena cava syndrome
version
viable
weight gain during pregnancy
zygote

Sexuality

anus
apocrine gland
bisexual
celibacy
clitoris
coitus
coitus interruptus
cunnilingus
dysparuenia
ejaculation
erection
fellatio
gender identity
hermaphroditism
heterosexual
homosexual
hymen
impotence
incest
intercourse
labia
lesbian

libido
lubricant
masturbation
oral sex
orgasm
penis
safe sex
scrotum
semen
sex chromosomes
sexual dysfunction
sexual response
transsexual
vagina
vaginismus

Sexually Transmitted Diseases

AIDS
cervicitis
chancre
chancroid
chlamydia
condom
condyloma acuminata
gonorrhea
granuloma inguinale
hemophilus vaginalis
hepatitis
herpes virus
hydrosalpinx
lymphogranuloma venerum
nit
ophthalmia neonatorum
pelvic inflammatory disease
pubic lice
safe sex
sexually transmitted disease
syphilis
trichomonas vaginalis
ureaplasma
urethritis
vaginitis
venereal disease

More books from the A-to-Z Series

THE *NEW* A-TO-Z OF WOMEN'S HEALTH: A Concise Encyclopedia by Christine Ammer

An up-to-date work that covers all aspects of women's health with over 1,000 expert entries; a cross-reference system and subject guide that make it easy to use; discussions of health topics that most affect women, including:

- Pregnancy, childbirth, and birth control
- Drugs, medication, fitness, and vitamins
- Cholesterol and diet
- Chronic disease, disabilities, and surgery
- Sexuality and sexually transmitted diseases

*"The coverage is more extensive than that of **The New Our Bodies, Ourselves** and more current than that of Felicia Stewart's **Understanding Your Body**.* — BOOKLIST

496 pages ... Paperback ... $16.95

THE A-TO-Z OF WOMEN'S SEXUALITY: A Concise Encyclopedia by Ada P. Kahn and Linda Hughey Holt, M.D.

This sensitively written book sorts out the information on women's sexuality in a clear, jargon-free style. Covers over 2,000 topics in an easy-to-use A-Z format with answers to questions about sexual partners, pregnancy, sex therapies, and legal and social issues affecting women of all ages. THE A-TO-Z OF WOMEN'S SEXUALITY has cross-referenced entries on:

- Sexual fears and disorders
- Menopause and estrogen replacement therapy
- The symptoms and complications of sexually transmitted diseases, including AIDS, PID, and chlamydia
- Female and male sexual response cycles
- Gynecological tests, medications, and contraception methods

"Easy to use. An ambitious attempt to compile a vocabulary of sexuality for a popular audience. The wide-ranging interdisciplinary coverage make it a good addition for ready reference." — BOOKLIST

368 pages ... Paperback ... $14.95

To order, please see last page

Hunter House Books on Pregnancy and Sexuality

GETTING PREGNANT AND STAYING PREGNANT:
Overcoming Infertility and Managing Your High-Risk
Pregnancy by Diana Raab, B.S., R.N.

This is a complete, accessible, and practical guide to the physical and emotional problems encountered during infertility and high-risk pregnancy. Fully updated with the most current medical information, it describes causes, symptoms, and possible treatments. Topics include infertility, Caesarean birth, miscarriage, premature birth, nutrition, tests, new technology, and genetic risks.

The author has experienced infertility and high-risk pregnancies herself, and discusses the emotional aspects of these problems: hope, frustration, depression.

336 pages ... 28 illustrations ... Paperback ... $14.95

THE FERTILITY AWARENESS HANDBOOK:
The Natural Guide to Avoiding or Achieving Pregnancy
by Barbara Kass-Annese, R.N., C.N.P. and Hal Danzer, M.D.

Do you know your fertility signs? Did you know that by charting the natural language of your body you can track the days of the month when you are most fertile and most likely to conceive? Or you can determine when you are definitely infertile and can safely have intercourse without conceiving? These noninvasive techniques have no side effects and teach you how to be more in touch with your body, more secure in your lovemaking, and more in control of your health and sexual well-being.

176 pages ... 47 illustrations ... Paperback ... $11.95

SEXUAL PLEASURE: Reaching New Heights of Sexual
Arousal and Intimacy   by Barbara Keesling, Ph.D.

This book is for all people who are interested in enhancing their sex lives and experiencing lovemaking as a deeply pleasurable physical and emotional exchange. It shows readers how to develop sensual awareness and learn to please themselves. A series of graduated sensual exercises reveal the three secrets of sexual pleasure: enjoying being touched, enjoying touching, and merging touching and feeling as an ecstatic experience. Sensual photographs add a note of artistic intimacy and make this book the perfect personal gift for caring partners.

288 pages ... Paperback ... $12.95 ... also available in hardcover

For our FREE catalog of books please call 510/865-5282

Other Books from Hunter House

ONCE A MONTH: The Original Premenstrual Syndrome Handbook by Katharina Dalton, M.D.

Surveys have shown that as many as 75% of women complain of at least one medical symptom of premenstrual syndrome. Once considered an imaginary complaint, PMS has at last gotten the serious attention it deserves, thanks largely to the work of Katharina Dalton, M.D. Dalton pioneered the diagnosis and treatment of PMS. This new fourth edition of her classic work is the first—and still the best—book about the symptoms, effects, medical and self-help treatments for premenstrual syndrome.

"Dalton is amply qualified to make the diagnosis."
— NEWSWEEK

272 pages ... Fourth Edition ... Paperback ... $11.95

HOW WOMEN CAN *FINALLY* STOP SMOKING
by Robert C. Klesges, Ph.D., and Margaret DeBon

While rates of smoking among men are now declining, rates among women are on the *increase*. Until recently, strategies on quitting were based exclusively on men, but what works for men does not necessarily work for women: women tend to gain more weight, their menstrual cycles and menopause affect the likelihood of success, and their withdrawal symptoms are different from those of men. This program is derived from the highly successful model at Memphis State University and is authored by pioneers in the work of women's health and smoking.

192 pages ... Paperback ... $8.95

RUNNING ON EMPTY: Living With Chronic Fatigue Immune Dysfunction Syndrome by Katrina Berne, Ph.D.

To many, Chronic Fatigue Immune Dysfunction Syndrome is a mystery disease, elusive and often misdiagnosed. To the thousands of people who suffer from it—and to their families —CFIDS is debilitating and frightening. This award-winning book combines the latest medical findings with insight and support covering: a history of CFIDS; its effects and how to live with it; medical and alternative treatment options.

"A solid package of thoroughly researched information that, for sufferers, could mean the difference between being virtually bedridden for years and being able to maintain an almost normal life." — NATURAL HEALTH

320 pages ... Paperback ... $14.95 ... also available in hardcover

Prices subject to change without notice

ORDER FORM

10% DISCOUNT on orders of $20 or more —
20% DISCOUNT on orders of $50 or more —
30% DISCOUNT on orders of $250 or more —
On cost of books for fully prepaid orders

NAME

ADDRESS

CITY/STATE   ZIP

COUNTRY [outside USA]   POSTAL CODE

TITLE	QTY	PRICE	TOTAL
The A-to-Z of Pregnancy & Childbirth *(pb)*		@ $ 16.95	
The A-to-Z of Pregnancy & Childbirth *(hc)*		@ $ 29.95	
The A-to-Z of Women's Health		@ $ 16.95	
The A-to-Z of Women's Sexuality		@ $ 14.95	
The Fertility Awareness Handbook		@ $ 11.95	
Getting Pregnant and Staying Pregnant		@ $ 14.95	
How Women Can *Finally* Stop Smoking		@ $ 8.95	
Once A Month (4th ed.)		@ $ 11.95	
Running On Empty		@ $ 13.95	
Sexual Pleasure		@ $ 12.95	

Shipping costs:
First book: $2.50
($3.50 for Canada)
Each additional book:
$.75 ($1.00 for
Canada)
For UPS rates and
bulk orders call us at
(510) 865-5282

TOTAL	___
Less discount @____%	(___)
TOTAL COST OF BOOKS	___
Calif. residents add sales tax	___
Shipping & handling	___
TOTAL ENCLOSED	___
Please pay in U.S. funds only	

❏ Check   ❏ Money Order   ❏ Visa   ❏ M/C

Card # _____ Exp date _____

Signature _____

Complete and mail to

Hunter House Inc., Publishers

PO Box 2914, Alameda CA 94501-0914
Phone (510) 865-5282 Fax (510) 865-4295
❏ Check here to receive our book catalog

ATP 11/93